Quality of Life in Asia

Volume 12

Series editors

This series, the first of its kind, will examine both the objective and subjective dimensions of life quality in Asia, especially East Asia. It will unravel and compare the contours, dynamics and patterns of building nations, offering innovative works that discuss basic and applied research, emphasizing inter- and multi-disciplinary approaches to the various domains of life quality. Thus, the series will appeal to a variety of fields in humanities, social sciences and other professional disciplines. Asia is the largest, most populous continent on Earth, and it is home to the world's most dynamic region, East Asia. In the past three decades, East Asia has been the most successful region in the world in expanding its economies and integrating them into the global economy, offering lessons on how poor countries, even with limited natural resources, can achieve rapid economic development. Yet while scholars and policymakers have focused on why East Asia has prospered, little has been written on how its economic expansion has affected the quality of life of its citizens. The series will publish several volumes a year, either single or multiple-authored monographs or collections of essays.

More information about this series at http://www.springer.com/series/8416

Daniel T. L. Shek · Grace Ngai
Stephen C. F. Chan
Editors

Service-Learning for Youth Leadership

The Case of Hong Kong

Springer

Editors
Daniel T. L. Shek
Department of Applied Social Sciences
The Hong Kong Polytechnic University
Kowloon
Hong Kong

Stephen C. F. Chan
Department of Computing
The Hong Kong Polytechnic University
Kowloon
Hong Kong

Grace Ngai
Department of Computing
The Hong Kong Polytechnic University
Kowloon
Hong Kong

ISSN 2211-0550 ISSN 2211-0569 (electronic)
Quality of Life in Asia
ISBN 978-981-13-0447-7 ISBN 978-981-13-0448-4 (eBook)
https://doi.org/10.1007/978-981-13-0448-4

Library of Congress Control Number: 2018943250

Printed on acid-free paper

This Springer imprint is published by the registered company Springer Nature Singapore Pte Ltd.
The registered company address is: 152 Beach Road, #21-01/04 Gateway East, Singapore 189721, Singapore

Foreword

The past 8 years have provided The Hong Kong Polytechnic University with a rare but golden opportunity to reshape our undergraduate curriculum as we underwent the move that led us from a 3-year undergraduate curriculum to a 4-year curriculum that was first implemented in the 2012/13 academic year. We boldly took the opportunity to develop a new model for nurturing graduates who are not only successful professionals, but also socially responsible citizens. I have vivid memories of the debate in the Senate meeting held in December 2010 when we decided to require all undergraduate students to take at least one three-credit Service-Learning subject before graduation. Although most Senate members supported the new 4-year undergraduate curriculum, roughly one-fourth expressed doubts about the necessity, value and feasibility of the Service-Learning requirement.

We faced three "zeroes" when we decided to require our undergraduate students to take a three-credit Service-Learning subject as a mandatory graduation requirement. First, at that time, we had "zero" credit-bearing subjects of a similar nature, although we did have some isolated community service projects. Second, although we had a handful of colleagues who had experience of non-credit-bearing Service-Learning programmes, we had "zero" teachers with relevant experience of teaching Service-Learning subjects. Third, as Service-Learning received "zero" points in major university ranking exercises, some colleagues doubted the value of our pursuing it. It was obviously a daunting challenge. However, after much soul searching, we were convinced that it was the right thing to do as we had a rare opportunity that might not offer itself again, and we had faith that our colleagues would enable us to achieve that vision. Hence, we decided to take the bold move.

We are very grateful to the small group of passionate staff who plunged into this challenge fearlessly from the outset and led the way. They started to pilot Service-Learning subjects in the summer of 2011, developing exciting projects in Hong Kong and beyond. Other colleagues began to join in and the community grew. The whole university learned together. I followed developments closely and did my best to be part of that community. I visited students and their teachers working in the field in Hong Kong. I went to Cambodia in 2014 and Kyrgyzstan in

2017 to see the teams work in challenging situations. I witnessed our students' admirable spirit and their ability to overcome obstacles, as well as how our teachers nurtured and supported them. We are justifiably proud of our teachers and students. All along, I reminded them that Service-Learning is an academic pursuit and we have to ensure the successful achievement of the learning outcomes. My feeling is that colleagues have done a good job and they have achieved beyond our expectations.

I believe that even we in the university leadership team might not at the time have fully realized the scale and complexity of the challenge ahead of us. However, we have faith in our will and ability to succeed. We had to build the programme from scratch, encouraging academic staff to buy in and write the syllabi, develop guidelines for subject proposals, design the approval mechanisms, build up a central supporting office, train teaching staff, train students in relevant practical skills and ensure the achievement of the learning outcomes. These are very demanding tasks.

In addition to developing the academic structure, we have had to learn how to manage and operate the projects. We need to solicit funding for Service-Learning projects and to develop new financial procedures specific to the context of the projects, some of which operate in developing countries that are not part of the global banking system. Furthermore, we have to build up a global network of partners: academic, non-profit and even medical and ensure that our students are challenged, but in a safe and healthy manner. We are grateful to the support from more than 150 partners, including NGOs, universities, schools and other organizations in Hong Kong, Mainland China and several overseas countries. They have helped much in identifying and providing opportunities for our Service-Learning projects over the years.

In the process, many academic staff members have been stimulated to discover new ways to apply their research in community service, and their research has, in turn, been informed by the challenges encountered in the field. The result is much more than the sum of the number of students and teachers involved in Service-Learning. It is no less than a change of culture at our university. We have mobilized the whole campus to support the students, and in turn, we have all been inspired. Everyone feels part of the effort. We are indeed becoming a more socially responsible university. This book is about what we have experienced. By publishing a book, we document our successes and challenges that have played a part in shaping the PolyU culture. I believe this book would be helpful to colleagues in the higher education sector when they wish to scale up their own Service-Learning initiatives.

Of course, we are far from perfect. There are still many challenging tasks we face. In the spirit of the digital age, we can refer to what we have done at PolyU so far as Service-Learning 1.0. We are now striving to further improve the quality of our subjects, deepen the impact of the service projects and experiment with more innovative ways to teach. We are also expanding our international cooperation, using Service-Learning as a vehicle to teach global leadership and competency, and sharing our experience with other institutions in order to promote Service-Learning outside PolyU, even outside Hong Kong and the Mainland. This is what we are referring to as Service-Learning 2.0. Readers can look forward to a future book along these lines.

Although Service-Learning still has a score of "zero" in major university ranking exercises, we strongly believe that it is a meaningful and impactful way to promote social responsibility in university students that helps a university to thrive. I am very proud to have played a part in laying the foundation for our new education model.

Professor Timothy W. Tong
President
The Hong Kong Polytechnic University

Preface

There are two issues surrounding the development of contemporary university students. The first issue concerns the attributes of university students. With the changing economy, there are views arguing that besides intellectual competence, university students should also possess skills cherished in the knowledge economy, such as critical thinking, resilience, cooperation with others and integrity. Unfortunately, the need for "soft skills" in university students is commonly overlooked by university administrators who are more interested in ranking exercises. At the same time, there are studies showing that university students are in fact more egocentric and less empathetic as compared to several decades ago. Hence, how universities can help to promote the holistic development of university students, including their social–emotional competence (e.g., resilience, emotional competence and social awareness), moral character and social responsibility is an important issue to be considered. Conceptually speaking, these holistic development attributes of university students can be regarded as indicators of student well-being.

The second issue is on the social responsibility of university students. With reference to the existence of social problems such as poverty and vulnerable groups, it is important to ask how we can nurture university students, who are "intellectuals", to help build a better society. Essentially, how can university students contribute to the quality of life of the vulnerable groups and the community should be considered. In fact, there are views suggesting that universities should help university students develop their civic engagement and social responsibility. This is especially the case when university education in the public sector is usually heavily subsidized by tax money.

How can we promote psychosocial competencies and social responsibility in university students? Traditionally, classroom learning with teachers delivering abstract materials is the main form of learning in university settings. While classroom learning can help students acquire knowledge in an efficient way, it is constrained by the lack of linkage to the real world. With the growing emphasis on the importance of experiential learning, which typically highlights the importance of student reflection, active learning and learning outside the classroom, teachers are encouraged to promote reflective learning in students. As a pedagogy, Service-Learning provides excellent experiential learning to promote student learning experience through emphasis on the active role of the learners, student reflection and application of knowledge in real-life settings with particular reference to the vulnerable groups.

There is a growing interest in Service-Learning in Western societies in the past few decades. Research findings show that Service-Learning can facilitate student learning by helping students to apply the learned materials to real life. Besides, it also promotes civic engagement and youth leadership by enriching students' understanding of the needs of the needy people and the community. Most important of all, research has shown that Service-Learning promotes quality of life of students and the service recipients. Unfortunately, although Service-Learning as a vehicle for student change has been emphasized in many North American universities, Service-Learning is just at the beginning in many Asian communities, including Hong Kong. While there are many community service projects in different Chinese societies, they are primarily related to volunteering in university students (i.e., serving without explicit intended learning outcomes). Besides, evaluation of Service-Learning in the Asian context is weak. Hence, there is a need to document experiences on Service-Learning and its impact on the well-being of different stakeholders.

Because of the curriculum reform taking place in Hong Kong, The Hong Kong Polytechnic University seized this valuable opportunity to revamp the undergraduate curriculum. One bold initiative in the new 4-year undergraduate curriculum, which is a pioneer in Hong Kong, is to require students to take a Service-Learning subject before graduation. There are several common intended learning outcomes in different Service-Learning subjects. In the Subject Proposal Form, it is stated that:

On completing the subject, students will be able to:

- *Apply the knowledge and skills they have acquired to deal with complex issues in the service setting,*
- *Reflect on their role and responsibilities both as a professional in their chosen discipline and as a responsible citizen,*
- *Demonstrate empathy for people in need and a strong sense of civic responsibility, and*
- *Demonstrate an understanding of the linkage between service-learning and the academic content of the subject.*

Obviously, the above intended learning outcomes are closely related to well-being on two levels. As far as the well-being of the students undertaking Service-Learning projects is concerned, the competencies and empathy developed in the study constitute enhancement in student well-being because psychosocial competence is commonly regarded as an indicator of well-being. Knowing the importance of serving and acquiring the skills of helping are reflections of the well-being of students. Concerning the well-being of the service recipients, it is expected that Service-Learning projects would promote their wellness.

Although the vision of Service-Learning (SL) at PolyU is grand, there are several questions that remain to be answered—is it possible to implement SL in a massive scale (around 4000 students undertaking Service-Learning projects every year at the steady state)? Do students welcome SL? How can SL subjects in different disciplines be developed? Does SL experience promote the well-being of the students? Does SL promote the well-being of the service recipients? As systematic research on Service-Learning in different Chinese communities is almost non-existent, there is a great need to document the related experience and distil the factors shaping the development of Service-Learning in Chinese communities.

In response to the lack of documentation of the experience and lessons learned in the implementation of Service-Learning projects in Hong Kong, this book attempts to outline the development and implementation experience of Service-Learning subjects at The Hong Kong Polytechnic University. This book is a pioneer attempt to look at Service-Learning with particular reference to the experience gained at The Hong Kong Polytechnic University. PolyU is the first university that makes Service-Learning requirement a graduation requirement in Hong Kong. In terms of students taking Service-Learning per year (around 4200 in 2017/18 academic year), it is probably the largest number in the world. In this book, we describe the background of the SL initiative at PolyU. Besides, selected Service-Learning projects in different disciplines are described. In each case, the subject being offered, service site(s), service projects completed, evaluation findings and reflections of teachers will be highlighted. The opportunities and future directions for SL development at PolyU are also discussed. It is our hope that this book will stimulate thinking and sharpen the thoughts of educators, administrators and those who want to promote quality of life of students and service recipients through Service-Learning.

Kowloon, Hong Kong

Daniel T. L. Shek
Grace Ngai
Stephen C. F. Chan

Contents

Contributors

Helena S. S. Au Global Youth Leadership Institute, The Hong Kong Polytechnic University, Hunghom, Hong Kong

Joe S. C. Au Institute of Textiles and Clothing, The Hong Kong Polytechnic University, Hunghom, Hong Kong

Yammy L. Y. Chak Department of Applied Social Sciences, The Hong Kong Polytechnic University, Hunghom, Hong Kong

Ann Chan School of Optometry, The Hong Kong Polytechnic University, Hunghom, Hong Kong

Henry H. L. Chan School of Optometry, The Hong Kong Polytechnic University, Hunghom, Hong Kong

Lily Y. L. Chan School of Optometry, The Hong Kong Polytechnic University, Hunghom, Hong Kong

Natalie Y. Y. Chan School of Optometry, The Hong Kong Polytechnic University, Hunghom, Hong Kong

Stephen C. F. Chan Office of Service-Learning, The Hong Kong Polytechnic University, Hunghom, Hong Kong

Mabel N. S. Cheng Department of Applied Social Sciences, The Hong Kong Polytechnic University, Hunghom, Hong Kong

Eugene L. P. Cheung Office of Service-Learning, The Hong Kong Polytechnic University, Hunghom, Hong Kong

Memory W. H. Chiu Department of Computing, The Hong Kong Polytechnic University, Hunghom, Hong Kong

Geoffrey Chu School of Optometry, The Hong Kong Polytechnic University, Hunghom, Hong Kong

Josephine M. Csete Educational Development Centre, The Hong Kong Polytechnic University, Hunghom, Hong Kong

Chi-wai Do School of Optometry, The Hong Kong Polytechnic University, Hunghom, Hong Kong

Wynants W. L. Ho Department of Applied Social Sciences, The Hong Kong Polytechnic University, Hunghom, Hong Kong

Patrick C. L. Hui Institute of Textiles and Clothing, The Hong Kong Polytechnic University, Hunghom, Hong Kong

Alison K. Y. Ip Office of Service-Learning, The Hong Kong Polytechnic University, Hunghom, Hong Kong

Kam-por Kwan Office of Service-Learning, The Hong Kong Polytechnic University, Hunghom, Hong Kong

Charlotte S. Y. Lai Institute of Textiles and Clothing, The Hong Kong Polytechnic University, Hunghom, Hong Kong

Cindy H. Y. Lam Office of Service-Learning, The Hong Kong Polytechnic University, Hunghom, Hong Kong

Jin C. H. Lam Institute of Textiles and Clothing, The Hong Kong Polytechnic University, Hunghom, Hong Kong

Chi Kin Lau Office of Service-Learning, The Hong Kong Polytechnic University, Hunghom, Hong Kong

Savio Lee School of Optometry, The Hong Kong Polytechnic University, Hunghom, Hong Kong

Pecky P. K. Li Department of Applied Social Sciences, The Hong Kong Polytechnic University, Hunghom, Hong Kong

Kenneth W. K. Lo Office of Service-Learning, The Hong Kong Polytechnic University, Hunghom, Hong Kong

Vivian W. Y. Lo School of Optometry, The Hong Kong Polytechnic University, Hunghom, Hong Kong

Ada H. T. Ma School of Optometry, The Hong Kong Polytechnic University, Hunghom, Hong Kong

Cecilia M. S. Ma Department of Applied Social Sciences, The Hong Kong Polytechnic University, Hunghom, Hong Kong

Kwok Wai Mui Department of Building Services Engineering, The Hong Kong Polytechnic University, Hunghom, Hong Kong

Frency S. F. Ng Institute of Textiles and Clothing, The Hong Kong Polytechnic University, Hunghom, Hong Kong

Peter H. F. Ng Department of Computing, The Hong Kong Polytechnic University, Hunghom, Hong Kong

Grace Ngai Department of Computing, The Hong Kong Polytechnic University, Hunghom, Hong Kong

Phyllis C. P. Pang School of Nursing, The Polytechnic University of Hong Kong, Hunghom, Hong Kong

Daniel T. L. Shek Department of Applied Social Sciences, The Hong Kong Polytechnic University, Hunghom, Hong Kong; Centre for Innovative Programmes for Adolescents and Families, The Hong Kong Polytechnic University, Hunghom, Hong Kong; Department of Social Work, East China Normal University, Shanghai, People's Republic of China; Kiang Wu Nursing College of Macau, Macau, People's Republic of China; Division of Adolescent Medicine, Department of Pediatrics, Kentucky Children's Hospital, University of Kentucky College of Medicine, Lexington, KY, USA

Barbara W. Y. Siu Department of Civil and Environmental Engineering, The Hong Kong Polytechnic University, Hunghom, Hong Kong

Horace H. Y. Wong School of Optometry, The Hong Kong Polytechnic University, Hunghom, Hong Kong

Ling Tim Wong Department of Building Services Engineering, The Hong Kong Polytechnic University, Hunghom, Hong Kong

Wing S. Wong Office of Service-Learning, The Hong Kong Polytechnic University, Hunghom, Hong Kong

Cynthia S. T. Wu Senior Teaching Fellow School of Nursing, The Polytechnic University of Hong Kong, Hunghom, Hong Kong

Kelly Y. Xing Department of Applied Social Sciences, The Hong Kong Polytechnic University, Hung Hom, Hong Kong

Jenny Yau Department of Educational Psychology, The Chinese University of Hong Kong, Shatin, Hong Kong

Lu Yu Department of Applied Social Sciences, The Hong Kong Polytechnic University, Hung Hom, Hong Kong

Walter W. Yuen Department of Mechanical Engineering, University of California, Santa Barbara, CA, USA

Chapter 1
Development of the New 4-Year Undergraduate Program in Hong Kong

Daniel T. L. Shek

Abstract To address the problems of the old 3-year undergraduate degree structure modeled after the British higher education system, a new 4-year undergraduate degree structure was implemented in 2012/13 academic year in Hong Kong. In this chapter, the background of the undergraduate curriculum reform is outlined. With reference to The Hong Kong Polytechnic University, the development of the new undergraduate degree program is described. For the extra undergraduate year, the General University Requirements (GUR) was developed. There are several components of the GUR, including Freshman Seminar, Language and Communication Requirements, Cluster Area Requirements, Leadership and Intrapersonal Development, Service-Learning, and Healthy Lifestyle Program. To evaluate the impact of the GUR on the students, a longitudinal evaluation study was conducted. Results showed that the GUR was able to promote the holistic development in students. In particular, the evaluation findings showed that the Leadership and Intrapersonal Development and Service-Learning Requirements are the signature programs which can help students develop in a holistic manner.

Keywords Curriculum reform · The Hong Kong Polytechnic University
Leadership · Service-learning · Holistic student development

1.1 Introduction

Before 1997, Hong Kong was a British colony. During this period, Hong Kong adopted the British education system. With specific reference to higher education, the duration of university education was 3 years preceded by 5 years of secondary education (Form 1–Form 5) and 2 years of matriculation education (Form 6 and Form 7). Under this system, students had to take two public examinations—the

D. T. L. Shek (✉)
Department of Applied Social Sciences, The Hong Kong Polytechnic University, Hunghom, Hong Kong
e-mail: daniel.shek@polyu.edu.hk

D. T. L. Shek et al. (eds.), *Service-Learning for Youth Leadership*,
Quality of Life in Asia 12, https://doi.org/10.1007/978-981-13-0448-4_1

Hong Kong Certificate of Education Examination at Form 5 and the Hong Kong Advanced Level Examination at Form 7.

Undoubtedly, the British higher education has produced many outstanding graduates and it is still very influential in the commonwealth countries. However, there are also many criticisms of the 3-year university system (Jaffee, 2012). Primarily, the British education system has been criticized for its early disciplinary training because students have to specialize in different streams when they reach Form 4. In the university years, students are commonly required to declare their major study very early, with some programs requiring the students to complete many major subjects in their freshman year. Second, because of the early streaming emphasis, students are not exposed to many non-major-related disciplines. This is in sharp contrast to the liberal arts education in North America where the students are encouraged to take general education subjects in their undergraduate years. Finally, as the students are not given adequate exposure, it can be argued that their development is not holistic in nature. The above problems are summarized in the report of the Hong Kong Education Committee that "learning effectiveness of students remains not very promising; learning is still examination-driven and scant attention is paid to 'learning to learn.' School life is usually monotonous; students are not given comprehensive learning experiences with little room to think, explore and create. The pathways for lifelong learning are not as smooth as they should be. To make up for these weaknesses, we need to uproot outdated ideology and develop a new education system that is student-focused" (Hong Kong Education Commission, 2000, p. 4). Obviously, there is a strong need to restructure the higher education system to address the above-mentioned issues associated with the old 3-year undergraduate program.

With the handover of Hong Kong back to China in 1997, there is a good opportunity to reconsider the possible changes in the education system with reference to three points. First, as the 4-year undergraduate degree structure is adopted in China, changing the education system in Hong Kong will create a better transition for students. Second, with the general shift from the manufacturing economy to the service economy in the global context, there is a need to rethink about whether the higher education system can nurture the attributes of ideal graduates, such as critical thinking and communication skills. Against the above background, Hong Kong Education Commission (2000) proposed a reform of education in the academic structure, curricula and assessment of secondary and higher education with the vision to promote lifelong learning, and holistic development in university students. Regarding the goal of higher education, it should not only enable "students (to) master the necessary knowledge and skills for specific professions/ disciplines", but also "give them exposure to other learning areas and help them develop a sense of integrity, positive attitude, a broad vision and important generic skills" (Hong Kong Education Commission, 2000, p. 9). Starting from 2012/13 academic year, all universities supported by government funding changed from a 3-year undergraduate program to a 4-year undergraduate program. For the additional year created, it is expected that it will be used for general education regardless of the specialization or career aspirations of the students.

The education reform was based on a thorough and comprehensive examination of the education system in Hong Kong, which attempted to tackle the issues such as specialization at an early stage (streaming at an early stage), morbid emphasis on examination, the practice of passive learning as well as the lack of emphasis on critical thinking, creative thinking, and lifelong learning. To broaden the learning experience of the students, the 4-year undergraduate education focuses on the breadth and depth of university education with an emphasis on holistic student development. According to the Hong Kong Education Commission (2000), the new 4-year higher education aims "to develop students' independent and critical thinking, creativity and ability to learn independently and to explore, in preparation for the mastering of knowledge in a certain discipline; to foster in students an aspiration for self-improvement, a positive attitude towards life and a commitment to their families, their society and their country; and to enhance students' ability to learn, live and work in a diverse social and cross-cultural environment" (p. 32–33) and it attempts to "strike the right balance between the breadth and the depth of such programs. This would, in addition to helping students master the necessary knowledge and skills for specific professions/disciplines, give them exposure to other learning areas and help them develop a sense of integrity, positive attitude, a broad vision and important generic skills" (p. 9).

According to the University Grants Committee (2002), higher education is "at the core of Hong Kong SAR's future economic development. Without a highly educated and capable workforce with the necessary developmental skills, there will be no success in building a knowledge economy, which is not simply appropriate for, but is essential to, Hong Kong's place as a developed, internationally focused community" (p. 4). While Hong Kong strives to be Asia's world city, "there is no doubt that realization of that vision is only possible if it is based upon the platform of a very strong education and higher education sector" (University Grants Committee, 2002, p. 1). Clearly, the education reform taking place in the higher education sector in Hong Kong can be regarded as a strategic move to develop a "strong" higher education sector which hopefully can positively respond to the changing economic and social environment across the globe. The new 4-year education is expected to nurture students with "generic and transferable skills" transcending specialization and will help the graduates to contribute to their work, Hong Kong, our nation and the world. Clearly, this echoes the global trend calling for strengthening the global perspective, critical thinking, and transferable skills through general education curricula in different regions, including the USA, Mainland China, Taiwan, and European countries (van der Wende, 2011; Xing, Ng, & Cheng, 2013).

1.2 New 4-Year Undergraduate Program at The Hong Kong Polytechnic University (PolyU)

The overall goal of the new 4-year undergraduate curriculum at PolyU is to promote holistic development in undergraduate students. The core vision is that as learned intellectuals, graduates should not be just expected to possess professional competence alone. Instead, they should also possess other qualities such as critical thinking, communication skills, and ethical leadership. In the new 4-year undergraduate curriculum, there are six major desired attributes for graduates, including professional competence, critical thinking, effective communication, problem-solving, lifelong learning, and ethical leadership (Shek, Yu, Wu, & Ng, 2015).

Against the above background, in addition to the disciplinary-specific requirements for the major study, a new component of the undergraduate curriculum entitled "General University Requirements (GUR)" was designed and implemented in 2012/13 academic year. There are several components in the new 4-year curriculum, including Freshman Seminar (3 credits), Language and Communication Requirements (9 credits), Cluster Area Requirements (12 credits), Leadership and Intrapersonal Development (3 credits), Service-Learning (3 credits), and Healthy Lifestyle (0 credit). Based on the official documents (such as the papers of the Senate and other working groups), the details are outlined in the following sections.

1.2.1 Freshman Seminar

One of the reasons for changing the undergraduate curriculum to 4 years is that we want the freshmen to make informed choices about their major study. Hence, Freshman Seminar is included in the GUR to enable the students to gain more understanding of the broad disciplines so that they can choose their major study after having some basic understanding about their potential major programs. Besides deepening the students' understanding, this requirement also fosters creativity, problem-solving skills, and global outlook in students and helps them understand professional career development and basic spirit of entrepreneurship. Finally, the subject facilitates students' smooth transition to the university life and promotes their independent learning. The content of this requirement includes inspiring lectures and talks by experts and renowned researchers to stimulate the students and the innovative curricular components or activities that foster the spirit of entrepreneurship and global outlook in the students. For the teaching and learning activities, seminar or workshop component in small groups and freshman projects on discipline-related issue/problem inquiry are commonly employed.

1.2.2 Broadening subjects via Cluster Area Requirements, China Study Requirement, and Reading and Writing Requirements via Cluster Area Requirements

Throughout the world, general education subjects have been regarded as a useful means to broaden the intellectual development and multidisciplinary perspective of students. In many places, the Harvard model with different clusters such as culture, history, society, and technology is employed. After considering different general education models, PolyU has developed a general education model with four clusters, with at least three credits from each of the four cluster areas. The common learning goals of the four cluster areas are extracted from the official document approved by the Senate and are described below.

CAR (A): Human Nature, Relations and Development (HRD). This cluster is intended to promote students' understanding of human nature and its development from different theoretical perspectives. Through the related subjects, students will develop skills and attitudes in understanding oneself and others. Subjects from a wide range of disciplines such as psychology, philosophy, anthropology, spiritual science, and arts fall within this cluster area.

CAR (B): Community, Organization and Globalization (COG). Humans do not live in a social vacuum. Subjects in this cluster area attempt to sensitize students to the nature and needs of the larger communities and societies. Through this cluster area, students will be nurtured to develop understanding in working with people in different organizations, community, and the world. Subjects related to sociology, political science, economics, management, business, and finance are relevant to this cluster area.

CAR (C): History, Cultures and World Views (HCW). In addition to human development and society, human beings develop in different cultures and there are historical changes involved. The subjects in this cluster attempt to help students inquire into the human condition in relation to others with reference to history and places. Besides, students are nurtured to appreciate ideas in other cultural traditions. Subjects in the areas of history, art, the literature, philosophy, religion, and culture fall within this cluster area.

CAR (D): Science, Technology and Environment (STE). Having a scientific mind and logical thinking is important. Hence, subjects in this cluster area attempt to help students understand scientific methods and their benefits. Besides, students are nurtured to apply scientific knowledge for sustainable development and dealing with real-life issues or problems.

There are two additional requirements within the CAR. First, to promote the communication competence of the students, students have to complete the English reading and writing requirements via one CAR subject. Similarly, to strengthen the

Chinese language skills of the students, they have to complete the Chinese reading and writing requirements. Besides, a China study-related requirement is included to help students understand the Chinese culture and Chinese society.

1.2.3 Leadership and Intrapersonal Development Requirement

As there are research findings showing that university students lack intrapersonal and interpersonal competencies, how to nurture university students in a holistic manner is a grave concern. To prepare the students to lead themselves and others, they are required to successfully complete a three-credit subject in the area of Leadership and Intrapersonal Development. The objectives of the subjects designed to fulfill this requirement are to promote intrapersonal and interpersonal competencies as well as ethical leadership in university students. Regarding the objectives of this requirement, a subject in this area helps the students to understand and integrate the theories, research, and concepts on the intrapersonal and interpersonal qualities of effective leaders in the Chinese context. Besides, it promotes self-awareness, self-understanding, interpersonal skills, and self-reflection skills in students. This requirement lays the foundation for the students to become lifelong learners and develop ethical leadership.

1.2.4 Service-Learning Requirement

As learned intellectuals, students are expected to have passion about needy people and the society. Besides, students should develop a sense of social responsibility and citizenship. As Service-Learning is regarded as a vehicle to nurture citizenship and civic-mindedness as an academic subject, PolyU is committed to providing holistic education to our students through the Service-Learning requirement.

In the new 4-year curriculum, all PolyU students must successfully complete one 3-credit subject designated to meet the Service-Learning requirement. They are required to participate in substantial community service or civic engagement activities that benefit the service users or the community at large in a meaningful way. In their Service-Learning projects, the students will apply the knowledge and skills acquired from their majors or other learning experiences at the university to the community service activities. Throughout the process, we expect the students to reflect on their Service-Learning experience in order to link the theories with practice for the development of a stronger sense of ethical, social, and national responsibility.

1.2.5 *Language and Communication Requirements (LCR)*

To promote biliteracy in written English and Chinese and trilingualism in spoken English, Mandarin, and Cantonese, enhancement of Chinese and English language knowledge and skills is indispensable. To achieve this overall objective, four major requirements are intrinsic to LCR, including requirements in English (6 credits) and Chinese (3 credits), writing and reading requirements via the CAR subjects, and Discipline-specific Language Requirements. Besides these mandatory requirements, other language enhancement initiatives such as Read@PolyU and English Across the Curriculum are also carried out.

1.2.6 *Healthy Lifestyle*

To study well and adjust well in university, good health is indispensable. As such, a noncredit-bearing Healthy Lifestyle Program was designed to promote all-round development in students, covering the concepts on health and fitness, sports skills acquisition, and exercise practicum via e-learning and lectures. The subject helps students to understand the positive contribution of training or participation in sports, acquire knowledge on health (physical, social, psychological, and spiritual), appreciate the factors affecting health, reflect on values and priorities in health, reflect on one's health, and consider self-improvement.

1.3 Review of the New 4-Year Program at PolyU

Although the GUR structure was well designed, it is not clear how well these different components worked and how effectively the GUR was able to help nurture the desired graduate attributes in the students. In addition, there is a need to examine whether improvement is needed for a better implementation of the GUR in the long run. Hence, since its inception, different mechanisms have been used to evaluate the impact of the new 4-year program on the students, including the routine student evaluation strategies. In particular, to evaluate the implementation effects and effectiveness of the GUR, a 5-year longitudinal evaluation project has been implemented with the funding support by the Teaching Development Grants from 2012 to 2015 (Shek, Yu, & Ngai, 2015).

In the longitudinal evaluation study, several research questions were investigated, including: (a) How are different GUR subjects and programs offered and managed? (b) How do students and teachers view the content, teaching, and benefits of GUR subjects and programs? (c) Are there changes in the desired graduate attributes over their undergraduate study? The findings presented in this chapter are extracted from the reports on the GUR study and the published papers on the effectiveness of the GUR study (e.g., Shek, Yu, Chai, Wu, & Ho, in press, a; Shek, Yu, & Merrick, in press, b).

To arrive at a more holistic picture about the effects of GUR on the students, seven evaluation methods based on different evaluation strategies were used. First, objective outcome evaluation was conducted. In particular, a longitudinal evaluation study using a pretest–posttest design with multiple posttest measures was carried out to look at the changes in the students. Besides looking at the developmental changes over time, two control groups (Year 3 PolyU students under the old 3-year program and Year 3 students under the new 4-year program from a sister institution) were used. Second, we used Collegiate Learning Assessment Plus (CLA +) to evaluate students' changes in effective communication, critical thinking, and problem-solving skills in the students. Third, the data collected from the routine student feedback questionnaires (SFQs) were analyzed to understand the views of the students on the GUR subjects. Fourth, we used the student focus group and qualitative evaluation form to conduct qualitative evaluation to understand the subjective experience of the students. Fifth, the views of teachers were collected via the teacher focus group and qualitative evaluation form. Sixth, a longitudinal case study was implemented to understand the views of the students throughout the undergraduate years. Finally, we used the repertory grid tests to understand the changes in the students after studying in the undergraduate program (Shek, Yu, Chai, Chan, & Ngai, in press; Shek, Yu, & Merrick, in press, d).

1.3.1 *Longitudinal Online Survey*

From the academic year of 2012/13–2015/16, a longitudinal online survey had been implemented on a sample of randomly selected students enrolled in the 4-year curriculum of PolyU in the academic year of 2012/13. The students were invited to respond to a survey questionnaire in each academic year to measure their performance with a set of developmental indicators corresponding to the five desired graduate attributes of PolyU. There were 543, 643, 566, and 538 students who completed the questionnaire in each of the 4 years, respectively. Four validated instruments were used, including Chinese Interpersonal Reactivity Index (C-IRI), Chinese Positive Youth Development Scale (CPYDS), Index of Learning Style (ILS), and National Survey of Student Engagement (NSSE). Based on the data collected over the 4 years, it can be concluded that the students developed in a positive manner over time (Shek, Yu, Wu, Zhu, & Chan, 2017).

To assess the changes in the students with reference to some comparison groups, two control groups were added to the study in 2014/15 academic year. Control Group 1 (CG1) comprised 300 students enrolled in the old 3-year curriculum of PolyU which would be phased out in the summer of 2015. Control Group 2 (CG2) consisted of 300 students enrolled in the 4-year curriculum in a comparable local university. The performance of experimental group (i.e., students participated in the four waves of the longitudinal survey) was compared with those of CG1 and CG2.

These studies showed that PolyU students in the 4-year program performed better than did these two control groups, thus giving support to the effectiveness of the new four-year program in promoting holistic development in university students (Shek, & Yu, 2017a, 2017b).

1.3.2 Collegiate Learning Assessment Plus (CLA+)

Before the beginning and near the end of the academic years of 2013/14 and 2015/16, four groups of 150 randomly selected students studying in the 4-year curriculum of PolyU participated in the CLA+ test. The CLA+ is a standardized online test to assess students' competencies in problem-solving, written communication, and higher-order thinking. Group 1 included 150 first-year students who took the test before the start of 2013/14 academic year. For Group 2, 150 second-year students took the test in Semester 2 of 2013/14 academic year. We then compared the performance of Group 1 and Group 2. To understand the changes of the students over time, 150 first-year students (Group 3) completed the test before the start of 2015/16 academic year. Finally, 150 senior-year students (Group 4) participated in the test in Semester 2 of 2015/16 academic year. The findings showed that the senior-year students (Group 2 and Group 4) performed better than did the control groups (Group 1 and Group 3), providing support that the senior-year students showed better performance than did the control groups (Shek, Yu, Chan, & Ho, 2016).

1.3.3 Secondary Data Analyses of the Student Feedback Questionnaire (SFQ) Data

As a mandatory quality assurance mechanism, PolyU students are invited to complete a student feedback questionnaire for each subject. From the academic year of 2012/13–2015/16, the data of SFQs for the GUR subjects offered in each semester were collected from the Educational Development Center (EDC). In the four academic years, 15,810, 17,463, 22,589, and 13,765 (Semester 1), SFQs were collected. Secondary data analyses were performed on six standardized items in SFQ, which assessed students' perceptions of the GUR subjects in terms of their understanding of the intended learning outcomes, effectiveness of teaching and learning activities and assessments, understanding of the grading criteria, and quality and effectiveness of teaching.

Overall speaking, the SFQ findings based on the subjective outcome evaluation approach are favorable, suggesting that students had positive perceptions of the GUR subjects, including Freshman Seminar (FS), Leadership and Intrapersonal Development (LIPD), Language and Communication Requirements (LCR), Cluster

Area Requirements (CAR), and Service-Learning (SL). The mean scores for all six SFQ items regarding students' learning experiences and perceived teachers' teaching in all of the four academic years were favorable, indicating students' positive learning experiences in different GUR components regarding the intended learning outcomes, perceived effectiveness of the teaching and learning activities and assessments, understanding of the grading criteria, and perceived quality and effectiveness of teaching. Particularly, students evaluated very positively the LCR component, CAR component, and Tomorrow's Leaders in the Leadership and Intrapersonal Development Requirements (Shek, Yu, Wu, & Ng, 2015; Shek, Yu, & Pu, 2017).

1.3.4 Student Focus Group and Qualitative Evaluation Form

To enrich the quantitative evaluation findings, qualitative evaluation was carried out. Forty-seven-student focus group interviews with 279 students were conducted in the four academic years from 2012/13 to 2015/16 to investigate students' views of the GUR in terms of the content, teaching and learning, implementation, and benefits. In the academic years of 2013/14 and 2014/15, to understand the students' views of the GUR subjects, 163 and 332 randomly selected students also completed a qualitative evaluation form. Generally speaking, the qualitative findings suggested that the students had positive perception of GUR and they found benefits of studying the GUR subjects (Shek, Yu, Wu, & Chai, 2015; Shek, Yu, Wu, Ng, & Chai, 2017).

1.3.5 Teacher Focus Group and Qualitative Evaluation Form

To complement the students' views, teachers' views were collected to triangulate the evaluation findings. In the four academic years from 2012/13 to 2015/16, 4 ($N = 20$), 8 ($N = 49$), 8 ($N = 52$), and 8 ($N = 50$) teacher focus groups were conducted with different GUR subject teachers, respectively. The focus group interviews explored teachers' perceptions of the subjects they taught in respective GUR components with reference to their rationale, content, teaching, implementation, and benefits. In addition, 75 and 78 GUR subject teaching staff completed a qualitative evaluation form on their views of the GUR components in 2013/14 and 2014/15 academic years, respectively. The findings generally suggested that the teachers endorsed the value of GUR subjects and had positive experience when teaching the GUR subjects (Shek, Yu, & Chai, 2017; Shek, Yu, Wu, & Chai, 2017; Shek, Yu, Wu, Zhu, & Chai, 2017).

1.3.6 Longitudinal Case Study

A group of first-year students, who were enrolled in the PolyU's 4-year curriculum in the academic year of 2012/13, were followed up for 4 years from 2012/13 to 2015/16. At the end of each academic year, the students were invited to attend an individual interview on their personal growth and adjustment under the 4-year curriculum and the GUR. In the 4 years, 71, 31, 20, and 23 students participated in the interviews, respectively. Despite the problem of attrition, the findings showed that the students changed in their undergraduate years and demonstrated positive changes (Shek et al., in press, e; Wu, Shek, Chai, & Zhu, in press).

1.3.7 Repertory Grid Test

To assess the change in students under the 4-year curriculum with reference to the five desired graduate attributes of PolyU, in the second semester of the academic year of 2015/16, 100 senior-year students, who had participated in the GUR longitudinal online survey, were selected using the random stratified sampling method to complete the repertory grid test. The findings were very positive, which suggested that the students changed in a positive direction in the undergraduate years.

With reference to the quantitative findings based on different evaluation strategies, several observations can be highlighted from the findings. First, the longitudinal study showed that the students displayed positive changes throughout the four undergraduate years. Besides, compared to the two control groups, the experimental group did better. These findings suggested that the students studying in the new 4-year undergraduate program had positive development. For the quantitative subjective outcome evaluation, the findings were also generally positive. The students showed positive views of the subjects, teachers, and benefits of the subject. For the repertory grid test, the quantitative findings showed that the students perceived positive changes after studying in the new 4-year undergraduate program.

With reference to qualitative evaluation, the findings based on the student focus groups, qualitative evaluation form, and longitudinal case study also suggested that students had positive perceptions of different GUR components. Besides, the data based on the student evaluation forms throughout the years generally indicated that students had positive impressions and feelings of the different GUR subjects they had studied, particularly for the SL and HLS subjects. They also had positive perception of the design of the LCR component and CAR component.

The qualitative findings also showed that the students had positive comments and experiences of different components of GUR, including the active, interactive and experiential nature of group projects (including group discussion, group presentation, and hands-on group workshop), fieldwork, service-learning, and multimedia teaching. These engaged them in active, collaborative, and deep learning, which is aligned with the intended learning outcomes of different GUR components. Similarly, many teachers of different GUR subjects opined that they engaged the students in a deep level of learning and perceived the subjects to be able to nurture the desired graduate attributes of PolyU. For example, the group discussions and presentations on Tomorrow's Leaders promoted students' critical thinking and the subject facilitated students' understanding of the leadership concepts and utilization of some intra- and interpersonal skills in daily life.

1.4 Leadership and Service-Learning as Signature Requirements at PolyU

In this chapter, we focus on the students' views of two signature requirements of the GUR. The first signature requirement is Leadership and Intrapersonal Development focusing on the subject entitled "Tomorrow's Leaders" (TL; Shek et al., in press, a; Shek et al., in press, c).

Several observations can be highlighted from the evaluation findings. First, the students had positive evaluation of the teachers. Second, some students perceived that the TL subject promoted their self-reflection and self-understanding skills. Third, a portion of students expressed that as a leadership subject, the TL subject effectively strengthened their understanding of the leadership attributes and developed their leadership awareness and skills, particularly for the attribute of self-leadership. The evaluation work of TL can be seen in different papers (Shek & Leung, 2014a; Shek & Leung, 2014b, 2016; Shek & Ma, 2014; Shek & Yu, 2014, 2016; Shek, Ma, & Merrick, 2016).

Some of the narratives of the students are as follows:

> The 'Tomorrow's Leaders' subject was very useful. It gave me a very detailed instruction about different attributes leading to leadership. This knowledge is very important and attractive to us.

> The GUR subjects were more vivid and diversified. In many subjects in my major, we just sit there and listen as passive learners. However, the design of the GUR subjects such as 'Tomorrow's Leaders' was more vivid and joyful. It did not just have us sit there and listen but have interactions.

> I used to be a person who tended to make blind conjectures … For example, I tended to make all kinds of conjectures of others' careless words or jokes, e.g., 'Why did she say in such a way?' or 'Does she not like me?' In this way, I would easily misunderstand others. After studying the 'Tomorrow's Leaders' subject, I realized that communication was so important. Since then, [when I met the similar circumstances,] I have been trying not to make any conjectures about others but directly ask them to explain their behavior. I feel much better after being more direct and open in interpersonal communication.

> It was when I studied the TL subject that I had more opportunities to do self-reflection and gain more self-understanding. Leadership was scarcely mentioned in the subjects in my secondary school. However, the TL subject not only asked us to write a term paper, but also incorporated the theories and self-reflections in the teaching and learning. Therefore, our learning in the TL subject was deeper and more advanced.

> Tomorrow's Leaders is a very good subject because it did not just teach us how to lead others, did not just teach group leadership, [it also let us know that] our self-leadership is also very important. It (self-leadership) means that we should be role models for others.

> I think one benefit (of the TL subject) would be the critical thinking. It is like Lucy [alias for confidentiality] who just mentioned that the topic of moral dilemma had facilitated students' thinking in a multi-perspective way. Meanwhile, basically, we had a lot of in-class discussions in each class. They (the students) improved a lot. They knew how to express their viewpoints. We never told the students that 'your thinking is wrong!' We encouraged them to discuss.

Besides the views of the students, valuable and highly positive views of the teachers teaching LIPD subjects, particularly the TL subject, were gathered from the teacher focus groups and qualitative evaluation conducted in the four academic years. The teachers generally had positive impressions of the TL subject. Based on the qualitative studies focusing on metaphors and descriptors, some high-frequency descriptors included "a sense of achievement," "enjoyable," "meaningful," "reflective," and "rewarding". These indicated that the teachers gained positive experiences and feelings through their teaching of LIPD subjects.

The teachers perceived that the TL subject facilitated students' development in a variety of important competences, including effective communication, critical thinking, and problem-solving. The content of interpersonal relationship and the active teaching and learning methods in the TL subject, such as group project involving students from different disciplines, promoted students' interpersonal communication skills. The content related to the value judgment, group discussion, and presentation also effectively facilitated students' critical thinking.

Some teachers perceived that the TL subject changed some students' prior conceptions of leadership and developed students' understanding of the concepts of "ethical leadership" and "self-leadership." For example, in the teacher focus group in 2012/13, one teacher shared her experience, where she observed that at the very beginning, many students thought the TL subject had no relationship with them because "they thought many leaders were born in that way and they did not have the inborn traits of leadership." However, at the end of the course, the teacher observed that "many students thought that actually every person could become a leader. Most importantly, they knew that they should 'take responsibility for their life,' which means they knew the importance of self-leadership." Some teachers also observed students applying the leadership skills they learned in the TL subject in their daily lives. The sharing of a teacher is as follows:

> The TL subject taught the students how to be a leader, particularly for the students who were taking leadership roles. … I remember there was a student from the Department of Radiography. He was the chairman of a student society. He said that he understood more about the functioning of teamwork, relationship building and problem-solving through studying the subject. He said that previously he easily ran into conflicts with some of his society members and felt tormented by that. Now he realized that conflict was a necessary journey to walk through. He also learned ways of conflict solving through our subject.

Another signature subject in the new 4-year undergraduate program is Service-Learning (SL). Primarily, the SFQ results suggested that the students' evaluation of SL component was generally positive, particularly in the first few years. Second, the findings based on student focus groups, student qualitative evaluation, and longitudinal case study were very positive. A number of students held the view that SL subjects were the GUR subjects with most engagement. Through the SL subjects, particularly those offered by one's own departments, the students gained more understanding of their majors and future professions. Third, the students generally perceived that the SL subjects helped them develop their problem-solving skills, communication skills, team spirit, critical thinking, leadership, and social responsibility. Besides, the students learned to be grateful for what they possessed and the opportunities to serve the needy (Ma, Shek, & Li, 2016).

Some narratives of the students are as follows:

> My service learning experience was very unforgettable as I went to a mountain area in Sichuan province to help rebuild a village damaged heavily by an earthquake. We attempted to help the village to develop some ecotourism projects based on the local resources. … The service process was very unforgettable … [Therefore,] I think the general education subjects should include more experiential learning like this. Why do I have very deep impressions of the subject? Because I really went to Sichuan and did something! … If the subject only lectured some 'empty-talk' knowledge to us, we will forget the knowledge quickly.

> Since I had never been a leader before, when I studied in mainland China, I wanted to change myself in this summer. So I took the initiative to be a group leader in my service learning subject. However, because of my avoidance of the responsibility, our group eventually failed [in our group project]. …So, although I have learned this concept (of leadership) since my freshman year, it was my sophomore year in this summer and from this lesson (in service learning) that I realized the importance of responsibility and team spirit. Otherwise, not only one person but the whole team will fail.

Similarly, the teachers of SL subjects had positive views and experiences of the SL subjects. The teachers generally had positive impressions of the SL subjects they taught as shown by positive descriptors and metaphors, such as "a (strong) sense of achievement," "a (strong) sense of satisfaction," "happy to witness the (personal) growth of students," and "co-walker." In addition, the teachers perceived that the SL subjects were able to nurture problem-solving skills, social responsibility, empathy, communication, teamwork, and leadership in students. Particularly, students' encounters with the underprivileged people exposed the students to the life and conditions of people in different classes of the society, which can help to develop empathy in students. An example of the sharing of a teacher is as follows:

> My students mentioned that the home visit or getting along with the elder people … this kind of … real touch, real feeling was crucial. This experience could not be provided by books. The sense of community of Hong Kong, the diversity, and empowerment, all these things are something different from the textbook knowledge. Students could feel this when they really get in touch with the old people and this contact provided them with genuine feelings [towards the needy].

> Students have developed a great sense of civic responsibility and realized the importance of a concerted effort by different stakeholders in the society to work towards environmental sustainability. For many students, the experience of working with students with different academic backgrounds not only created synergy in problem-solving, but also enabled them to polish their teamwork skills, and to appreciate the strengths of other professionals.

1.5 Summary and Conclusion

To summarize, the 4-year undergraduate program in Hong Kong was developed as a response to the limitations and problems of the previous British 3-year undergraduate program. Starting from 2012/13 academic year, all institutions funded by the University Grants Committee launched the 4-year new undergraduate program. At The Hong Kong Polytechnic University, the General University Requirements (30 credits) with six components was developed to broaden the horizons of undergraduate students and promote their holistic development.

To understand the impact of the 4-year undergraduate program on the students, many evaluation studies have been conducted, including the longitudinal GUR evaluation study which was conducted to answer four research questions. Regarding the first two research questions, the data from different evaluation methods including objective outcome evaluation, subjective outcome evaluation, secondary data analyses of the SFQ data, student focus group and qualitative evaluation, longitudinal case study, and teacher focus group and qualitative evaluation indicated a generally smooth and successful implementation of different GUR components and this conclusion holds for students and teachers. With regard to the third research question, the data from different evaluation methods including the four-year longitudinal online survey, the Collegiate Learning Assessment Plus (CLA+), student and teacher focus groups and qualitative evaluations, and longitudinal case study congruently suggested that the GUR subjects were helpful to students' development in the five desired graduate attributes of PolyU: critical thinking, effective communication, innovative problem-solving, lifelong learning, and ethical leadership. In particular, the active and engaging teaching and learning methods adopted in different GUR subjects were perceived as highly beneficial to the development of the graduate attributes. For the two signature requirements, there was support for Leadership (TL) and Service-Learning.

While disciplinary-specific knowledge is basic, there is a call to broaden the perspective of the students and to strengthen their soft skills, including emotional management skills, resilience, communication skills, conflict resolution skills, and leadership.

References

Hong Kong Education Commission. (2000). *Learning for life, learning through life: Reform proposals for the education system in Hong Kong*. Hong Kong: Hong Kong Education Commission. https://www.e-c.edu.hk/doc/en/publications_and_related_documents/education_reform/Edu-reform-eng.pdf

Jaffee, D. (2012). The general education initiative in Hong Kong: Organized contradictions and emerging tensions. *Higher Education, 64*(2), 193–206.

Ma, C. M. S., Shek, D. T. L., & Li, P. (2016). *Promoting service leadership through service learning among Chinese University students.* Paper presented at 2016 Proceedings of the Second International Conference on Service-Learning (pp. 6–8). Hong Kong: The Hong Kong Polytechnic University.

Shek, D. T. L., Chai, W. Y., Lu, H., Yu, L, Chan K. H. W., Ho, W., … Law, M. (in press, e). Development of undergraduate University students: A 4-year longitudinal case study in Hong Kong. *International Journal of Child and Adolescent Health, 12(1).*

Shek, D. T. L., & Leung, H. (2014a). Post-lecture subjective outcome evaluation of a university subject on leadership and positive youth development in Hong Kong. *International Journal on Disability and Human Development, 13*(4), 465–472.

Shek, D. T. L., & Leung, J. T. Y. (2014b). Perceived benefits of a university subject on leadership and intrapersonal development. *International Journal on Disability and Human Development, 13*(4), 481–488.

Shek, D. T. L., & Leung, J. T. Y. (2016). Developing social competence in a subject on leadership and intrapersonal development. *International Journal on Disability and Human Development, 15*(2), 165–173.

Shek, D. T. L., & Ma, C. M. S. (2014). Do university students change after taking a subject on leadership and intrapersonal development? *International Journal on Disability and Human Development, 13*(4), 451–456.

Shek, D. T. L., Ma, C. M. S., & Merrick, J. (Eds.). (2016). Special issue: Promoting leadership and intrapersonal development in university students. *International Journal on Disability and Human Development, 15(2)*, 125–231.

Shek, D. T. L., & Yu, L. (2014). Post-course subjective outcome evaluation of a subject on leadership and intrapersonal development for university students in Hong Kong. *International Journal on Disability and Human Development, 13*(4), 457–464.

Shek, D. T. L., & Yu, L. (2016). Student feedback on a subject on leadership and intrapersonal development for university students in Hong Kong. *International Journal on Disability and Human Development, 15*(3), 339–346.

Shek, D. T. L., & Yu, L. (2017a). General University Requirements and holistic development in university students in Hong Kong. *International Journal of Adolescent Medicine and Health, 29*(1), 41–48.

Shek, D. T. L., & Yu, L. (2017b). The impact of 3-year and 4-year undergraduate programs on university students: The case of Hong Kong. *International Journal of Adolescent Medicine and Health, 29*(1), 49–55.

Shek, D. T. L., Yu, L., & Chai, W. (2017). Qualitative evaluation of a new general education program at a university in Hong Kong: Teachers' experiences. *International Journal of Child and Adolescent Health, 10*(1), 73–89.

Shek, D. T. L., Yu, L., Chai, W., Chan, K. H. W., & Ngai, J. (in press, c). General education at The Hong Kong Polytechnic University: A comprehensive evaluation study. *International Journal of Child and Adolescent Health.*

Shek, D. T. L., Yu, L., Chai, W., Wu, F. K. Y., & Ho, W. W. L. (in press, a). Achievement of desired university graduate attributes through a new 4-year undergraduate program. *International Journal of Child and Adolescent Health.*

Shek, D. T. L., Yu, L., Chan, K. H. W., & Ho, W. W. L. (2016). Assessing learning gains of university students in Hong Kong adopting the Collegiate Learning Assessment Plus (CLA+). *International Journal on Disability and Human Development, 15*(3), 331–337.

Shek, D. T. L., Yu, L., & Merrick, J. (in press, b). Special issue: Promotion of holistic development of university students in Hong Kong. *International Journal of Child and Adolescent Health.*

Shek, D. T. L., Yu, L., & Merrick, J. (in press, d). The impact of a new 4-year undergraduate program in Hong Kong. *International Journal of Child and Adolescent Health.*

Shek, D. T. L., Yu, L., & Ngai, J. (2015). Evaluation of a general education program in Hong Kong: Secondary data analyses based on student feedback questionnaires. *International Journal on Disability and Human Development, 14*(4), 401–406.

Shek, D. T. L., Yu, L., & Pu, X. (2017). Evaluation of a general education program in Hong Kong based on student feedback questionnaires. *International Journal of Child and Adolescent Health, 10*(1), 91–98.

Shek, D. T. L., Yu, L., Wu, F. K. Y., & Chai, W. (2015). General university Requirements at The Hong Kong Polytechnic University: Evaluation findings based on student focus groups. *Assessment & Evaluation in Higher Education, 40*(8), 1017–1031.

Shek, D. T. L., Yu, L., Wu, F. K. Y., & Chai, W. (2017). Teachers' views of a new general education program in Hong Kong: A qualitative study. *International Journal of Adolescent Medicine and Health, 29*(1), 57–65.

Shek, D. T. L., Yu, L., Wu, F. K. Y., & Ng, C. S. M. (2015). General education program in a new 4-year university curriculum in Hong Kong: Findings based on multiple evaluation strategies. *International Journal on Disability and Human Development, 14*(4), 377–384.

Shek, D. T. L., Yu, L., Wu, F. K. Y., Ng, C. S. M., & Chai, W. (2017). Qualitative evaluation of general university requirements in a new 4-year university curriculum: Findings based on experiences of students. *International Journal of Adolescent Medicine and Health, 29*(1), 91–102.

Shek, D. T. L., Yu, L., Wu, F. K. Y., Zhu, X., & Chai, W. (2017). Teachers' views on a new general education program in Hong Kong: Qualitative data collected over two years. *International Journal of Child and Adolescent Health, 10*(2), 233–243.

Shek, D. T., Yu, L., Wu, F. K. Y., Zhu, X., & Chan, K. H. W. (2017). A 4-year longitudinal study of well-being of Chinese university students in Hong Kong. *Applied Research in Quality of Life, 12*(4), 867–884.

University Grants Committee. (2002). *Higher education in Hong Kong: Report of the university Grants Committee*. Hong Kong: University Grants Committee. https://www.ugc.edu.hk/doc/eng/ugc/publication/report/her/hereport.pdf

van der Wende, M. (2011). The emergence of liberal arts and sciences education in Europe: A comparative perspective. *Higher Education Policy, 24*(2), 233–253.

Wu, F. K. Y., Shek, D. T. L., Chai, W., & Zhu, X. (in press). Well-being of university students in Hong Kong: A longitudinal case study. *International Journal of Child and Adolescent Health.*

Xing, J., Ng, P. S., & Cheng, C. (Eds.). (2013). *General education and the development of global citizenship in Hong Kong, Taiwan and Mainland China: Not merely icing on the cake*. New York: Routledge.

Chapter 2
Service-Learning as a Vehicle for Youth Leadership: The Case of the Hong Kong Polytechnic University

Stephen C. F. Chan, Grace Ngai, Jenny Yau, Walter W. Yuen, Daniel T. L. Shek and Helena S. S. Au

Abstract At PolyU, we instituted service-learning as an effective experiential pedagogy to nurture social responsibility which is also strongly related to youth leadership, leading ultimately to improvements in the quality of life of the students themselves, as well as the communities that they serve. While designing an effective program to integrate service-learning into our undergraduate academic programs, we aim to address the well-known motivational needs of human behavior: autonomy, competence, and relatedness, as well as the desirable qualities of leadership and global outlook. We have also taken into consideration the specific cultural characteristics of higher education in Hong Kong. The result is an academic

S. C. F. Chan (✉)
Office of Service Learning, The Hong Kong Polytechnic University,
Hunghom, Hong Kong
e-mail: stephen.c.chan@polyu.edu.hk

G. Ngai
Department of Computing, The Hong Kong Polytechnic University,
Hunghom, Hong Kong
e-mail: grace.ngai@polyu.edu.hk

J. Yau
Department of Educational Psychology, The Chinese University of Hong Kong,
Shatin, Hong Kong
e-mail: jyau@cuhk.edu.hk

W. W. Yuen
Department of Mechanical Engineering, University of California,
Santa Barbara, CA, USA
e-mail: yuen@engineering.ucsb.edu

D. T. L. Shek
Department of Applied Social Science, The Hong Kong Polytechnic University,
Hunghom, Hong Kong
e-mail: daniel.shek@polyu.edu.hk

H. S. S. Au
Global Youth Leadership Institute, The Hong Kong Polytechnic University,
Hunghom, Hong Kong
e-mail: helena.ss.au@polyu.edu.hk

D. T. L. Shek et al. (eds.), *Service-Learning for Youth Leadership*,
Quality of Life in Asia 12, https://doi.org/10.1007/978-981-13-0448-4_2

service-learning program which is compulsory yet includes a wide selection of subjects, structured instructions balanced with student-based learning, challenging as well as meaningful service projects, and a growing set of boundary-crossing, international projects in far away radically different cultures. This chapter discusses the design of the program in some details.

Keywords Autonomy · Competence · Relatedness · Leadership
Boundary-crossing · Self-determination theory

2.1 Introduction

Leadership development has been attracting much attention in higher education. In the East Asia region, in particular, there is growing awareness that a university education should be more than simply about career and vocational training. At the same time, the rapidly changing face of society resulting from increasing urbanization, globalization, automation, and digitization has made the world a more complex place in which to live and maneuver. The world in which today's university graduate will have to navigate is a much different environment than it was only a decade ago. It was once assumed that university studies would train a student in a particular discipline, which would stay relevant for at least a decade after graduation. Many of today's graduates may not work in a field related to their area of study, are likely to change career directions more than a few times before their tenth reunion, and are most likely to return to school to obtain an advanced degree for career development or advancement. In short, they will have to learn to make and find their own opportunities; to be sensitive to and aware of their context; and to reflect and learn from their own experiences and mistakes.

These are skills and attributes that leadership education cultivates. It is also obvious that many of these are common with the attributes that service-learning aims to cultivate. Many of these attributes are best learned in an experiential learning environment, such as service-learning projects and reflections. Simultaneously, there is also growing realization that the interconnectedness of society and the world makes it important that young people are taught to make ethical choices, and to be socially aware and socially responsible. These are also obviously attributes that are cultivated by service-learning programs. Therefore, service-learning is increasingly being recognized as an effective pedagogy for the training of leadership development.

For the last six years, the Hong Kong Polytechnic University (PolyU) has made academic service-learning part of its institutional strategy to cultivate students' generic attributes in social responsibility, community engagement, and ethical behavior. For many years, PolyU has encouraged students to engage in community service, mainly through the Community Service-Learning Program (CSLP). Hundreds of students participated voluntarily in dozens of community service projects each year. The learning elements of these service projects, however, were not strong, and there were many constraints which limited the effectiveness of the program, both in terms of the impact of the service to the clients and the learning outcomes for our students. The students' enthusiasm in voluntary service often could not be sustained because of academic and other demands. The student turnover rate was naturally high, making it difficult to sustain projects. Without systematic training, it was difficult for the students to tackle more challenging and impactful projects. Without purposeful, intentional teaching and structured reflections, learning was often superficial.

Around the year 2000, triggered by a change in the Hong Kong education system, the university had an opportunity to revamp all undergraduate curricula. It made the decision to greatly strengthen the general education components in the form of the General University Requirements (GUR). Part of the "backbone" of the GUR is the Service-Learning Requirement—each undergraduate student is required to pass at least one 3-credit subject in service-learning. Participation in the program is compulsory, but the students can choose a service-learning subject from a wide range of disciplines, serving very different communities with diverse needs. Each subject combines lectures, workshops, a purpose-designed community service project of at least 40 hours, structured reflection, and continuous assessment of all aspects of the subject. Currently, each year, roughly 4000 undergraduate students enroll in over 60 such subjects. These subjects challenge the student to engage with an unfamiliar community, empathize with people who look, speak, feel, and think differently, and learn to work out practical solutions for real benefits with fellow students.

To maximize their exposure and to challenge them to learn to lead, we strive to take students outside Hong Kong, to remote places in Mainland China, to foreign countries like Vietnam, Cambodia, Myanmar, Indonesia, Kyrgyzstan, and Rwanda. We provide opportunities for our students to work together with students from different places.

2.2 Major Design Features of the Program

In the review of our undergraduate programs, it was realized that the university needed to strengthen certain intangible learning outcomes such as social responsibility and global outlook. Based on reading of the literature and study on the experience of leading universities, the university was convinced that service-learning is an effective pedagogy to nurture social responsibility and other desirable qualities.

The design of the SL program was guided by established theories of human motivation and personality, in particular, the Self-Determination Theory (Deci & Ryan, 1985; Deci, Vallerand, Pelletier, & Ryan, 1991). This stresses the importance of autonomy, competence, and relatedness, which have been corroborated by many other researchers.

We have hence designed the service-learning program with critical features to address these qualities. Figure 2.1 shows the overall design. For example, the

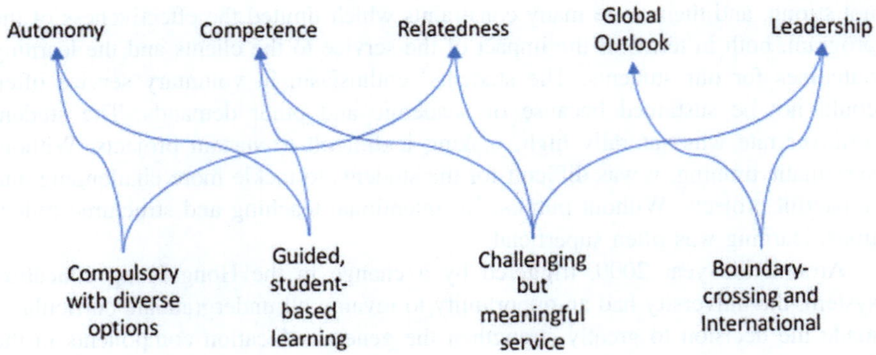

Fig. 2.1 Desired qualities and features of service-learning designed to engender them

program is compulsory and yet encompasses a diverse selection of subjects and projects—for autonomy and relatedness. The general outlines of the service projects are designed by the teachers, with plenty of room for students to learn and exercise leadership—for autonomy and competence. The service projects are challenging yet meaningful—for competence and relatedness.

Global competence with a global outlook is a necessity for university education in today's world. This is particularly true for a small place such as Hong Kong, which was built on import–export trade and even today is reliant on commerce, tourism, and similar interactions with external communities for survival and development. There are surely plenty of underprivileged groups in Hong Kong; hence, a large number of our service projects are carried out in Hong Kong. But we make it a priority to take our students to Mainland China and foreign countries for SL. Our students work closely with local students at these offshore sites, and we also strive to learn and serve with students from foreign universities, so that our students can learn and practice a global outlook first hand.

Service-learning subjects are like other typical academic subjects and hence must be equally rigorous. They must have well-defined learning objectives and expected student learning outcomes, clearly defined syllabus teaching methods, and assessment. A committee of experienced academic staff was appointed to vet SL subject proposals, and their decisions are accountable to the committee on General University Requirements, which is overseen by the Associate Vice President. Major design features are discussed in the following subsections.

2.2.1 Compulsory with Diverse Options—Autonomy and Relatedness

The vision of providing an all-rounded education to our students applies to all students. Since social engagement is considered a critical aspect of responsible citizenship, and service-learning has been chosen as the key pedagogy to nurture responsible citizenship, it was decided, after much debate, to make service-learning compulsory. Each undergraduate student is required to take at least one 3-credit subject in service-learning. An important consideration was that, in contrast to places such as the USA, the culture of civic engagement was not very strong among the youths in Hong Kong, including students at our university. Hence, it was necessary to promote a stronger incentive for the students to get engaged. At the same time, we were aware of the possible negative consequences, such as resentment at being compelled to engage in something undesired, and the distortion of the motivation to serve as it is compulsory rather than voluntary.

Hence, the university decided to provide a diverse range of service-learning subjects across multiple disciplines, targeting diverse clients, in widely different locations. The rationale behind this was that while students were required to fulfill their service-learning requirement, they still had a choice of subject and project nature that is in line with their abilities and interests. Another rationale behind this was to promote inclusivity in service-learning across all professions and disciplines represented at the university. PolyU is a comprehensive university with 30 academic units from across 8 faculties and schools. The academic disciplines represented range from engineering to applied sciences, health sciences, social sciences, business, design, textiles, hospitality, and humanities.

Over the last 7 years, we have successfully developed almost 70 SL subjects, and today SL subjects are offered by almost all ($\sim$95%) of the academic departments. We have deliberately aimed at developing service projects serving a diversity of client communities: children, youths, elderly, handicapped, ethnic minorities, people with special needs, immigrants, and so on. Our projects cover all the 18 districts in Hong Kong, many provinces in Mainland China ranging from the Maritimes to the remote mountains, Taiwan, and several foreign countries in Southeast Asia, Central Asia, and Africa. This provides the students a lot of room to exercise their autonomy in choosing a suitable subject with which to fulfill their graduation requirement. They can also take the opportunity to engage with communities that they wish to connect with, for personal, cultural, faith, and other reasons.

The offering of service-learning subjects from across all disciplines brings a lot of academic, teaching, and supporting staff into the community of social responsibility. We have now $\sim$170 staff members engaged in teaching these subjects and many more assisting in the teaching and training of students, financing, administering, advising, health checking, arranging of logistics, and myriad other functions. In some ways, the development of service-learning is nothing short of starting a culture and paradigm shift at the university. The impact on the teaching staff is no less significant than the impact on the students. In fact, even though there is a lot of attention on students doing service, the culture of a university is seen to be embodied in the staff even much more than the students. Students come and go. They usually stay for no more than 4 years and are generally available for active service for no more than two—since they are probably too inexperienced in the first year, and too occupied with graduation, job hunting, or applying for graduate studies in the final year. It is the staff and the support infrastructure that enable the generations of students to carry on the culture of social engagement.

If the objective of service-learning is to cultivate a lifelong civic responsibility and engagement in our students, it is imperative that all disciplines recognize that they can contribute to community and serve the community in some way. At a more fundamental level, we strongly believe that practically every academic discipline can offer some meaningful community service—given sufficient will and creativity. Our own experience and experiences we have witnessed at other leading universities have borne this out. In particular, PolyU's own historical background as a vocational training institute means that our academic departments in general tend to put great emphases on applied science, engineering, and other professional disciplines. These disciplines exist to solve practical problems in the community, and therefore, it is logical to expect that these disciplines actually have a lot to offer the underprivileged. In the rest of this book, there are many creative and possibly surprising examples.

2.2.2 Guided, Student-Based Learning—Competence and Autonomy

Since PolyU's model of service-learning encompasses all the disciplines and is graded for academic credit, it was necessary for parity and comparability to define a service-learning subject. To this end, a set of core learning outcomes was developed to cover all service-learning subjects. These learning outcomes ensure that students understand a *societal issue* that underpins the project that they are working on, apply their *academic knowledge and skills* to address the issue, and develop their *affective and civic competencies* through experience and reflection (Fig. 2.2).

Upon completing the subject, students should be able to:

1. *Academic Knowledge and Skills*: Apply the knowledge and skills they have acquired to deal with complex issues in the service setting.
2. *Affective and Civic Competencies*: Reflect on their roles and responsibilities both as a professional in their chosen discipline and as a responsible citizen.
3. *Affective and Civic Competencies*: Demonstrate empathy for people in need and a strong sense of civic responsibility.
4. *Societal Issue*: Demonstrate an understanding of the linkage between service-learning and the academic content of the subject.

When designing their subject, teachers are free to insert additional learning outcomes as they see appropriate or to rephrase these common learning outcomes in a manner that better matches their course content. However, the existence of a set of common learning outcomes ensures that all service-learning subjects achieve their intended objectives and hence any student graduating from PolyU would have fulfilled certain outcomes. As have been frequently pointed out, service-learning is

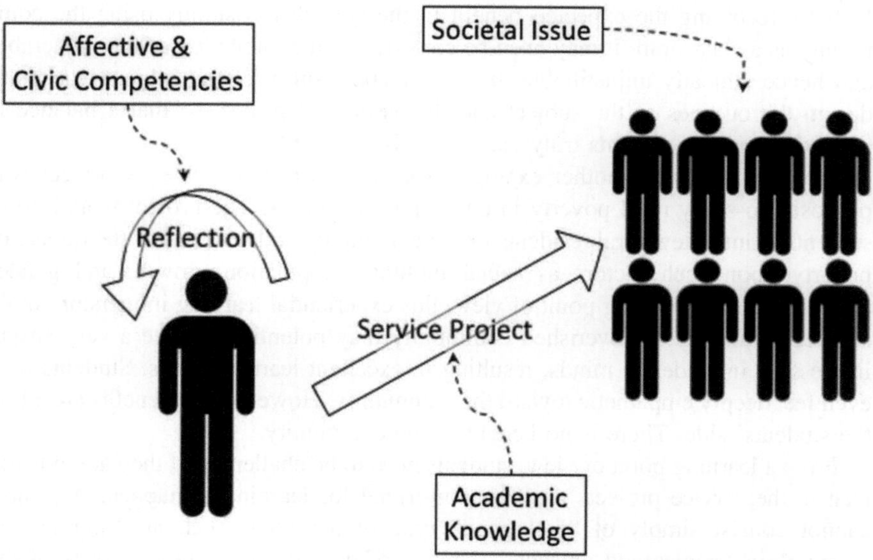

Fig. 2.2 Relationship between the common intended learning outcomes of a service-learning subject and the teaching and learning components

balanced integration of learning and community service. It is very easy to shift the balance one way or the other. One common pitfall is to put too much emphasis on the community service and not enough on the students' learning. This can easily happen when the students are given too much autonomy, or the partner community's desires are given too much emphasis. It is highly desirable from certain point of view. Unfortunately, it then distorts service-learning and makes it difficult to achieve some of the key expected outcomes.

We illustrate with an example from our own experience. A project was organized to install solar panels to produce electricity for a village in a developing country. From the point of the NGO, and even the community, it is very desirable to maximize the number of solar electrical systems installed and the number of villagers helped, to achieve maximal benefit for the community. From their point of view, interaction with the community residents is unnecessary and indeed detrimental to the progress of the project, as it takes away time that could have been spent installing an additional system for an additional household. This, however, results in the students spending all of their time and energy on the technical aspects and the numerical targets of the project, and they would learn very little about the community and the socioeconomic issues involved, such as the impact of energy poverty.

On the other hand, if too much is focused on the students' learning, it becomes a learning tour, and the benefits to the local community may be in doubt. This needs to be considered in light of the investment, the time and cost that the community has invested in receiving and providing assistance to the team of teachers and students.

Without receiving the expected benefit in the end, this is simply using the community as a classroom. It may even be considered an exploitation of the vulnerable and hence ethically unjustifiable. It is the responsibility of the subject teacher to design the outlines of the subject and the associated project so that a balance is achieved, and the students truly learn what is expected.

We illustrate with another example from our own experience. A project was proposed to study rural poverty in developing countries. The project would bring students to interview rural residents of the community and learn about the impact of poverty upon such factors as social mobility, population growth, and gender equality. From a learning point of view, this experiential learning immersion into a socioeconomically impoverished community may potentially create a very strong impression in students' minds, resulting in excellent learning gains. Students may even feel deeply empathetic toward the community. However, the benefits are all on the students' side. There is no benefit to the community.

From a learning point of view, students need to be challenged if they are to learn. Hence, the service projects must be non-trivial for learning to happen. A project cannot consist simply of "feel good" type of activities, such as "singing and dancing" or "games and presents." Unless, of course, the academic focus of the subject relates to singing and dancing, for example, in the form of performance therapy. In that case, the students should understand the reason and the benefit of these singing and dancing activities and be taught to sing and dance well, as well as the skills needed to teach their service recipients to sing and dance well. This clearly requires careful planning and preparations prior to the service and is obviously non-trivial. In all cases, the teacher must use lectures and workshops to teach the student the relevant knowledge and skills, and to provide guidance to the students in carrying out the service. The students gain competence in the process. It is partly this teaching and guidance that makes service-learning an academic endeavor.

On the other hand, it is important for the students' learning and growth that they have a certain degree of autonomy. It is possible for a project to be useful to the community and yet has no room for students to exercise problem solving. An example would be a health assessment project that follows a very prescribed protocol in which there is no room for deviation. Hence, we require that our teachers design only the outlines or boundaries of the project, leaving sufficient room for the students to apply their skills and knowledge in real settings and to learn to exercise their creativity, adaptability, teamwork, and leadership.

We illustrate with another example. One project requires students to design clothes for and together with people recovering from mental illness, as a form of art therapy. But it is up to the students to decide how the team should work together and with the client, how to engage the client to create their design, how to realize their design within the feasible parameters, and finally how to model the product garment for the public, which can do wonders for the self-image of the recovering client. It is a challenge to balance guidance and autonomy, but when it works, the results can be quite satisfying for all parties involved. This subject is one of the most popular among the students and other stakeholders.

2.2.3 Challenging but Meaningful Service—Competence and Relatedness

A service project has to be challenging for the students to truly learn from it. Students may feel good about passing an easy examination. By the same token, students may feel good about successfully carrying out an easy community service project. But they do not learn much from the experience if it does not pose a real challenge. The maxim "no pain, no gain" applies just as much in service-learning as it applies in other contexts. Worse, they may develop a fixed mindset—that they possess already a certain inborn talent which enables them to cruise through life; henceforth, they just need to preserve this talent and their own position of superiority, rather than appreciating their own capacity to work hard, overcoming challenges, and growing—developing a growth mindset (Dweck, 2008). The task of the teacher is to design a service project that requires the students to learn something new, to motivate them to work hard, and to apply it in the service project. On the other hand, the project should not be so hard that it is beyond the capacity of the students to learn within a reasonable time frame. That would only result in frustration on all three sides—student, teacher, and community.

The project also has to be meaningful—to the students, not only to the teacher. This is a common fallacy. As teachers, we often fall into the trap of feeling that since the project is meaningful to me, hence it must be naturally meaningful to my students. An example is community-based research projects that involve students in collecting data from the community, and this data will then be analyzed for potential improvements to, for example, community infrastructure or support. There is no doubt that these projects often result in sustained, long-term benefit for the community. However, in the time span of a single class over a single semester, or even during the 4-year study period of a group of students, these projects often seem like "toy" projects that result in "yet another study" or "yet another analysis." Without ample communication and facilitation from the teacher, these types of projects may create a sense of cynicism and distrust in students, who may perceive that what they are doing is meaningless and just for show, or worse, that they are being used as cheap labor to support some larger research or political agenda.

In the best-case scenario, a project would provide some immediate tangible benefit to the community as well as open up avenues for longer-term, sustainable development for a deeper, structural betterment of the community. To achieve this, projects need to be developed between the subject teachers and community partners aiming at building a long-term relationship. Often, it takes a number of years to develop a good mutual understanding. We have to understand the community and their needs; the community has to develop an appreciation of our capabilities and commitment, and the consequent trust in us. Here having the stable infrastructure of an academic subject that is run year after year has the big advantage of continuity and sustainability. Then, our students can engage with the community based on this long-term relationship that the subject leaders have developed. The fact that we offer a comprehensive set of subjects and associated projects providing a wide range of options so that the students can surely find something that they can relate to. And their teachers will then help them build on that relationship.

We have a number of "offshore" service projects outside of Hong Kong. The value of sending students on service projects of $\sim$40 hours to a foreign country has sometimes been queried—the perception is that the period is too short to learn about the community and the problem, and to devise and implement a solution. However, it is our experience—and we have demonstrated—that rigorous preparation and intense execution can generate significant benefit to the community, even with just 40 hours of service.

We illustrate with another example. In 2016 and 2017, teams of 15 students from our university have collaborated with an equal number of local youths and students to build 4 solar electrical systems for charging car batteries, besides wiring up 100+ village houses for LED lighting powered by those batteries. This has been achieved in 10 days of service. These systems have been consistently providing electrical power to the whole villages who had never seen electricity before. It was made possible in such a short period of time because the SL course was designed that our students would go through one full semester of training and preparations; then a two-week trip was planned systematically and thoroughly; the students work their heart out to make full use of the time. This is also a demonstration that large impact in a short period of time is doable when the team is committed because they care about the community. This is also a demonstration of competence driven by relatedness.

Some of our projects involve collaboration between multiple teams. This makes sense as community needs are complex and interdisciplinary. In one of our projects, multiple teams work together for one week to turn a used cargo container into a community learning center. The container was purchased, and the teams designed and painted a colorful mural on the outside, paneled the inside, built furniture for it, installed a library of books, set up computers and a network, installed solar panels for electricity, and installed LED lighting and electric fans, all in one week. The whole process required intricate planning to make sure that the teams would not be getting in each other's way, intense preparation to ensure that the teams would be effective and efficient when working, and meticulous coordination to shuffle the teams in and out of the site. This was possible because of our long-term working relationship in the community, which was anchored by repeated offering of the service-learning subject. This enhanced our understanding of the local issues and built up the trust with the local community.

2.2.4 Boundary-Crossing and International—Global Competence and Leadership

Service-learning is boundary-crossing almost by definition. In most cases, students serve populations different from themselves. The differences may be in terms of age, health, ability, ethnicity, color of skin, language, history, culture, etc. In general, the more differences between the service recipients and the students, and the more challenges they encountered, the more they would learn.

To this end, we strive to take the students to different communities in Hong Kong. This is not too difficult if the boundary is largely socioeconomic or age. Racially, however, Hong Kong, despite its reputation as an international city, is a largely homogeneous society. The general population demographics in 2018 have 94% of the population as Han Chinese speaking Chinese; 1.9% Indonesian; 1.9% Filipino; 0.78% white; 0.40% Indian; 0.25% Pakistani; 0.23% Nepalese; 0.18% Japanese; 0.16% Thai, etc. For many of our students, growing up in Hong Kong means that they do not have previous experience interacting with individuals of a different race as peers.

This obviously puts our students at a disadvantage in this increasingly globalized world. Hong Kong's economy is becoming more and more closely integrated with Mainland China, and Hong Kong's primary economic activity is trading. Therefore, it is easy to see the importance of global competence to our students. To compensate for the racial homogeneity of Hong Kong, we make an effort to provide them with opportunities to learn and serve outside of Hong Kong. We are currently sending 16% of our students ($\sim$640) to Mainland China and 6% ($\sim$240) to foreign countries such as Vietnam, Cambodia, Myanmar, Kyrgyzstan, and Rwanda. We are planning to gradually increase that to 20% for Mainland China and 10% for foreign countries.

We wish for our students to be able to see people of different races and ethnicities as peers. As part of that strategy, in most of our projects in foreign countries, we partner with major local universities in those countries. This is partly out of necessity—most of the time our students do not speak the local language and are not familiar with the local customs. Hence, we rely on local student collaborators to interpret for them and to interact appropriately with the local community.

This relationship between our students and these local students is at least twofold. On the one hand, they are partners in the service. On the other hand, our students, together with their teachers, are training the local students in the technical aspects of the project, transferring their knowledge to the local community, as well as passing on the culture of social engagement to the local students. That is also part of our students' service and sometimes arguably more impactful in the long run than the visible service itself.

This partnership, which was first created out of practicality, has led to an exciting development. Increasingly, we discover that many local universities are also eager to adopt service-learning as an effective pedagogy. Hence, our students are learning from working with their students, while their students are learning service-learning, among other things, from our students. The teachers and staff also gain from this collaboration. During the process of planning and leading service projects for the students, our teachers and staff need to work with their local counterparts, who are from a different culture and often a different discipline than their own. This cross-institution sharing and learning among the staff and administrators also builds up their own global competency and broadens their perspective.

This cross-institutional sharing and collaboration has brought about unexpected results. In small scales for now, but which hopefully can be further developed in future, we are partnering with foreign universities in service projects, often executed in a third country. For example, one of our engineering courses partners with a leadership studies course in a US institution. The two groups of students learn about the global leadership and cross-cultural competencies, about the digital poverty and the impact of technology through digital technologies, such as shared lectures broadcasted on Skype and digital collaboration tools such as Slack. The students then collaborate on a digital inclusion project in Cambodia, where they will meet face-to-face for the first time.

This project obviously crosses the boundary between two very different cultures—Chinese and American. It also brings together two very different disciplines—engineering and education. Not only do the students need to learn to adapt to each other's learning styles, but the teachers also need to adapt to each other's teaching styles and the idiosyncrasies of the different disciplines. More importantly, they need to learn to see the relevancy of their discipline content in the context and space of another. This has been a tremendous challenge which took a lot of time and effort to pull off, but it has also brought along very intense learning gains on the part of both teacher and student.

Setting up an overseas site takes time and effort as we navigate the contexts of a new location, new partners, new financial arrangements, and so on. To consolidate efforts, we have set up an offshore base in Cambodia in collaboration with the Royal University of Phnom Penh (RUPP). This offshore base hosts upward of 100 students per year, working in multiple service projects in the same community in rural Cambodia. These projects are done in collaboration with students and teachers at RUPP, which is gradually building up its own service-learning and leadership program.

Service-learning has also facilitated boundary-crossing through student exchanges. Many of our strategic partners send their students to Cambodia to work in service projects together with our students. Often these students, from USA, Israel, etc., have very different background and cultures compared to our students, who come mainly from Hong Kong and Mainland China, but increasingly also from Taiwan, Malaysia, Singapore, Indonesia, Kazakhstan, etc. Many exciting opportunities are being explored.

2.3 Balanced Implementation Approach

The program has been achieved at PolyU with a balanced centralized-distributive approach. On the one hand, service-learning subjects are academic subjects, which are properly the domain of academic departments. Hence, academic departments are encouraged through policies and incentives to design and offer academic subjects in service-learning, with a very large degree of autonomy. On the other hand, this is a new initiative where many departments have little or no expertise and experience. The university also needs to articulate the vision clearly and consistently, and provides the primary driving force to move forward such a tremendous endeavor.

Hence, the university set up a central unit, Office of Service-Learning (OSL), to direct and coordinate the endeavor. A committee of experienced academics is also set up to ensure the academic vision, and standards are upheld. The OSL can be seen as the operational arm of the infrastructure and the committee the quality control arm. The OSL has been working very closely with academic departments, experimenting with innovative pedagogies, co-developing and co-teaching some of the key subjects, and instrumental in building up an affective community of practice with a critical mass. For example, the OSL has set up practically all the international service project sites with a number of adventurous colleagues and even created an offshore base in Cambodia. These would probably not have been possible without the close collaboration between the visionary central office and a number of courageous academics. It is clear that the close collaboration between the central office and the academic departments is a critical factor in the success of the program. More details can be found in a subsequent chapter on Engaging Teachers (Chap. 17).

2.4 Conclusion

In the process of designing and implementing service-learning at our university, we have learned a lot from leading universities around the world, particularly those from the USA, such as University of San Francisco, University of California, Los Angeles, University of Pennsylvania, Purdue University, and Tufts University. We have also learned much from University of Manchester of the UK, University of Pretoria of South Africa, and Pontifical Catholic University of Argentina at Buenos Aries. That said, however, we also have to make many adaptations due to the particular environment that is Hong Kong and our own university's heritage of an application-oriented technical university. The result is a model of service-learning that suits ourselves particularly, but which may also have certain degree of applicability for universities with some similarity to ours.

References

Deci, E. L., & Ryan, R. M. (1985). *Intrinsic motivation and self-determination in human behavior*. New York: Plenum Press.

Deci, E. L., Vallerand, R. J., Pelletier, L. G., & Ryan, R. M. (1991). Motivation and education: The self-determination perspective. *Educational Psychologist, 26*(3&4), 325–346.

Dweck, C. S. (2008). *Mindset: The new psychology of success*. New York: Ballatine Books.

Chapter 3
Perceived Changes and Benefits of a Service-Learning Subject for Underprivileged Children in Shanghai: Views of University Students

Daniel T. L. Shek and Yammy L. Y. Chak

Abstract Over the past two decades, service-learning has become popular in university education. As such, service-learning subjects are developed at The Hong Kong Polytechnic University to help students develop positive personal understanding and self-identity, critical thinking ability, social awareness, and social responsibility. The purpose of this chapter is to examine the perceived changes and benefits from the perspectives of 86 students who had taken a 3-credit service-learning subject entitled "Promotion of Children and Adolescent Development" which provided 40 hours of service for more than 300 underprivileged children in Shanghai. Both quantitative and qualitative findings showed that the students benefited from this 2-semester course. A number of positive perceived changes were recognized, including enhancement of their interpersonal effectiveness, team building, problem-solving ability, and social responsibility. The findings also demonstrate the advantages of having mandatory service-learning subject requirement.

Keywords Service-learning · University students · Perceived changes
Reflection · Mandatory requirement · Hong Kong

D. T. L. Shek (✉) · Y. L. Y. Chak
Department of Applied Social Sciences, The Hong Kong Polytechnic University, Hunghom, Hong Kong
e-mail: daniel.shek@polyu.edu.hk

Y. L. Y. Chak
e-mail: yammy.chak@polyu.edu.hk

D. T. L. Shek et al. (eds.), *Service-Learning for Youth Leadership*,
Quality of Life in Asia 12, https://doi.org/10.1007/978-981-13-0448-4_3

3.1 Introduction

The number of service-learning (SL) courses offered in higher education is increasing globally. It is "a form of experiential education in which students engage in activities that address human and community needs together with structured opportunities intentionally designed to promote student learning and development" (Jacoby, 1996, p. 5). It has been well documented that the service-learning pedagogy goes beyond traditional classroom teaching to enable students to combine subject matter knowledge and a set of complementary skills, to serve the community and obtain a fuller understanding of the society. Based on the growing body of research, SL can also positively promote student learning, positive values, personal growth as well as development through experiential and reflective learning (Astin, Vogelgesang, Ikeda, & Yee, 2000; Nokes, Nickitas, Keida, & Neville, 2005; Reising et al., 2008; Warren, 2012).

3.2 Mandatory Service-Learning

There is an active debate concerning whether SL courses in university should be a mandatory requirement. It is assumed that while voluntary service-learning could increase the likelihood that students will contribute with a higher degree of intrinsic motivation and enthusiasm, mandatory requirement would lead to reluctance or even resentment of students which would eventually lead to poor emotional state and undesirable service. Students may also perceive mandatory SL requirement as a burden and negative external control. However, since SL has been found to be a powerful pedagogy for promoting student learning and development (Bringle & Hatcher, 1996; Burnett, Long, & Horne, 2005; Eyler & Giles, 1999; Eyler, Giles, Stenson, & Gray, 2001; Simons & Cleary, 2006), it can be argued that the advantage of inviting those who are least motivated (initially less-inclined to take part in volunteer or community service) in mandatory service-learning can enable them to "taste" and realize the intrapersonal and interpersonal benefits in their involvement.

The major argument against mandatory SL is that those being forced to join the required SL courses, their future intentions to volunteer would be negatively affected, especially when the purpose and rationale of the requirement were not clearly explained (Dienhart et al., 2016). However, there is evidence showing that students who take part in compulsory SL courses continue to volunteer at greater levels (Nicholls & Schimmel, 2012). In addition, students' previous experiences in service involvement will influence their interest in future service involvement in a positive way (Moely & Ilustre, 2011). From the discussion, the crucial factor for future intentions to volunteer is whether the students can find their meaning, motivation, and satisfaction fulfilled in the service experiences, not simply about "compulsory" versus "voluntary" involvement. Basically, if students are not aware of the rationales of the mandatory learning, or they cannot identify personal fulfillment or benefits of their service experiences, negative outcomes would occur. To this end, Nicholls and Schimmel (2012) concluded in their study that perceived attitude change toward service and satisfaction are the main drivers for future volunteering intentions. As long as the SL subject is well designed, explained, and implemented, the students have a clear understanding on why they need to "learn to serve," and they are provided with enough guidance and support, mandatory SL should not be that problematic. In this regard, to promote reflection in service-learning can facilitate better SL implementation and outcome.

3.3 Learning Through Purposeful and Continuous Reflection

Kolb's (1984) experiential learning theory suggested that learning from experience follows a cycle. Particularly, reflective observation is essential in the four-stage process. The foundation of service-learning stems from the experiential approach, in which purposeful reflection about concrete service experiences can enable students to make connections to their past or current learning from different perspectives and to make judgments as well as drawing meaning to guide their future behavior.

Reid (1993) defined reflection as "a process of reviewing an experience of practice in order to describe, analyze, evaluate and so inform learning about practice" (p. 306). Eyler and Giles (1999) emphasized the importance of having reflection in service-learning as it is the hyphen that links service to learning. Incorporating purposeful and continuous verbal and/or written reflection after having concrete service experiences can stimulate students' cognitive processing and facilitate them to consolidate their experiences, internalize learning, and generate new insights or even transformation (Eyler & Giles, 1999; Kolbs, 1984). In this regard, the SL course entitled "Promotion of Children and Adolescent Development" intentionally gives emphasis to "learning through reflection" and treats continuous reflection as a vehicle of transformation.

3.4 Service-Learning at The Hong Kong Polytechnic University

In Hong Kong, The Hong Kong Polytechnic University (PolyU) is the first local university to introduce a mandatory SL requirement for all full-time undergraduate students from 2012–2013 academic year onward, in which they are required to complete a 3-credit SL subject before graduation. With such requirement, we expect to nurture every student of every degree with five desirable graduate attributes, including critical thinking, innovative problem-solving, effective communication, ethical leadership, and lifelong learning, which go beyond the disciplinary expertise and knowledge (Shek, Yu, Wu, & Ng, 2015). In addition, all SL subjects at PolyU are designed with three key components, including (1) purpose-designed academic teaching, (2) challenging, meaningful, and demanding services, and (3) structured reflection and assessment (Office of Service-Learning, 2016). By engaging in a more inclusive reflection of their service-learning experiences, PolyU students are expected to develop positive personal understanding and self-identity, stronger critical thinking ability, and social awareness.

"Promotion of Children and Adolescent Development" is one of the service-learning courses offered by the Department of Applied Social Sciences of PolyU, with one of the service sites in Shanghai. We have collaborated with the Wujing Town government, the East China Normal University, the Starfish Saver (a local non-governmental organization) to hold a 5-day summer camp (40 hours) entitled "Journey of Hope" for third to fifth graders in Shanghai's Minhang District, Wujing, with most of them being children of migrant workers. This subject was first implemented in the academic year 2012–2013 with 40 participants being provided service. To date, 393 PolyU students took this subject and they have served more than 1800 underprivileged or migrant children in Shanghai. This 2-semester subject aimed at (1) introducing different psychosocial perspectives on children and youth development as well as the needs and challenges of their living in underprivileged circumstances; (2) cultivating the positive values and strengths orientation among university students; (3) enhancing the competencies of students in the areas of problem-solving, decision-making, communication, and teamwork; (4) nurturing students' sense of social responsibility, social awareness and promote prosocial behaviors; and (5) nurturing students' sense of care and compassion.

Based on the positive youth development and strength-based approaches that emphasize on assets, competencies, aspirations, abilities, and potential of children and adolescents (Damon, 2004; Rapp & Goscha, 2012; Shek, Siu, & Lee, 2007), multiple teaching and learning approaches have been adopted to engage PolyU students in two consecutive semesters. In the 6 months before the service trip, all students have to learn about service-learning through the e-learning platform, as well as by attending lectures and workshops. During the service trip, PolyU students are required to offer different programs and activities to the underprivileged children in the summer camp, with various themes such as Living English, Interesting Science, Health, and Personal Development. Through the design and implementation of service projects, college students are expected to acquire knowledge on the different perspectives on child and adolescent development which could enhance their own competencies of problem-solving, decision-making, communication, and teamwork. They are also expected to learn and understand the developmental needs and challenges of children living in disadvantaged circumstances in Mainland China, in order to help the children improve their personal development and strengthen their confidence by encouraging them to participate in class and affirming their abilities.

The SL course under focus on this chapter was offered in the academic year 2013–2014, with 87 students enrolled in this subject. Structured reflective activities and assignments (both verbal and written) were arranged before, during, and after completion of the service delivery and at the end of the course. By examining the perceived changes and benefits from the perspective of 86 students, the purpose of the current study is to understand the overall evaluation of the service-learning experience and the effectiveness of the SL subject. Three research questions are addressed: (1) How did the students perceive their performance and learning experience in the subject? (2) What is the subjective evaluation of the students on the perceived benefits after completion of the SL subject? (3) What are the perceived changes in the students after completion of the SL subject?

3.5 Method and Data Analyses

A total of 87 students participated in this subject across two semesters in the 2013–14 academic year. These students came from different disciplines including accounting, marketing, hotel management, nursing, and engineering. To address the research questions and to gauge students' perceptions of their learning experience, all enrolled students were invited to (i) complete the pre- and post-surveys developed by the Office of Service-Learning of PolyU and (ii) write several reflective journals on what they had learnt from the service and the course.

For the pre- and post-survey questionnaires, it aims to examine students' overall learning and development from the beginning to the end of the course. A total of 84 questionnaires were received, and the response rate was 96.6%. The data collected were analyzed by the SPSS. The questionnaire consists of four parts. It starts with some general information (Part 1), followed by 20 generic/soft skills questions (Q1 to Q22 in Part 2) to analyze students' generic competencies. In Part 2, all students were asked to respond to 20 questions concerning the four domains of generic competencies by indicating on a 5-point Likert scale the extent to which they agree with each item, ranging from 1 (never) to 5 (always) in the pre- and post-surveys. Each domain contains five sub-questions. To determine the statistical significance of changes on the four generic competencies, summation rating method was performed under each domain to reconstruct a new scale to capture students' attitudes. Paired samples t-tests were performed on students' learning mean scores on the four generic competencies. Part 3 of the post-project survey consists of 12 questions. Students are asked to rate their self-perceptions of their performances on a Likert scale of 1–5, where 1 represents "strongly disagree" and 5 represents "strongly agree." In Part 4, students are asked to give their comments and suggestions for improvement on the SL subject.

For the qualitative data, it was one of the reflective assignments which was submitted at the end of the course. Students were required to write reflective journals with around 1000 words on their service experiences. They were required to reflect on: (i) their ability in integrating the knowledge into practice; (ii) their roles, responsibility, and contribution as a professional and as a citizen; (iii) their own strengths and potentials; (iv) their passion in helping the underprivileged children and adolescents; (v) their problem-solving and decision-making capacities; and (vi) their social competence and interpersonal skills in collaboration with others. A general qualitative orientation was adopted in this study. The collected data were analyzed by using the general techniques proposed by Miles and Huberman (1994). First, 86 reflective papers were read once and relevant raw codes were developed from students' work. Then, the codes were further categorized into different patterns. Lastly, the categories of codes were revealed to broader themes for further analyses.

3.6 Results

3.6.1 Characteristics of the Students and Their Reasons of Taking the Subject

It is shown that most of the students had prior experience in voluntary service (92.9%). Concerning the reasons for taking the course, 86.9% of the respondents reflected that "they would like to gain more experiential learning experience outside the classroom" and the majority of them "believe it will broaden my horizon on understanding the life of the underprivileged people inside or outside Hong Kong" (82.1%). Interestingly, 78.6% of respondents reflected that they took the course because of other reasons. Based on the teachers' understanding and observation, roughly one-third of the students joined the course because this course was an offshore project and they simply wanted to fulfill the university requirement.

3.6.2 Changes in Generic/Soft Skills After Completion of the Course

Table 3.1 shows the mean score (min = 5; max = 25) and the results of the paired samples t-tests of the 20 items revealing the changes in students. Overall speaking, the mean score is high in general and the results showed statistically significant enhancement in the four generic competencies measured, i.e., interpersonal effectiveness (mean difference = 1.62, effect size = 0.694, $p < 0.001$), teamwork (mean difference = 1.36, effect size = 0.540, $p < 0.001$), problem-solving (mean difference = 1.42, effect size = 0.528, $p < 0.001$), and social responsibility (mean difference = 1.24, effect size = 0.495, $p < 0.001$). In particular, positive change in the domain "interpersonal effectiveness" is the most substantial.

Table 3.1 Changes in generic/soft skills after completion of the course ($N = 84$)

Generic/soft skills	Students' SL learning status	Mean scores	Differences in mean scores	Sig. 2-tailed	Effect size
Interpersonal effectiveness	Pre-SL Post-SL	19.81 21.43	1.620	<0.001	0.694
Teamwork	Pre-SL Post-SL	20.48 21.84	1.360	<0.001	0.540
Problem-solving	Pre-SL Post-SL	19.59 21.01	1.420	<0.001	0.528
Social responsibility	Pre-SL Post-SL	20.27 21.51	1.240	<0.001	0.495

3.6.3 *Overall Evaluation of Students' Learning Experience*

Table 3.2 is about the students' self-perceptions of their performances and learning experience after completion of the course. Generally, the findings revealed that the perception of the students was highly positive. The mean score of the items ranged from 4.08 to 4.60. In terms of learning experience, the majority of students reflected that they learnt better from the service project than traditional classroom learning mode. Almost all of them treasured the learning experience throughout the service project (96.4%). In addition, the students agreed that they should have the responsibility to serve the community (97.6%). With particular reference to the future intention to serve, 94% of the students stated that they would continue their involvement in community services and 90.5% of the students reflected that they are willing to participate in SL activities in the future and there is only one student (1.2%) disagreed that he/she will have further SL participation.

3.6.4 *Qualitative Data from the Reflective Journals*

With reference to students' reflection, the findings are highly consistent with the quantitative evaluation. Three observations can be highlighted. First, the content of all journals collected can be defined as positive and encouraging. It is remarkable that there is no negative reflection received. All students mentioned their own self-evaluation, the perceived benefits, and changes in the reflection journals constructively. Second, students stated that SL course is important to their personal growth and development. Most of the students reported that their capacity of "team building" had been improved chiefly. In addition, they reflected that there is enhancement in the areas of "interpersonal communication", "social responsibility", and "problem-solving" after they have participated in the SL course and delivered the service in Shanghai. Third, a number of cases have shown that the mindsets of

Table 3.2 Students' self-perceptions of their performances and learning experience

After completing the SL subject	*N*	Mean	Std. dev.	Strongly agree (5) (%)	Agree (4) (%)	Neutral (3) (%)	Disagree (2) (%)	Strongly disagree (1) (%)
I applied the professional knowledge/skills that I learnt from class at the service-learning project/trip	84	4.15	0.591	26.2	63.1	10.7	0.0	0.0
I will continue my involvement in community services	84	4.31	0.580	36.9	57.1	6.0	0.0	0.0
I feel that the work I did through service-learning benefited the community	84	4.36	0.573	40.5	54.8	4.8	0.0	0.0
Service-learning helped me become more aware of the needs in the community	84	4.45	0.648	52.4	41.7	4.8	1.2	0.0
I believe that I have a responsibility to serve the community	84	4.51	0.549	53.6	44.0	2.4	0.0	0.0
I think I can make a difference in the community	84	4.25	0.618	34.5	56.0	9.5	0.0	0.0
I treasured the learning experience throughout the service project	84	4.60	0.562	63.1	33.3	3.6	0.0	0.0
The service project was well prepared and organized	84	4.42	0.625	47.6	47.6	3.6	1.2	0.0
Generally speaking, I learn better from the service project than traditional classroom learning mode	84	4.50	0.631	56.0	39.3	3.6	1.2	0.0
I will participate in service-learning activities in the future	84	4.37	0.690	47.6	42.9	8.3	1.2	0.0
I can get enough support from the NGO in carrying out the project	84	4.08	0.698	28.6	51.2	20.2	0.0	0.0
I can get enough support from the PolyU staff in carrying out the project	84	4.43	0.566	46.4	50.0	3.6	0.0	0.0

[a]Total percentage of each statement may not be equal to 100%. The difference is due to rounding

students toward SL course have changed positively after they participated in the service.

Students had experienced positive changes in team building, as many of them mentioned that they could learn to be a good team player. They also shared that there were a lot of chances to learn how to build good rapport and teamwork with their group mates as well as other groups. For example, two PolyU students shared and reflected as follows:

> I learnt about the importance of team work. I have built up a sense of mutuality with my group mates during the trip. Actually, many sudden situations occured during the service, if there was only me or we did not cooperate well, we cannot overcome these difficulties. For example, I felt sick during service, my group mates were so nice that they were willing to take over my lesson. We reallocated the workload quickly and finally we could still finish the lesson successfully. Apart from that, I also needed to cooperate with people from other groups during the farewell ceremony. The group work in this service trip made me notice the importance to work as a team. The cooperation and meetings with different people also enhanced my confidence and interpersonal skills in collaboration with others.

> It was a great chance to train my collaboration with others as we needed to make decision rapidly under some unexpected situations.

Some other students also made the following remarks in their reflective journals:

> I gained a lot from cooperating with my group mates. I saw the changes during the service. When we started to conduct lessons, our unspoken consensus was building up…… Another group consensus was that when facing emergency situation, we could cooperate and handle…… I realized that we must cooperate. No one can work alone and become successful. We need to be interdependent when working as a team.

> I have learnt that if we want to succeed as a team, each one of us should play our role accordingly.

> When a primary student vomited during the lesson, one of us went to the teacher in-charge and called for help, one helped to take care of the primary students and the remaining group of us helped to pacify the crowd. We did not have to communicate but all of us knew our own positions and helped to manage the class. I can feel that every group member is part of the team and I appreciate our efforts and cooperation.

To sum up, through taking part in a range of activities and group tasks, students believed that smooth and close collaboration within and between the group(s) made them feel proud and became parts of the team. With strong physical, emotional, and psychological support from peers, PolyU students also learnt the importance of "connectedness and togetherness"—how to effectively manage and cope with difficulties together.

Besides, a group of students reported that effective communication is essential to communicate well with others. It also showed that through service-learning, PolyU students had learnt how to effectively communicate with people from different age groups and background. For example, some students claimed that:

> The cooperation between teammates and meeting different people also enhanced my confidence and interpersonal skills in collaboration with others.

I learned the skills to communicate with the primary children and listen to their feelings…… Primary school students learned from us and we also learned from the kids.

I also used some (communication) skills to manage students during class, for example, I-message…… This kind of real life practice has deepened my understanding towards those theories and improved my ability to apply theories and knowledge into real life situation.

Another student has realized that her interpersonal and communication skills were greatly improved after the service trip. She also reflected further as follows:

From this 5-day intense service, I realized that my interpersonal and communication skills were improved. Now I listen attentively and try to put myself into others' shoes before making decisions or comments. I could do so when I am working with other people, why can't I apply when I communicate with my family, friends and future colleagues? I believe our arguments will be reduced a lot.

In addition, SL course has given a chance for students to get involved in the community. One of the students recalled and shared the following:

One of them (the kid) even wants to study at The Hong Kong Polytechnic University and find us in the future. These messages moved me deeply…… Some of them we served were living in poor environment and were allocated few resources. This leads me to think about underprivileged group in Hong Kong. Many people may hesitate to help them, including me. However, now my passion is growing. If I have chances, I may try to serve the needy in Hong Kong.

Some other members also shared similarly as follows:

The SL course has enhanced my awareness towards the minorities in the society. I think that the contribution is just a beginning of my journey and would like to do more in the future.

After this trip, I would like to make a promise here. As a university student, we have the knowledge and ability to serve the underprivileged communities. I will join more voluntary activities to help them, especially children. The opportunities of helping them is everywhere.

As a professional, I should apply the knowledge I acquired to make changes to the society. Though my major is nursing, how I can help should not be limited to building sense of hygiene in children's minds since I am a citizen……. I believe that we should be the change agent and changes in attitude and mindsets can transform the life. That is why I should be the powerful push which makes people believe the change can be seen someday by behaving ourselves and attending more to social issues. I used to escape from politics but it is now my turn to manage the social issues, to take care of the underprivileged, to take part in the revolution process.

Obviously, SL is not only a course but also helping students to reflect their roles in the society and their responsibilities in the community. The SL experiences also nurture "ethical leadership" in students.

During the service delivery process, PolyU students encountered various unanticipated problems when providing services. In particular, many students had spotted that there were challenges when they were being the role as a "teacher" to manage the class and the kids. From these lessons, many students reported that their problem-solving skills had improved. They highly realized the importance of having contingency plans as unexpected incidents happened and they had learnt to think carefully and eliminate the chance of being panic and making mistakes under stress. These experiences could help students to enhance their creative as well as critical thinking skills, and promote innovative problem-solving in the process. Two students shared as follows:

> I tried to incorporate both simple and difficult words in my PowerPoint, so that the more capable students would not feel boring, while the kids with lower English levels could learn something new. I thought that this practice has improved my problem-solving skills, to deal with situation that did not go with what I had expected or planned.

> During this trip, we have encountered many difficulties…… I have learnt that in a group, we can solve problems more easily by cooperating with each other…… We found out that the computers provided by the NGO were not working…… I have learnt that with collaboration and flexibility, we can beat the difficulties. I have also realized that contingency plans are always needed because you will never know what will happen next and always bring extra materials just to be safe.

Other than the benefits mentioned, a number of cases have shown that the mindsets of students toward volunteer work or SL course have changed in a positive way after they participated in the service. Some students have claimed that:

> In my past experience, the general way to deal with group assignments within a team was dividing the workload into equal pieces and finally combining the individual parts together. From this service, I had learnt not only dividing the burden, but more vitally, was to share each other's burden.

> I didn't have passion to serve the children at first so I did not have any expectations from the course. However, after the service, I positively changed my attitude because I could unexpectedly learn something important from the children, but not only contributing in one direction.

Two students were also aware of the meaning of serving:

> I have found the meaning of doing volunteer service!!! I am a business student and my belief is to do things that are beneficial to me. Honestly, the purpose for me to do volunteer work is to make my curriculum vitae become richer and have something to say during interview…… However, in this service trip, I have the feeling that is totally different from before.

> In the very beginning, I chose to join this course because I would like to fulfill the graduation requirement. However, I have learnt more about myself during this meaningful service. I would like to say thank you to the children and my teacher who cheered me up in the process. Their encouragement is invaluable and it motivated me. I would like to follow their trace to enlighten others in the world…… If I can let more people think positively, I can plant the seed of happiness in the public and more people will follow it. The world would be better in that way.

Based on the students' sharing and reflection, we strongly believe that the SL experience has positively changed students' perceptions toward community service and the SL course, a mandatory requirement.

3.7 Discussion

The present study evaluated the perceived effectiveness of the SL course. Based on the positive qualitative and quantitative feedback, the majority of the students perceived the subject favorably and they valued the experiential learning experience. It has shown that the SL exposure was helpful to cultivate students' positive values, improve, and strengthen their generic competencies, including both their intrapersonal and interpersonal competencies (specifically their teamwork, interpersonal communication, and problem-solving) and nurture stronger sense of social responsibility among them. In particular, students greatly benefited from the SL experience, as constructive self-perceived insight, growth, and changes were significantly observed. Additionally, the qualitative findings show that the SL subject was also effective in promoting the five graduate attributes (i.e., critical thinking, innovative problem-solving, effective communication, ethical leadership, and lifelong learning) in students. The encouraging results also shed some light on the effectiveness of the mandatory service-learning and the importance of incorporating reflection in the process.

Although the current study did not directly investigate the effectiveness of mandatory SL in the long run, the findings revealed that this SL experience did not undermine the future intention of the students to serve the community or to participate in SL. Most of the students identified their personal fulfillment or benefits of their service experiences and highly treasured the learning experience of "learn to serve and serve to learn." As proposed by Greene (1998), "an observant student, especially if guided by service-linked educational objectives, stands ready to learn from the service recipient empowered by the service rendered. Both server and served provide and receive. In the process, the student more clearly sees the recipient as one who has something to give instead of one only in a position to receive. This realization itself is an important lesson in valuing others." (p. 411). With reference to the qualitative results, there is a good impact on those who were least inclined to take part in the course. For some students who did not have any prior experience in voluntary service, they eventually realized the tremendous power of SL as well as the benefits of SL activities. They were contented about their participation, social interaction, empathic involvement, and personal changes. Generally speaking, the current mandatory SL experience had apparently opened our students' mind and broadened their horizons.

Regardless of the fact that the SL requirement is structured, experience itself cannot produce learning. Bringle and Hatcher (1999) stated that "experience becomes educative when critical reflective thought creates new meaning and leads to growth and the ability to take informed actions" (p. 180). Jacoby (1996) indicated that reflection is one of the key components of service-learning. Thus, provision of purposeful and continuous reflective activities and assignments is essential as students are given the chances to examine the critical issues related to their projects, and to evaluate as well as reflect on their own attitudes toward learning, values, and life. In addition, reflective activities could help orienting the students to the same philosophical and practical emphasis of the SL project. These reflective tasks could also develop a positive culture with shared vision and ownership. Therefore, learning through reflection should be treated as the crucial component to strengthen the power of service-learning pedagogy.

Despite the positive findings observed in the present study, there are limitations that need to be addressed. First, the current evaluation was solely based on the data of the self-rated assessment and self-reflection, without having any control groups for objective comparison. Second, as only one class of students (around 86 students) was involved in the study, the views and data collected may not represent the whole picture of the university's condition and thus its generalizability is restricted. It is suggested that future research should be carried out in order to provide stronger evidence for the impacts and causal relationship of implementing mandatory service-learning subjects in university. Nevertheless, the positive evaluation findings are generally consistent with those based on other cohorts of students. Even with these limitations, the present study successfully used both qualitative and quantitative methods to investigate what students have gained after taking a SL subject. These findings also demonstrate the advantage of having mandatory SL subject that attempts to promote the student development and cultivate their civic responsibility. Obviously, learning through reflection helped to promote a more positive attitude and healthier personal development in students.

3.8 Personal Reflections and Conclusions

Traditional pedagogy is about imparting knowledge to learners, and service-learning is about learning and understanding through experience and reflection. Being the subject teachers, we witnessed the positive changes that the PolyU students have made throughout their SL experience. Their involvement, motivation, and proactive attitudes showed in the summer camp were impressive. With reference to the field observation, we found that some of the PolyU students who used to be egocentric had undergone lots of meaningful self-reflections and self-exploration in the process and then begun to care about others and be more altruistic. These changes also strengthened their capacities of relationship building and team building. And for some of them, they might be overprotected in the past but they took initiatives to overcome difficulties and their resilience was greatly enhanced. In addition, after participating in the subject and service projects, they also have great changes in their attitudes toward life, moral conscience, and sense of social responsibility. From the SL teaching experiences, we can observe that the service-learning effectively helps our students to reflect deeply on their strengths and weaknesses and encourages them to think what they can give back to the community. We were proud of the excellent performance of PolyU students and greatly moved by the effectiveness of the service-learning program. It helps us become even more optimistic, confident, and passionate in organizing the mandatory service-learning programs at PolyU. Besides, this teaching experience stimulates us to reflect and reconsider our roles, expectations, and commitment as "educators." In fact, this SL project "Journey of Hope" has great impacts on sowing the seed of competence, resilience, and aspiration among the students as well as teachers. It is our hope that more people in different corners of Hong Kong and China could enjoy the fruits of this project.

References

Astin, A. W., Vogelgesang, L. J., Ikeda, E. K., & Yee, J. A. (2000). *How service learning affects students*. Los Angeles, CA: Higher Education Research Institute, University of California.

Bringle, R. G., & Hatcher, J. A. (1996). Implementing service learning in higher education. *The Journal of Higher Education, 67*(2), 221–239.

Bringle, R. G., & Hatcher, J. A. (1999). Reflection in service learning: Making meaning of experience. *Educational Horizons, 77*(4), 179–185.

Burnett, J. A., Long, L. L., & Horne, H. L. (2005). Service learning for counselors: Integrating education, training, and the community. *The Journal of Humanistic Counseling, Education and Development, 44*(2), 158–167.

Damon, W. (2004). What is positive youth development? *The Annals of the American Academy of Political and Social Science, 591,* 13–24.

Dienhart, C., Maruyama, G., Snyder, M., Furco, A., McKay, M. S., Hirt, L., & Huesman, R. Jr. (2016). The impacts of mandatory service on students in service-learning classes. *The Journal of Social Psychology, 156*(3), 305–309.

Eyler, J., & Giles, D. E. Jr. (1999). *Where's the learning in service-learning?* San Francisco, CA: Jossey-Bass.

Eyler, J., Giles, D. E. Jr., Stenson, C. M., & Gray, C. J. (2001). *At a glance: What we know about the effects of service-learning on college students, faculty, institutions and communities, 1993–2000*. Washington, DC: Learn and Serve America National Service Learning Clearinghouse.

Greene, D. (1998). Reciprocity in two conditions of service-learning. *Educational Gerontology, 24* (5), 411–424.

Jacoby, B. (1996). Service-learning in today's higher education. In B. Jacoby (Ed.), *Service-learning in higher education: Concepts and practices* (pp. 3–25). San Francisco, CA: Jossey-Bass.

Kolb, D. A. (1984). *Experiential learning: Experience as the source of learning and development.* Englewood Cliffs, NJ: Prentice Hall.

Miles, M. B., & Huberman, A. M. (1994). *Qualitative data analysis: An expanded sourcebook* (2nd ed.). Thousand Oaks, CA: Sage.

Moely, B. E., & Ilustre, V. (2011). University students' views of a public service graduation requirement. *Michigan Journal of Community Service Learning, 17*(2), 43–58.

Nicholls, J., & Schimmel, K. (2012). Match/mismatch of the college business student service-learning experiences: Drivers of perceived attitude change, satisfaction, and future volunteering intentions. *Journal of Higher Education Theory and Practice, 12*(6), 91–99.

Nokes, K. M., Nickitas, D. M., Keida, R., & Neville, S. (2005). Does service-learning increase cultural competency, critical thinking, and civic engagement? *Journal of Nursing Education, 44*(2), 65–70.

Office of Service-Learning. (2016). *Learn to serve, serve to learn—The Hong Kong Polytechnic University's experience of mandatory service-learning*. Hong Kong: The Hong Kong Polytechnic University.

Rapp, C. A., & Goscha, R. J. (2012). *The strengths model: A recovery-oriented approach to mental health services* (3rd ed.). New York: Oxford University Press.

Reid, B. (1993). "But we're doing it already!" Exploring a response to the concept of reflective practice in order to improve its facilitation. *Nurse Education Today, 13*(4), 305–309.
Reising, D. L., Shea, R. A., Allen, P. N., Laux, M. M., Hensel, D., & Watts, P. A. (2008). Using service-learning to develop health promotion and research skills in nursing students. *International Journal of Nursing Education Scholarship, 5*(1), 1–15.
Shek, D. T. L., Siu, A. M. H., & Lee, T. Y. (2007). The Chinese positive youth development scale: A validation study. *Research on Social Work Practice, 17*(3), 380–391.
Shek, D. T. L., Yu, L., Wu, F. K. Y., & Ng, C. S. M. (2015). General education program in a new 4-year university curriculum in Hong Kong: Findings based on multiple evaluation strategies. *International Journal on Disability and Human Development, 14*(4), 377–384.
Simons, L., & Cleary, B. (2006). The influence of service learning on students' personal and social development. *College Teaching, 54*(4), 307–319.
Warren, J. L. (2012). Does service-learning increase student learning?: A meta-analysis. *Michigan Journal of Community Service Learning, 18*(2), 56–61.

Chapter 4
Impact of a Service-Learning Programme in Mainland China: Views of Different Stakeholders

Lu Yu, Daniel T. L. Shek and Kelly Y. Xing

Abstract This paper describes the evaluation findings about a service-learning programme offered in a public university in Hong Kong based on the data collected in 2015–2016 academic year. The programme aims to nurture generic competences, positive values, and social responsibilities in university students and to promote the positive development of migrant children in Mainland China through the service. Evaluative findings based on different stakeholders including service providers (i.e. university students), service recipients (migrant children), project collaborators (teachers of the local primary school), and service observers (local university students) converged to suggest that this programme was implemented smoothly and there were multiple benefits to not only university students but migrant children in the served community. Both service providers and recipients also showed very positive perceptions about the programme content and the service. Ratings of the programme by community collaborators and observers further suggested that the quality of service provided by university students was high. The present findings add to the limited literature that provides scientific evidence for the impact of service-learning programmes on the community. The usefulness of including different informants in programme evaluation has also been demonstrated.

Keywords Service-learning · Migrant children · Programme evaluation
University student · Stakeholder

4.1 Introduction

Service-learning as an experiential teaching and learning pedagogy has been increasingly adopted in university education worldwide to promote both students' growth and the common good of the community (Jacoby, 2014). Through applying

L. Yu (✉) · D. T. L. Shek · K. Y. Xing
Department of Applied Social Sciences, The Hong Kong Polytechnic University, Hung Hom, Hong Kong
e-mail: lu.yu@polyu.edu.hk

D. T. L. Shek et al. (eds.), *Service-Learning for Youth Leadership*,
Quality of Life in Asia 12, https://doi.org/10.1007/978-981-13-0448-4_4

knowledge and skills to service settings and guided self-reflection, students are provided with opportunities to nurture their real-world skills, develop civic responsibility, and bring positive changes to the society (Eyler & Giles, 1999). In the USA, a wealth of research has documented the benefits of service-learning programmes to different stakeholders in various aspects. Important evidence supporting service-learning as a high-impact educational practice has also been provided (e.g. Astin, Vogelgesang, Ikeda, & Yee, 2000; Clayton, Bringle, & Hatcher, 2012; Eyler, Giles, Stenson, & Gary, 2001).

In contrast, systematic investigation on the effectiveness of service-learning programmes is insufficient in Asia, where service-learning remains a relatively new concept (Xing & Ma, 2010). With specific reference to Hong Kong, the first service-learning programme was developed and implemented in 2000 (Ngai, 2006). Since then, while more and more service-learning subjects and programmes have been offered in different higher educational settings, published academic work in the field remains focusing on discussion of theoretical framework of service learning (e.g. Ngai & Chan, 2016), and case studies that either describe the implementation processes or report performance and learning gains by university student participants (i.e. service providers). For example, researchers have reported benefits of service-learning programmes to university students based on survey data (Ngai, 2006; Ma, Shek, & Li, 2016; Yu, Shek, Liu, Chen, & Zhi, 2016), students' reflection on related learning experiences (Chak et al., 2016; Pang & Wu, 2016), and teachers' observations of students' performance (Wu, Shek, Mok, & Shek, 2016). On the other hand, the impact of service-learning programmes on the community being served and service recipients has not been rigorously examined. In particular, it is unclear whether the service provided by student participants based on their academic study in service-learning programmes really benefits the communities where they served. As service learning has gained increased popularity in the past ten years in Hong Kong (Xing & Ma, 2010), the question of whether service recipients and the related organizations may also gain from service-learning programmes must be addressed.

Being one of the eight public universities in Hong Kong, The Hong Kong Polytechnic University (PolyU) always places great importance on nurturing students into socially responsible professionals with a heart to serve the community (Chan, Ngai, & Shek, in press). Consistent with this mission, service learning has been incorporated into the university's formal curriculum as a compulsory component starting from 2012/13 academic year. Students studying in the four-year undergraduate degree programme are required to complete one 3-credit service learning subject during their studies as part of the General University Requirements (The Hong Kong Polytechnic University, 2013). Different departments are encouraged to propose subjects that fulfil the service-learning requirements. To understand the impact of these service-learning programmes on university students, several studies have been conducted to examine students' learning gains through self-report ratings of learning experiences (e.g. Office of Service Learning, 2015; Shek, Yu, Wu, & Chai, 2015; Shek, Yu, Wu, & Ng, 2015). The results generally showed that students had positive changes and meaningful reflection after participating in these programmes. While the findings are encouraging and provide evidence for the effectiveness of these programmes on university students, the influence of such programmes on the served community has not been scientifically investigated. In fact, previous studies (e.g. Tryon & Stoecker, 2008) indicated that it was not uncommon that community collaborators expressed difficulties in working with students in service learning due to various reasons, such as inconsistent communication with faculty, inappropriate service activities, and limited service hours. To obtain a complete picture of the impact of service learning, voices of different stakeholders must be heard and examined.

The present study attempted to fill this gap through evaluating the impact of a service-learning programme based on subjective outcomes obtained from different stakeholders, including service providers (university students), service recipients (migrant children in the served primary school), and service collaborators (teachers of the primary school). The programme entitled “Promotion of Child and Adolescent Development” is amongst the first batch of service-learning subjects approved by PolyU. The focus of the subject is to nurture university students’ generic competences, positive values, social responsibilities, and sense of care and compassion towards people in need through designing and providing direct service for children and adolescents living in underprivileged conditions in Mainland China. Since launching in 2012/13, the subject has received highly positive feedback from participating students, and the number of students enroled increases every year. To cater for the growing needs of students, a new service-learning site was formed in 2014 at the Hangzhou Shuren Primary School, which exclusively serves children of migrant workers. PolyU students designed and implemented a five-day summer camp for migrant children in the school to promote their resilience, aspirations, and various competences based on knowledge and skills learned in the lectures and workshops. A pilot study based on survey data from 37 university student participants in 2014/15 academic year suggested that the first-year implementation of this service-learning programme in Hangzhou was smooth, and the programme contributed to the holistic development of university students. Despite this, less is known about possible effects of this programme on the served community and service recipients. To address this issue, the present study was conducted to have a more comprehensive evaluation based on the second year implementation (2015/16 academic year) of this subject in Hangzhou.

Specifically, three major research questions would be answered: (1) How do university students perceive their learning experience in this subject? (2) What are the subjective evaluations of migrant children as service recipients of this programme? (3) How do the teachers of the served school as collaborators perceive the implementation and benefits of this programme? In addition, observations by trained observers from a local university were described to provide additional information on quality of the service provided by Hong Kong university students.

4.2 Methods

4.2.1 *Participants and Procedure*

Participants consisted of 79 PolyU students who successfully enrolled in the subject in 2015/16 academic year. The students provided service in Hangzhou to 355 migrant children from the primary school who participated in the summer camp with the involvement of 18 teachers of the primary school where students served. Besides, to evaluate PolyU students' performance in providing service, 19 students at either undergraduate or postgraduate level with social sciences backgrounds were recruited from Zhejiang University as observers. A training workshop was provided to all observers before the service started to introduce the major content of the service-learning subject, purposes of the provided service, and how to assess students' performance using the standard observation form developed by the research team. For each class, there was at least one observer to rate PolyU students' performance. In the five days of service, a total of 275 sessions were evaluated in 16 classes.

All participants were invited to complete a subjective outcome questionnaire upon completion of the programme in different settings. PolyU students filled in the questionnaire in the last workshop of the subject. Both migrant children and school teachers completed another questionnaire on the last day of the summer camp. While the children were instructed to complete the survey in classroom settings administered by trained student helpers (Zhejiang University students), school teachers finished the questionnaire in a self-administrative way. It took around 20 min to complete the whole questionnaire. In addition, a standardized rating scale was used by observers to evaluate the quality of service and performance of PolyU students.

4.2.2 *Instruments*

4.2.2.1 Subjective Outcome Evaluation Form

Three subjective outcome evaluation forms were used in the present study to measure the respective perceptions of service providers (i.e. PolyU students, Form A), service recipients (i.e. primary school students, Form B), and collaborators (i.e. teachers of the primary school, Form C) about the implementation and impact of the service-learning programme. Form A consists of four subscales completed by service providers: (1) views about the service programme (10 items); (2) views about their own performance (8 items); (3) perceived effectiveness of the programme on service recipients (9 items); and (4) perceived effectiveness of the programme on their own development (10 items). Form B has 26 items which measure service recipients' (1) views towards the service programme (8 items);

(2) views about the service providers (8 items); and, (3) perceived benefits of the service programme to their development in different aspects (10 items). Form C is similar to Form B, except that in the third part, collaborators are asked to evaluate their perceived benefits of the programme to service recipients (i.e. migrant children of the primary school). All items were rated on a six-point Likert scale with higher scores representing more positive evaluation. In each form, there are two open-ended questions to further illicit respondents' feelings, perceptions, and experiences related to the service programme. The present study focuses on the quantitative evaluation findings. All scales and subscales showed good internal consistencies with Cronbach's alpha coefficients ranging from 0.75 to 0.83.

4.2.2.2 Observation Form

The standardized observation form has 13 items that assess the quality of the provided service and PolyU students' performance in the following areas: service attitude, sense of responsibility, awareness of needs, sense of care, cultural sensitivity, teamwork and problem-solving skills, communication skills with service targets, teaching skills, ability to apply the discipline-related knowledge, reflective attitude, punctuality, and overall performance. Cronbach's alpha coefficient for this rating form in the present study was 0.81, indicating good internal consistency.

4.3 Results

4.3.1 Subjective Outcome Evaluation by Service Providers (PolyU Students)

Service providers' subjective evaluation about the programme is reflected in PolyU students' responses to Form A. The numbers and percentages of students who reported positive ratings (i.e. rating of 4 or above) for all items of the four subscales are summarized in Table 4.1. First, the majority of the service providers had positive views about the service-learning programme. For example, all respondents showed overall positive evaluation and were satisfied with the programme. All respondents were satisfied with the programme and perceived the learning experiences as pleasant. Second, more than 98% of the service providers had positive evaluations about their own performance in terms of preparation of service, attitude and behaviours towards service recipients, and commitment to service. Third, most service providers agreed that the programme benefited the migrant children they served (i.e. service recipients). Specifically, all service providers agreed that the programme helped improve migrant children's self-confidence, broadened their horizon, and promoted the overall development of these children. Fourth, service providers perceived significant effects of the programme on their own development.

Table 4.1 Subjective outcome evaluation by service providers ($N = 79$)

Item	Positive		Negative	
	n	%	*n*	%
Views about the service programme				
1. This service programme was well-designed	76	96.2	3	3.8
2. The form of the service we provided was appropriate	78	98.7	1	1.3
3. The process of delivering the service activities was pleasant	79	100.0	0	0.0
4. There was much peer interaction amongst the clients	79	100.0	0	0.0
5. The clients participated actively during our service	79	100.0	0	0.0
6. The clients were encouraged to do their best	78	98.7	1	1.3
7. We had good collaboration with different parties (school teachers, staff, etc.) during the service	78	98.7	1	1.3
8. The service experience I encountered enhanced my interest in this subject	79	100.0	0	0.0
9. The service experience increased my passion in helping people in need	78	98.7	1	1.3
10. Overall speaking, I have positive evaluation of the service programme	79	100.0	0	0.0
Views about the service providers (i.e. yourself)				
1. I prepared well for the service	79	100.0	0	0.0
2. I showed good professional attitudes in my service	78	98.7	1	1.3
3. I understood the needs and potentials of my clients	79	100.0	0	0.0
4. I was very involved in the service	79	100.0	0	0.0
5. I cared for the clients I served	79	100.0	0	0.0
6. I was ready to offer help to the clients whenever needed	79	100.0	0	0.0
7. I had much interaction with the clients	79	100.0	0	0.0
8. Overall speaking, I have positive evaluation of myself in serving the clients	78	98.7	1	1.3
The extent to which the service-learning programme has helped the clients				
1. It has strengthened our clients' resilience	77	97.5	2	2.5
2. It has helped our clients face the future with a positive attitude	78	98.7	1	1.3
3. It has improved our clients' self-confidence	79	100.0	0	0.0
4. It has broadened our clients' horizon	79	100.0	0	0.0
5. It has reinforced our clients' interest in learning	78	98.7	1	1.3
6. It has strengthened our clients' ability to care for other people	78	98.7	1	1.3
7. It has helped our clients build up good relationships with healthy adults	78	98.7	1	1.3
8. It has promoted our clients' aspirations in life	79	100.0	0	0.0
9. It has enriched the overall development of our clients	79	100.0	0	0.0

(continued)

Table 4.1 (continued)

Item	Positive		Negative	
	n	%	*n*	%
The extent to which the service-learning programme has helped the service providers				
1. It has enabled me to understand the needs and potentials of the service recipients	79	100.0	0	0.0
2. It has helped me integrate the academic knowledge into real-life situation through service delivery	79	100.0	0	0.0
3. It has enhanced my competences in problem-solving and decision-making	79	100.0	0	0.0
4. It has helped me appreciate and respect people from diverse backgrounds	79	100.0	0	0.0
5. It has helped me develop the sense of care and compassion towards other people	79	100.0	0	0.0
6. It has improved my interpersonal skills	79	100.0	0	0.0
7. It has boosted my self-confidence	79	100.0	0	0.0
8. It has enabled me to apply the knowledge and skills I acquired in university to solve complex issues in the service	78	98.7	1	1.3
9. It has inspired me to reflect on my roles and responsibilities as both a professional and a responsible citizen	79	100.0	0	0.0
10. On the whole, I am satisfied with this service programme	79	100.0	0	0.0

Note *Positive* = ratings of 4 or above on a 6-point scale, *Negative* = ratings of 3 or below

For instance, all student participants thought that the service programme enabled them to understand the needs and potentials of the service recipients and helped them integrate the academic knowledge into real-life situation through service delivery. They also agreed that the service enhanced their problem-solving competences, sense of care and compassion towards other people, and appreciation and respect to others from diverse backgrounds.

4.3.2 *Subjective Outcome Evaluation by Service Recipients (Primary School Students)*

Service recipients' perceived outcomes of the programme are summarized in Table 4.2. Several observations based on the descriptive findings can be highlighted. First, service recipients held overwhelmingly positive views about the service programme. Of the 355 respondents, more than 99% agreed that the programme was well designed and the process of service delivery was pleasant; 97.7% of the participating children perceived this experience as having enhanced their interest in this programme; and 99.4% of service recipients had an overall positive evaluation of the programme. Second, a large percentage of service recipients had quite favourable perceptions about the service providers. They highly appreciated PolyU students' "professional attitudes", "involvement in the service", "care", "readiness to offer help", which echoed the evaluative findings obtained from service providers. Third, almost all service recipients perceived that they had benefited from the programme in

Table 4.2 Subjective outcome evaluation by service recipients (N = 355)

Item	Positive		Negative	
	n	%	*n*	%
Views about the service programme				
1. This service programme was well-designed	354	99.7	1	0.3
2. The form of the service provided was appropriate	351	98.9	4	1.1
3. The process of delivering the service activities was pleasant	352	99.2	3	0.8
4. There was much peer interaction amongst us	348	98.0	7	2.0
5. I participated actively during the service	350	98.6	5	1.4
6. I was encouraged to do my best	353	99.4	2	0.6
7. The learning experience I encountered enhanced my interest in this programme	347	97.7	8	2.3
8. Overall speaking, I have positive evaluation of the service programme	353	99.4	2	0.6
Views about the service providers (i.e. PolyU students)				
1. The tutors prepared well for the service	354	99.7	1	0.3
2. The tutors showed good professional attitudes	352	99.2	3	0.8
3. The tutors understood my needs and potentials	351	98.9	4	1.1
4. The tutors were very involved in the service	354	99.7	1	0.3
5. The tutors cared about me	349	98.3	6	1.7
6. The tutors were ready to offer help to me whenever needed	354	99.7	1	0.3
7. The tutors had much interaction with us	352	99.2	3	0.8
8. Overall speaking, I have positive evaluation of the tutors in the service	352	99.2	3	0.8
The extent to which the service programme has helped the clients				
1. It has strengthened my resilience	349	98.3	6	1.7
2. It has helped me face the future with a positive attitude	350	98.6	5	1.4
3. It has improved my self-confidence	350	98.6	5	1.4
4. It has broadened my horizon	355	100.0	0	0.0
5. It has reinforced my interest in learning	351	98.9	4	1.1
6. It has strengthened my ability to care for other people	345	97.2	10	2.8
7. It has helped me build up good relationships with healthy adults (e.g. tutors, teachers, parents)	351	98.9	4	1.1
8. It has promoted my aspirations in life	352	99.2	3	0.8
9. It has enriched my overall development	350	98.6	5	1.4
10. On the whole, I am satisfied with this service programme	351	98.9	4	1.1

Note *Positive* = ratings of 4 or above on a 6-point scale, *Negative* = ratings of 3 or below multiple areas. Particularly, all respondents endorsed that participating in this programme had broadened their horizon. A large majority of service recipients reported improvements in "aspirations in life" (99.2%), "interest in learning", "ability to build up good relationship with healthy adults" (both at 98.9%), "ability to face the future with a positive attitude", "self-confidence" (both at 98.6%), "resilience" (98.3%) and "the ability to care for other people" (97.2%). Furthermore, 98.9% of the migrant children were satisfied with this programme.

4.3.3 *Subjective Outcome Evaluation by Service Collaborators (Primary School Teachers)*

Table 4.3 further showed the subjective outcome evaluation by the programme collaborators, i.e. 18 teachers of the served school. In general, the collaborators had quite positive views about the service programme, the performance of the service providers, and the beneficial impact of this programme on the served migrant children and the community. For example, all respondents agreed that the programme promoted a positive culture in the community and that the service programme was beneficial to the service recipients. All collaborators concurred in the effectiveness of the programme in helping migrant children face the future with a positive attitude, broadening their horizon, and enriching their overall development. None of them showed dissatisfaction with the service programme. Despite these encouraging findings, several issues reflected in collaborators' evaluation are worth noting. First, two collaborators (11.1%) disagreed that the service catered for the needs of the clients. Second, 16.7% of the respondents showed negative views about PolyU students' understanding of the needs and potentials of the service recipients. Third, in terms of the impact of the programme, a small proportion of the collaborators did not think that the service promoted migrant children' resilience (22.2%), strengthened service recipients' ability to care for other people (16.7%), and helped the children build up good relationships with healthy adults (16.7%). Although these findings are inconsistent with service providers' evaluation, they point to important directions for the improvement of the programme.

4.3.4 *Ratings of Service by Programme Observers (Zhejiang University Students)*

A total of 275 observers' assessment forms were collected, and the ratings showed that students performed quite well in the five days of service. As shown in Table 4.4, the percentages of positive responses (rated as "fair", "good" or "very good") ranged from 83.3% to 99.6% across the 13 items. In particular, service providers' "punctuality" and "service attitude" were rated positively in almost all

Table 4.3 Subjective outcome evaluation by service collaborators (N = 18)

Item	Positive		Negative	
	n	%	*n*	%
Views about the service programme				
1. This service programme was well-designed	18	100.0	0	0.0
2. The form of the service provided was appropriate	17	94.4	1	5.6
3. The process of delivering the service activities was pleasant	18	100.0	0	0.0
4. The service provided catered to the needs of the clients	16	88.9	2	11.1
5. The service programme promoted a positive culture in the community (e.g. school)	18	100.0	0	0.0
6. The observation I had in this programme enhanced my interest in participating in similar projects	18	100.0	0	0.0
7. On the whole, the service programme was beneficial to the clients	18	100.0	0	0.0
8. Overall speaking, I have positive evaluation of the service programme	18	100.0	0	0.0
Views about the service providers (i.e. PolyU students)				
1. PolyU students prepared well for the service	17	94.4	1	5.6
2. PolyU students showed good professional attitudes	18	100.0	0	0.0
3. PolyU students understood the needs and potentials of the service recipients	15	83.3	3	16.7
4. PolyU students were very involved in the service	18	100.0	0	0.0
5. PolyU students cared about the clients	18	100.0	0	0.0
6. PolyU students were ready to offer help to the clients whenever needed	18	100.0	0	0.0
7. PolyU students had much interaction with service recipients	18	100.0	0	0.0
8. Overall speaking, I have positive evaluation of PolyU students in the service	18	100.0	0	0.0
The extent to which the service programme has helped the clients				
1. It has strengthened the clients' resilience	14	77.8	4	22.2
2. It has helped the clients face the future with a positive attitude	18	100.0	0	0.0
3. It has improved the clients' self-confidence	16	88.9	2	11.1
4. It has broadened the clients' horizon	18	100.0	0	0.0
5. It has reinforced the clients' interest in learning	16	88.9	2	11.1
6. It has strengthened the clients' ability to care for other people	15	83.3	3	16.7
7. It has helped the clients build up good relationships with healthy adults	15	83.3	3	16.7
8. It has promoted the clients' aspirations in life	16	88.9	2	11.1
9. It has enriched the overall development of the clients	18	100.0	0	0.0
10. On the whole, I am satisfied with this service programme	18	100.0	0	0.0

Note *Positive* = ratings of 4 or above on a 6-point scale, *Negative* = ratings of 3 or below

Table 4.4 Quantitative ratings collected from observers ($N = 275$)

Item	Positive		Negative		N/A	
	n	%	*n*	%	*n*	%
1. Service attitude	273	99.3	0	0.0	2	0.7
2. Sense of responsibility	271	98.5	2	0.7	2	0.7
3. Awareness of needs	269	97.8	0	0.0	6	2.2
4. Sense of care	272	98.9	1	0.4	2	0.7
5. Cultural sensitivity	229	83.3	0	0.0	46	16.7
6. Teamwork	269	97.8	3	1.1	3	1.1
7. Problem-solving skills	262	95.3	3	1.1	10	3.6
8. Communication skills with service targets	268	97.5	3	1.1	4	1.5
9. Teaching skills	269	97.8	3	1.1	3	1.1
10. Application of discipline-related knowledge	267	97.1	2	0.7	6	2.2
11. Reflective attitude	257	93.5	3	1.1	15	5.5
12. Punctuality	274	99.6	0	0.0	1	0.4
13. Overall performance	271	98.5	2	0.7	2	0.7

Note *Positive* = rating of 3 or above, *Negative* = rating of 1 or 2, *N/A* = rating of 0

service sessions (99.6% and 99.3%). Their "sense of responsibility" and "overall performance" also received positive ratings in 98.5% of the service sessions. On the other hand, service providers' "cultural sensitivity" (83.3%) and "reflective attitude" (93.5%) were rated less positively as compared to other aspects of the service.

4.4 Discussion

The current study examined the impact of a service-learning programme based on subjective outcome evaluation by service providers, service recipients, collaborators, and observers in the community being served. Together with the findings of observers' ratings, the results showed that the current service-learning programme was welcomed by university student participants, migrant children, and teachers of the served community. Different stakeholders expressed very positive views about the programme and the service. They perceived the programme as having beneficial impact on not only service providers, but also the recipients as well as the community, which suggests an overall successful implementation of this service learning programme in 2015/16 academic year and provides preliminary evidence for the impact of the programme on different stakeholders. The study also highlights the utility of understanding the views of different stakeholders in the evaluation exercise.

Consistent with previous findings on the positive influence of service-learning programmes on student participants (Billig, 2009; Conway, Amel, & Gerwien, 2009), university participants as service providers in the present study favoured the programme and perceived that they had personal, social, and academic gains from the experience. Several characteristics of the programme may contribute to these encouraging findings. First, the programme is embedded in a credit-bearing subject with a well-designed curriculum, clear objectives, and explicit intended learning outcomes for the students. The teaching and learning activities and service are thoughtfully arranged in alignment with these goals. Students are required to apply what they have learned in lectures and workshops in the service context. Such a linkage between academic study and service practices has been found associated with improved learning outcomes in students (e.g. Billig, Root, & Jesse, 2005). For example, students expressed that the learning experience in the subject enhanced their interest in this programme. Second, with the guidance of subject teachers, students have the flexibility to design and implement their own service plan, which may contribute to students' active learning and engagement in the programme. Third, students' reflection has been consistently highlighted throughout the programme. In addition to various reflective activities in classroom teaching, students are asked to submit two reflective journals in this subject that help them to systematically review and reflect on the knowledge learned and the service they provided. During the five-day direct service, a reflection meeting was held every day in which university students and observers shared their service experiences, feelings, and observations, analysed problems they encountered, and found out solutions together. These reflective practices greatly deepened students' self-understanding, expanded their understanding and knowledge about their service recipients, and improved their problem-solving skills, self-confidence, and other intra- and interpersonal competences. In fact, these characteristics are aligned with the recommended practices for service-learning programmes by the National Service-Learning Cooperative (1998) in the USA. The present findings support that these elements may also help strengthen the outcomes of service-learning programme in university participants in a different cultural context.

Compared to the large amount of studies on service providers' learning gains, very few published papers have focused on the impact of service-learning programme on the community and direct recipients of the service. In the present study, findings based on subjective outcome evaluation by different stakeholders converged to suggest a positive impact of the service-learning programme on its recipients, and the served community. Multiple benefits have been endorsed by migrant children who received the service provided by university students, and school teachers as the programme collaborators. Specifically, all collaborators agreed that the service programme promoted a positive culture in the community, enhanced their interest in participating in similar projects, and was beneficial to the clients. For service recipients, they perceived that the programme broadened their horizon, enhanced their resilience and aspirations in life, and promoted their development of various competences. These findings help fill the gap in the literature with regard to the benefits of service-learning programme to community members. In addition, as support and partnership of community have been identified as an important element in service-learning programmes (Celio, Durlak, & Dymnicki, 2011), the positive views and satisfaction about the programme by

collaborators and service recipients identified in the present study may contribute to the desirable outcomes of this programme.

It should be noted that service providers' "understanding about the needs and potentials of the service recipients" has been rated less positive by collaborators as compared to other aspects. Similarly, observers' ratings also suggest that university students' cultural sensitivity in providing service to migrant children is relatively weak. This may be because most service providers have grown up in Hong Kong where the cultural and societal characteristics are quite different from Mainland China. Therefore, in future preparation of this service-learning programme, more background knowledge about migrant children in Hangzhou, as well as local culture, shall be provided to the university students. Moreover, although different theories about the needs and characteristics of child and adolescent have been introduced to the service providers in lectures and workshops, many of them do not have real experiences in serving and interacting with children prior to the service. We may consider adding a few preparation sessions to help university students better understand their service recipients before the five-day direct service formally starts. For example, university students can meet with master teachers of different classes in the school to have a basic understanding about the group of children they will serve. A half-day warm-up party may be arranged for university students and migrant children to get to know about each other. These new practices can be tried out in the future.

Despite the positive findings, several limitations of the present study must be acknowledged. First, only subjective outcome evaluation findings are reported to reflect the impact of the programme. It would be important to include more objective outcome measures in future studies, such as assessment of participants' competences (e.g. civic engagement, social skills, academic performance). Besides, paired samples t-tests shall also be used in the future to compare students' performance at pre- and post-tests. Second, only quantitative data were analysed which may not provide an in-depth understanding about how the service-learning programme makes an impact, facilitating factors and barriers encountered during the service by different stakeholders, as well as other possible positive or negative impacts of the programme which are not included in the questionnaire. Future studies may adopt a mixed-method approach that involves focus groups, individual interviews, or other qualitative methods with service providers, collaborators, and recipients to further explore the impact of the service-learning programme. Third, with regard to the collaborators, only teachers of the local school were invited to provide their subjective evaluation, while the views of subject teachers and other stakeholders (such as parents of the served children, administrators of the school) were not investigated. As their perceptions and evaluation would provide additional information about the impact of the programme, this must be taken into account in further studies. Finally, we need a large sample to make the findings more generalizable.

Despite these limitations, the present findings suggest that the implementation of the service-learning subject entitled "Promotion of Child and Adolescent Development" in Hangzhou can be regarded as successful. The findings add to the limited literature that provides scientific evidence for the effectiveness of service learning programmes. To further illustrate the merits of this programme, this programme was awarded an Excellent Project Award by the Communist Youth League in 2016.

References

Astin, A. W., Vogelgesang, L. J., Ikeda, E. K., & Yee, J. A. (2000). How service learning affects students. *Higher Education, 144*. https://digitalcommons.unomaha.edu/slcehighered/144.

Billig, S. H. (2009). Does quality really matter: Testing the new K–12 service learning standards for quality practice. In B. E. Moely, S. H. Billig, & B. A. Holland (Eds.), *Advances in service-learning research: Vol. 9. Creating our identities in service-learning and community engagement* (pp. 131–158). Greenwich, CT: Information Age.

Billig, S. H., Root, S., & Jesse, D. (2005). The relationship between quality indicators of service-learning and student outcomes: Testing the professional wisdom. In S. Root, J. Callahan, & S. H. Billig (Eds.), *Advances in service learning research: Vol. 5. Improving service-learning practice: Research on models that enhance impacts* (pp. 97–115). Greenwich, CT: Information Age.

Conway, J. M., Amel, E. L., & Gerwien, D. P. (2009). Teaching and learning in the social context: A meta-analysis of service learning's effects on academic, personal, social, and citizenship outcomes. *Teaching of Psychology, 36*(4), 233–245.

Celio, C. I., Durlak, J., & Dymnicki, A. (2011). A meta-analysis of the impact of service-learning on students. *Journal of Experiential Education, 34*(2), 164–181.

Clayton, P. H., Bringle, R. G., & Hatcher, J. A. (2012). *Research on service learning: Conceptual frameworks and assessment*. Sterling: Stylus Publishing LLC.

Chak, Y., Shek, D. T. L., Mok, B. P. W., Han, X. Y., Chen, J. F., Zhang, J. L., & Jiang, H. (2016). *Students' perceived changes and benefits in a mandatory service learning course*. Paper presented at the second international conference on service-learning organized by The Hong Kong Polytechnic University, University Social Responsibility Network together with Office of Service-Learning, Hong Kong.

Chan, S. C. F., Ngai, G., & Shek, D. T. L. (in press). Service-learning as a mandatory credit-bearing subject at The Hong Kong Polytechnic University. *International Journal of Child and Adolescent Health*.

Eyler, J., & Giles, D. E., Jr. (1999). *Where's the learning in service-learning? Jossey-Bass higher and adult education series*. San Francisco, CA: Jossey-Bass Inc.

Eyler, J., Giles Jr, D. E., Stenson, C. M., & Gray, C. J. (2001). At a glance: What we know about the effects of service-learning on college students, faculty, institutions and communities, 1993–2000 (Third Edition). *Higher Education, 139*. https://digitalcommons.unomaha.edu/slcehighered/139.

Hong Kong Polytechnic University. (2013). *General University Requirements (GUR) at PolyU*. Hong Kong: The Hong Kong Polytechnic University. http://www.polyu.edu.hk/ous/student_GUR.html.

Jacoby, B. (2014). *Service-learning essentials: Questions, answers, and lessons learned*. Hoboken, NJ: Wiley.

Ma, C. M. S., Shek, D. T. L., & Li, P. (2016). *Promoting service leadership through service leadership learning among Chinese university students*. Paper presented at the second international conference on service-learning organized by The Hong Kong Polytechnic University, University Social Responsibility Network together with Office of Service-Learning, Hong Kong.

National Service-Learning Cooperative. (1998). *Essential elements of service-learning*. St. Paul, MN: National Youth Leadership Council.

Ngai, S. S. Y. (2006). Service-learning, personal development, and social commitment: A case study of university students in Hong Kong. *Adolescence, 41*(161), 165–176.

Ngai, G., & Chan, S. C. F. (2016). *A two-dimensional classification framework for service-learning*. Paper presented at the second international conference on service-learning organized by The Hong Kong Polytechnic University, University Social Responsibility Network together with Office of Service-Learning, Hong Kong.

Office of Service Learning. (2015). *Service Learning Newsletter* (Vol. 6). Hong Kong: The Hong Kong Polytechnic University. https://www.polyu.edu.hk/osl/files/slNewsletter/OSL_Newsletter_Issue06.pdf.

Pang, P., & Wu, C. (2016). *Learning through reflection: students' service learning experiences in Cambodia*. Paper presented at the second international conference on service-learning organized by The Hong Kong Polytechnic University, University Social Responsibility Network together with Office of Service-Learning, Hong Kong.

Shek, D. T. L., Yu, L., Wu, F. K. Y., & Chai, W. Y. (2015a). General University Requirements at Hong Kong Polytechnic University: Evaluation findings based on student focus groups. *Assessment & Evaluation in Higher Education, 40*(8), 1017–1031. https://doi.org/10.1080/02602938.2014.960362.

Shek, D. T. L., Yu, L., Wu, F. K. Y., & Ng, C. S. (2015b). General education program in a new 4-year university curriculum in Hong Kong: findings based on multiple evaluation strategies. *International Journal on Disability and Human Development, 14*(4), 377–384. https://doi.org/10.1515/ijdhd-2015-0459.

Tryon, E., & Stoecker, R. (2008). The unheard voices: Community organizations and service-learning. *Journal of Higher Education Outreach and Engagement, 12*(3), 47–60.

Wu, F. K. Y., Shek, D. T. L., Mok, B. P. W., & Shek, V. K. F. (2016). *In search of meaning: novice teachers' perceptions on a service-learning subject through narrative inquiry*. Paper presented at the second international conference on service-learning organized by The Hong Kong Polytechnic University, University Social Responsibility Network together with Office of Service-Learning, Hong Kong.

Xing, J., & Ma, C. H. K. (Eds.). (2010). *Service-learning in Asia: Curricular models and practices*. Aberdeen, HK: Hong Kong University Press.

Yu, L., Shek, D. T. L., Liu, Q., Chen, H., & Zhi, H. (2016). *Promoting positive development of migrant children in Hangzhou: Pioneering experience and preliminary evaluation findings*. Paper presented at the second international conference on service-learning organized by The Hong Kong Polytechnic University, University Social Responsibility Network together with Office of Service-Learning, Hong Kong.

Chapter 5
Serving Clients in a Drug Rehabilitation Agency as a Vehicle to Promote Service Leadership in University Students

Daniel T. L. Shek and Wynants W. L. Ho

Abstract A credit-bearing service-learning (SL) subject from The Hong Kong Polytechnic University (PolyU) was developed with the aim of nurturing students' service leadership through engaging them in quality service projects in real-life contexts. Based on the responses of 193 students, this chapter reports how the SL experience at Christian Zheng Sheng College promoted the well-being of PolyU students. The findings, based on the students' written reflections and metaphors, revealed that their overall learning experience was positive and they were able to change their worldviews as well as their personal development.

Keywords Service leadership · Service-learning (SL) · Reflection
Metaphor · Christian Zheng Sheng College

Authorship is equally shared between the two authors.

D. T. L. Shek (✉) · W. W. L. Ho
Department of Applied Social Sciences, The Hong Kong Polytechnic University,
Hunghom, Hong Kong
e-mail: daniel.shek@polyu.edu.hk

W. W. L. Ho
e-mail: wynants.ho@polyu.edu.hk

D. T. L. Shek
Centre for Innovative Programmes for Adolescents and Families,
The Hong Kong Polytechnic University, Hunghom, Hong Kong

D. T. L. Shek
Department of Social Work, East China Normal University, Shanghai
People's Republic of China

D. T. L. Shek
Kiang Wu Nursing College of Macau, Macau, People's Republic of China

D. T. L. Shek
Division of Adolescent Medicine, Department of Pediatrics, Kentucky Children's Hospital,
University of Kentucky College of Medicine, Lexington, KY, USA

D. T. L. Shek et al. (eds.), *Service-Learning for Youth Leadership*,
Quality of Life in Asia 12, https://doi.org/10.1007/978-981-13-0448-4_5

5.1 Overview of the Subject

The credit-bearing service-learning (SL) subject entitled "Service Leadership through Serving Children and Families with Special Needs" was introduced in the 2013/14 academic year to foster the development of service leadership for students of The Hong Kong Polytechnic University (PolyU). Students are provided with opportunities to acquire service leadership skills through attending lessons and participating in quality service projects in authentic life settings. In the context of Christian Zheng Sheng College, the PolyU students applied knowledge of service leadership in providing quality service to Zheng Sheng students. There were several challenges faced by the students. First, the age range of Zheng Sheng students was similar to that of the PolyU students, which was more of a challenge for the PolyU students to demonstrate leadership roles than it would be if they were serving children and youths. Second, the worldviews of the Zheng Sheng and PolyU students were very different. Third, the developmental history of the Zheng Sheng students was complicated. Consequently, the PolyU students had to invest a great deal of effort in understanding the needs of the Zheng Sheng students and in building up relationships with them.

5.1.1 Service-Learning (SL) Subject—The Curriculum

The PolyU students first attended lectures to acquire a basic understanding of the definitions, theories, and concepts of service leadership. Subsequent workshops were provided for them to develop their service proposals. After that, the students were required to engage in service projects with the Zheng Sheng participants for at least 40 hours, providing leadership training, sharing sessions, and a few hours of labor. Reflection time was provided for the PolyU students in the evenings during the service camp to solicit feedback from both peers and teachers.

The curriculum of this subject was based on the service leadership model (SLAM) (Chung, 2011). According to the SLAM, service leadership "…is about satisfying needs by consistently providing quality personal service to everyone one comes into contact with, including one's self, others, groups, communities, systems and environments" (Chung, 2011). Service leaders not only provide service to others but also satisfy their own needs through the service because "a leader is unable to optimize his or her ability to lead others well unless he or she is healthy in mind, body, and spirit" (Chung, 2010). Seven transformative paradigm shifts underpin the frame of reference in service leadership education, which was included in the subject as the overarching framework for the curriculum (Chung, 2012). On top of the paradigm shifts, service leadership emphasizes that leadership is a service aimed at ethically satisfying the needs of one's self, others, groups, communities, systems, and environments (Chung, 2011).

Service leadership is a function of leadership competencies, moral character, and care. This can be illustrated by the equation: effective service leadership = MC^2, where M refers to moral character (Chung, 2012). In the Hong Kong community, a great deal of importance is placed on the moral characters of leaders, as integrity is regarded as the golden thread supporting a fair and just society. According to Shek and Chung (2015), an ethical service leader should display moral qualities such as integrity, respect, humility, and fairness. The two Cs in the equation are leadership competence and caring disposition. Leadership competence consists of intrapersonal and interpersonal competencies. Intrapersonal competencies should include the ability to solve problems, manage, and be aware of one's own and others' emotions. Interpersonal competencies should include the ability to communicate with others and to resolve conflicts. In addition to leadership competencies and moral character, a caring disposition is indispensable to a service leader. A caring service leader demonstrates empathy, consideration, and sincerity toward the service participants while attending to their needs. A key trait is agreeableness, defined as being helpful, generous, friendly, and altruistic. Past research has suggested that agreeableness is associated positively with job and learning performance (e.g., Cortina, Doherty, Kaufman, & Smith, 1992; Mohammed, Mathieu, & Barlett, 2002). In a longitudinal study of the relationship between personality traits and psychological health of medical students during stressful periods, there was a negative, albeit weak, association between agreeableness and stress levels (Yusoff, Pa, Mey, Aziz, & Rahim, 2013).

The model of service leadership developed by the Hong Kong Institute of Service Leadership and Management proposes several attributes of effective service leadership: leadership competence (intrapersonal and interpersonal competencies), moral character, caring disposition, self-leadership and continuous self-improvement, and self-reflection. These are important because service leadership is about inspiration through utilizing intra-/interpersonal competences, rather than by only smartness and hard power (SLAM education, 2013). Within the service leadership framework, the importance of generic leadership competencies, morality and competencies are addressed. In addition, intrapersonal competencies, interpersonal competencies, and caring disposition were addressed in the subject (Shek, Yu, Ma, Sun, Liu, 2013). Specifically, this subject was designed to enable students to: (i) understand the core attributes of service leaders; (ii) apply the core components of service leadership through the engagement of community-based service activities; (iii) develop self-awareness of sharing with and empathy to others and the community; and (iv) reflect on their service leadership qualities, particularly intrapersonal and interpersonal competencies. Service-learning has been highlighted in tertiary education in recent years to uphold the belief that experiential learning theory will foster student learning through providing service to the community.

Table 5.1 Number of PolyU students providing service since 2014 summer

Cohort	Number of PolyU students
2014 summer	60
2015 summer	47
2016 summer	41
2017 summer	45
Total	193

5.2 Description of the Service Site—Christian Zheng Sheng College

Christian Zheng Sheng College is a private school in Hong Kong established by the Christian Zheng Sheng Association (ZSA). By means of life education in the Christian faith, the College is committed to helping students with drug offenses and/or other behavioral problems such as theft and smuggling. Among the programs and schemes offered by the Correctional Services Department, Social Welfare Department, Department of Health, Hospital Authority, and non-governmental organizations (NGOs), Christian Zheng Sheng College is the only agency providing schooling for drug offenders to participate in the rehabilitation treatment programs (Narcotics Division, 2014). Since the summer of 2014, 193 PolyU students have provided services there (Table 5.1).

Christian Zheng Sheng College upholds the power of Christian faith that can transform lives through cultivating Christian values and beliefs in daily life experiences. The daily life in the College is simplistic. Regular schooling with a high school curriculum is provided for Zheng Sheng students to continue their academic studies. In addition, the College provides vocational training for the students to acquire skill sets such as haircutting and media production that can prepare them with skills to reenter society in future. Apart from studying and skills training, Zheng Sheng students have to undertake daily tasks such as doing laundry, cooking in rotation, and laboring. According to the teachers of the College, labor is essential. First, the College is located in a remote area surrounded by trees and plants. There is a need to clear up the plants regularly in order to maintain suitable living conditions. Second, the labor can help to discipline the Zheng Sheng students, which in turn can be beneficial in correcting their problematic behaviors. To cultivate their Christian faith, Zheng Sheng students are required to have thanksgiving prayers at every meal and they are encouraged to pray to God in the process of transformation of their lives.

5.3 Service Projects Conducted at the Site

Three major activities were conducted by the PolyU students during the service camps, namely laboring, leadership training, and sharing of life experiences. The major objective of the labor was to enable the PolyU students to have first-hand experience of the daily lives of the students in the College. Through engaging in the daily routines, the PolyU students had the opportunity to "put-on the shoes of others." Besides, as highly recommended by Zheng Sheng staff, laboring together could help to break the ice between the two groups of students so as to help develop rapport. Based on the above rationale, there were three specific objectives for the laboring activity: (1) developing PolyU students' empathy toward the service targets; (2) triggering a caring disposition for PolyU students; and (3) providing the opportunity for PolyU students to reflect on their physical strength, which is important for effective service leaders. Examples of the labor undertaken are clearing moss along the pavement from the pier to the site, clearing grass and rubbish near the female hall, cooking in the female hall kitchen, helping with organic farming, refurbishing lockers in the male hall, and cutting grass around the campus. Usually, the labor was for three hours in the whole service project.

For the leadership training activity, PolyU students were set the task of raising the Zheng Sheng students' awareness of specific leadership competencies at understanding, application, and synthesis levels, based on the SOLO taxonomy (Biggs & Collis, 1982). They were encouraged to introduce the basic concepts and theories related to the specific competence and then help the service targets to understand the antecedents and consequences of each particular leadership attribute. Then, the PolyU students attempted to help the service targets to generate new ideas based on the application of the attribute. Finally, a variety of ways to promote the attribute were suggested to the service targets for future sustainability. Topics were listed based on selected positive youth constructs (Shek, 2012), such as:

1. Cognitive competence;
2. Emotional competence;
3. Mental health;
4. Spirituality;
5. Positive and healthy identity;
6. Effective communication;
7. Relationship building, team building, and conflict management; and
8. Resilience.

For sharing of life experiences, PolyU students were required to design some prompting questions/activities related to intra- and/or interpersonal development. Since the worldviews of the two groups of students were very different, this was a valuable opportunity for the PolyU students to understand the needs of the Zheng Sheng students, to build up relationships with them through listening actively to each other's stories. More importantly, the sharing of life experiences was beneficial to develop the well-being for both Zheng Sheng students and PolyU students.

5.4 Evaluation of the Service-Learning Subject

The impact of the SL about leadership at Christian Zheng Sheng College was evaluated qualitatively by means of students' metaphorical writing, and quantitatively by looking at the pre-/post-survey to help us understand more about the students' attitudes and behaviors before and after their SL experiences. Conventionally, the effectiveness and impact of teaching and learning in higher education are assessed by using Likert scale questionnaires (Starr-Glass, 2005). Although this is efficient to view the impact in a quantitative way, the complexity of subjective experiences of learning cannot be identified easily out of the figures (Thomas & Beauchamp, 2011). Furthermore, Parlett and Hamilton (1972) argued that many formal evaluations are unable to provide a real picture of education life. In view of the above criticisms, it was necessary to adopt qualitative methods to evaluate the teaching and learning experience of this SL subject.

5.4.1 Metaphor Writing

From the various forms of qualitative evaluation approaches and methods such as focus groups, interviews, and written reflections, written descriptors and metaphors were adopted to understand the perception of student learning experience in the SL subject. In fact, metaphor has been used effectively in the field of educational evaluation (Patton, 2002; Kaminsky, 2000; Smith, 1988). It can be used to help people to understand, express, construct, and organize their worlds (Smith, 1988; Lakoff & Johnson, 2003). There are several benefits to using metaphor. First, it provides new perspectives and innovative ideas and insights (Smith, 1988). Second, it helps people to explain unknown experiences through reflecting on known ones (Munby, 1987). Third, it enables understanding of important features in a simple form from a complex idea (Crider & Cirillo, 1991; Morgan, 1980). Fourth, it provides dynamic and dramatic views beyond the surface of things and reveals their deeper meanings (Marchant, 1992). In the field of educational evaluation, Madaus and Kellaghan (2000) argued that metaphors "influence the way we understand and talk about education; they create mind-sets and influence behavior towards school and teachers; they also influence the kinds of questions we ask about educational programs" (pp.19–32). As such, metaphor is not only an evaluation method but also serves as a useful communication channel to turn ideas into actions. In spite of the advantages of adopting the metaphor as an evaluation method, there are some drawbacks of using metaphor in the field of education evaluation (Leavy, McSorley, & Boté, 2007). First, the conceptual framework is limited, due to the assumptions and predispositions reflected. This is because the metaphors can only reflect on the phenomena the author intends to cover. Second, metaphors may create distortions because they are "a way of seeing" and "ways of not seeing" at the same time (Morgan, 1986).

In view of the benefits and despite the drawbacks of using metaphors in education, they play a vital role in conceptualizing the process of teaching and learning (Leavy, McSorley, & Boté, 2007). For instance, Thomas and Beauchamp used metaphors in semi-structured interviews to understand new graduates' perceptions of their professional identity (Thomas & Beauchamp, 2011). Levin and Wagner used them to explore eighth-grade students' views on writing in science classrooms (Levin & Wagner, 2006).

During the reflection time at the end of each day of the service camp, the PolyU students were asked to write three descriptors and a metaphor which could stand for their SL experience of the day. They were asked to use three words or phrases (i.e., interesting, helpful to my development) to describe their feelings, perceptions, and experiences (i.e., descriptors). Upon completion of the SL subject, they were invited to complete a personal reflection form to conclude their overall learning experience by using the three descriptors and a metaphor, with a brief justification.

5.4.2 *Student Pre- and Post-experience Questionnaire*

The student pre- and post-experience questionnaires developed by the Office of Service-Learning (OSL) at PolyU contain 15 items used to measure students' attitudes and behaviors before and after their SL experience. The post-experience questionnaire contains an additional fourteen items focusing on the amount of learning students have gained, twenty items addressing student motivation and learning experiences of the SL subject and project, and three open-ended questions.

5.5 Results and Discussion

5.5.1 *Metaphor Writing*

From the 2015 and 2017 summer cohorts, 69 personal reflection forms were collected describing the overall learning experience (response rate = 72.6%, $N = 95$). Of the 207 descriptors written, 197 were positive about the overall learning experience. The top four descriptors, with high frequencies, were, "unexpected/amazing" ($N = 22$), "surprising" ($N = 12$), "satisfying" ($N = 12$), "meaningful/thought-provoking/valuable" ($N = 11$). The second tier of high-frequency descriptors was "energetic" ($N = 10$), "empathic" ($N = 10$), "inspiring/learning from ZS students" ($N = 10$), "delightful/joyful/happy/cheerful/enjoyable/pleasurable" ($N = 10$). The rest of the descriptors were scattered and their frequencies were in single digits.

The PolyU students used diverse metaphors, such as "sponge," "durian," "ship/ferry," and "magic stone." Each of the metaphors was supported by a brief justification. The majority of the justifications were single-theme, but a few referred to more than one theme.

> On the first day, it was quite uncomfortable to have a lot of straight restrictions for us to follow and we were not allowed to do a lot of things during the service. I finally felt how painful it is for you to have no freedom. And secondly, it was very happy and unexpected that the students were very welcoming and willing to share their lives with us which we could never have experienced and made me reflect on the way that I am living and my life.

Another PolyU student used "durian" as the metaphor and wrote the following with the themes of "fruitful out of hardness" and "paradigm shift":

> Before the PolyU visit and ZS camp, I didn't know much about Zheng Sheng students. I was afraid about what was going to happen and how I should communicate with them just like the outlook of the durian makes people scared. However, after I knew more about them, I loved to talk to them and made good friends with them like a tasty durian.

The metaphors and the corresponding justifications were examined to identify the common themes. Among the justifications written, four major themes were identified, namely "fruitfulness out of hardness" ($N = 23$), "caring disposition" ($N = 13$), "paradigm shift" ($N = 12$), and "reflection of self" ($N = 9$).

Theme 1: Fruitfulness out of hardness

The majority of the PolyU students perceived that the service was challenging in terms of the preparation for their activities, their physical fitness to cope with the natural environment, such as hot weather, rainfall, or even mosquito bites, and the face-to-face facilitation:

> The first two days were very tiring and challenging because of the labor. However, the sharing helped us to be more familiar with what Zheng Sheng students do and their feelings. Like bitter gourd which will finely taste the bitter taste then a sweet taste.

> At first, I was afraid of facing people in Zheng Sheng. When I arrived at Zheng Sheng, I was surprised by their passion. When people around me became passionate, I was also eager. It was like a magic stone, the stone used to be hard and cool, and I became a soft one.

> Rainbows usually occur after heavy rain (the bad weather) and I could feel how hard we tried to finish the labor and the whole course. However, we did feel satisfied and proud of ourselves as we worked together as a team, and it was just like a rainbow behind the cloud. What a beautiful thing!

Theme 2: Caring disposition

During the interaction with the service targets, the PolyU students learned more about how different their developmental histories were in comparison with those of the service targets. The sharing from the service targets triggered caring dispositions in the PolyU students as they demonstrated their empathy and active listening, and responded to the call to love (Barbuto & Wheeler, 2002; Spears, 2010):

> It was an unforgettable experience for me to come across the students in Zheng Sheng College. This course has provided a chance for us to have a better understanding about

> those teenagers with different backgrounds. We could really use what we learnt in the university to help them. We helped each other and shared our stories. It was just like meeting different people when you are traveling. Each day was a brand new tour full of excitement and surprises for us.
>
> When they shared their experiences and thoughts, I related to them. I couldn't help but think we are all on parallel roads going through life together. It's just that Zheng Sheng students have experienced rougher waters.
>
> Today our workshop's main part was conflict management, through role play and sharing their stories. However, the process was bitter because they share their sad pasts. We gave positive feedback in order to encourage them.

Theme 3: Paradigm shift

The influx of two groups of adolescents from quite different worldviews fostered vigorous reflections about themselves. The PolyU students indicated their paradigm shifts about their worldviews:

> The lunch had no seasoning (no salt, no oil), it looked like Zheng Sheng college is in a natural place, and ZS students had pure hearts to let me feel the most true and pure side of humans. This course gave me a chance to walk out of the city to enjoy the life.
>
> I enjoyed the process of this subject. It gave me a chance to meet and talk with ZS students. If I did not take this course, I may not have an opportunity to meet and understand them more and make friends with them. Therefore, this course was meaningful and very helpful to my development.
>
> In chemistry, chemical reaction refers to putting the reactants together and then yielding some products. In the course, we, the PolyU students and Zheng Sheng students, were like the reactants. When we met, through the conversations, sharing and the leadership training, we produced some positive messages and encouragement. These products, the positive energy, belonged to the ZS students and us. It was a really fruitful experience to learn how to respect each other and reflect about our lives.

Theme 4: Reflection of self

As reflection was one of the key elements in this subject to foster student learning, the PolyU students were aware of the importance of reflecting before, during, and after the service project. Some of them even showed deep reflection on their personal development and some concepts associated with service leadership:

> This course has provided me with an opportunity to reflect on myself and my life, like looking into a mirror, I was able to look closely at what I am like in the moment through knowing Zheng Sheng students' stories and reflections. It was a fruitful experience overall.
>
> I thought in this course I would only need to serve the children, like teaching them some new knowledge or technique, but actually we needed to weed and clean the moss, which is something I never did before. This is like the universe, you think there are only nine planets, but in fact, it has more that you have not discovered yet. I learnt some new methods to regulate my emotions, and tried to find more I had not tried before.

> The world is not as small as it looks, it can be bigger and bright when you head in the right direction. This course, just like a ferry, took me to have a look at the world. In this course, I could evaluate myself related to interest, leadership skills, team building, improve my strengths and amend my weaknesses. A wonderful course to make me reflect more about myself!

In summary, the four major themes reflected the effective learning gains of the PolyU students in terms of "fruitfulness out of hardness," "caring disposition," "paradigm shift," and "reflection of self." The four themes echo the intended learning outcomes of the subject and the development of their social responsibility through SL. Moreover, the subject was intended to introduce the concepts and theories of service leadership for students to apply and/or synthesize, such as caring disposition and moral character. The authentic scenario in Zheng Sheng College can provide PolyU students with the opportunity to develop their leadership skills to liaise with different parties during the preparation and implementation stages. After all, the use of serving learning pedagogy, service leadership as the subject content and Zheng Sheng College as the service collaborator was intended to cultivate the well-being of the PolyU students. Their vigorous reflection contributed to a paradigm shift in their worldviews, which in turn can deepen their personal development.

Despite the learning gains, the metaphors also reflected their challenges in serving the service targets. First, it was difficult for the PolyU students to take a leadership role with service targets of a similar age. It is interesting to observe that 23 out of the 69 metaphors showed the same theme, "fruitful out of hardness." On one hand, the PolyU students perceived that the service was difficult during the preparation and implementation process. On the other hand, they attained reflective, positive learning gains after having interacted with the service targets and group reflection activities. In fact, it is not surprising that the PolyU students perceived the service to be hard. First, was the above-mentioned challenge associated with the similarity in ages. Second, the metaphors reflected that different worldviews required the PolyU students to adjust their expectations and ways to deliver services to the service targets. One student reflected that discrimination had to be eliminated by sincere communication. Third, the complicated developmental history of the Zheng Sheng students caused challenges for the PolyU students. The nature of the College is to cater for teenagers/adolescents with drug and/or criminal offenses, so the developmental histories are quite different from those of the PolyU students. The PolyU students reflected that they were different from the service targets in a sense that they had different living patterns and personalities. They also viewed the service targets as much tougher than themselves and observed that they were persistent with hard work and treasured everything they had in the College, such as education, food, and nature. This was a good opportunity for both parties to learn from each other through sharing their life stories.

5.5.2 Student Pre- and Post-experience Questionnaires

Student Pre- and Post-Experience Questionnaires were used to measure the students' experiences of their service-learning subject and project across the 2014/2015 and 2015/2016 academic years. The first section was to compare students' learning before and upon completion of the subject in terms of intellectual and civic development. For intellectual development, the mean differences for "application of knowledge and skills" ($p = 0.208$), and "understanding of the linkage between service-learning and academic learning" ($p = 0.285$) were not significant. For civic development, there were no significant differences for "self-reflection" or "demonstration of empathy." Having said that, for "self-reflection" there were positive changes in both cohorts (see Table 5.2). In all, there were no significant differences in students' intellectual and civic development. One of the reasons is that the sample size was too small in each cohort ($N = 46$ in 2014/15 cohort, and $N = 41$ in 2015/16 cohort), which means it may not have been representative of students' learning experiences in general. Another possible reason is that quantitative figures cannot explain the complexity of students' subjective learning experiences in direct service (Thomas & Beauchamp, 2011). Moreover, there was a time lag factor that may have contributed to the discrepancy. The post-survey was conducted by the end of the semester, which was two months after the service activity.

Despite the discrepancy between the results analyzed quantitatively and the metaphors analyzed qualitatively, the statistical results showed that the students generally had favorable views about their SL experiences. The majority of the respondents across the 2 years agreed that the overall experience of the SL subject was useful and rewarding (range from 63.3 to 85.4%). Positive feedback was received for different aspects of their learning experiences. The mean ratings of the items in 2014/15 ranged from 4.32 to 5.73, with 46.7 to 80% of the students giving ratings of 5 or above on all items. In 2015/16, the average ratings of the items ranged from 4.22 to 5.63, with 46.3 to 82.9% of the students also giving ratings of 5 or above. The percentages of students giving negative feedback (e.g., ratings of 3 or

Table 5.2 *p* values of students' learning

Cohort	Learning gain from SL	Intellectual development		Civic development	
		Application of knowledge and skills	Understanding of the linkage between SL and academic learning	Self-reflection	Demonstration of empathy
2015 summer	*p* value	0.208	0.285	0.718	0.167
2016 summer	*p* value	0.852	0.174	0.929	0.525

below) on the items were quite low. The following four items received relatively higher ratings (over 76%) across the 2 academic years, in terms of the percentages of respondents giving a rating of 5 or above: “my teammates in the SL project were generally motivated and supportive,” “there was a lot of opportunities for me to meet and interact with the people I served,” “I developed a good personal relationship with my teammates,” and “in my SL project, I carried out tasks that were mainly designed by me/my team rather than following instructions.” The results suggested that the majority of the students were satisfied with their learning experiences in the SL subjects and projects. Through serving people, the students were able to develop interpersonal and intrapersonal skills and also to acquire and improve on necessary leadership skills required of them upon graduation.

To further understand the impacts of SL on students’ learning and development, the students from this aforementioned academic terms were asked to rate their learning with respect to the outcomes stipulated in the questionnaire on a 7-point scale (1 = very little; 4 = a fair amount; 7 = very much). In both academic years (2014/15 and 2015/16), the students generally had very positive views regarding their overall learning gains, with over 85% indicating that they had learned “a fair amount” or “very much” (mean = 5.72; mean = 5.38). In general, the students responded positively regarding their achievement of personal learning outcomes. The mean ratings of the items for 2014/15 ranged from 5.07 to 5.49, with 95.6 to 100% of the respondents giving ratings of 4 (a fair amount) or above. Similarly, the average ratings of the items for 2015/16 ranged from 4.98 to 5.41, with 75.6 to 80.5% of the respondents giving ratings of 4 (a fair amount) or above. The three most highly rated items, in terms of the percentage of respondents giving ratings of 5 or above, were “solving challenging real-life problems,” “communicating effectively with peers, collaborators, and service recipients,” and “better understanding of my own strengths and weaknesses.” Also, for the item “increased interest/commitment to serve people in need,” the students’ responses from both academic years were reasonably high, ranging from 5.17 to 5.37, with 80.5 to 83%. In conclusion, the statistics showed positive trends toward the impacts of student learning. However, there were no significant changes in their perceptions of their learning experiences.

As promoting paradigm shift is one of the major goals of service leadership education, it is essential to establish a very different authentic context as the learning environment for leadership development. In this subject, SL was used as a vehicle to promote leadership qualities in the students. The evaluation components showed that the students were able to achieve the intended learning outcomes and that they felt the subject helped them to achieve the qualities of service leaders. The findings of the present study demonstrated a paradigm shift in the students’ perceptions. The findings are consistent with previous studies in showing that SL provides an opportunity for students to learn to serve and serve to learn and they demonstrate how these experiences nurtured the students’ competencies and character strengths (Bringle & Hatcher, 1996; Mitchell, 2008; Warren, 2012). Also, the survey and qualitative analyses indicate self-reported positive gains for the PolyU students in terms of increased capacity for social learning, civic responsibility, critical thinking, personal learning, and the ability to collaborate with others, as well as developing a positive relationship with others. The integration of SL and learning communities will enable first-year students to gain valuable leadership skills when serving those in need, such as the Zheng Sheng students. Through participation in service-learning, students are enabled to develop problem-solving, critical thinking, public speaking, and interpersonal skills that can equip them for their professional development in future and continue to serve and to learn via SL. Hence, the implementation of SL to address the needs of communities definitely helped to refine the students' communication, team building, and leadership skills through effective feedback.

5.6 Personal Reflections on the Impact of the Subject on the Development of Well-Being

As the second author was the teacher responsible for this subject, it is appropriate to consider his experience, as follows:

"Teaching this SL subject was a great opportunity for me to respond to the calling to help people around. I have had this calling, from a Christian perspective, for almost 30 years. In the past decades, I have continually testified and verified this vocation to help people by observing and doing. The passion to serve drives me to contribute my time, effort, money, and skills to children, adolescents, adults, and the elderly. The most rewarding thing is to see the development of well-being of those whom I have served. The development of well-being is not necessarily materialistic, such as living conditions and wealth. Rather, this is about the intrinsic nature of human beings to restore the beauty of being human. The restoration of the beauty is inside out from knowing the God or higher being of one's religious belief or personal beliefs and values for atheists. However, such a knowing process requires a vigorous search of the inner heart in order to construct the personal knowledge. In order to have this vigorous search to know oneself, the affection of personal life is essential. The affection of personal life, as I perceive, is to take religious or personal beliefs seriously with the mind and heart through action and therefore life will undergo a transformation with an enlightened soul and renewed heart. Johnathan Edwards defined affections as "the vigorous and sensible exercises of the inclination and will of the soul" (Smith, 1987, p. 6). To define affections in detail, Edwards pointed out that they belong to the heart, not the body. Also, affections have to be exercised practically. Moreover, they come from an intensive inclination of the mind. Since affections are matters of the heart rather than of the body, they are different from the bodily emotions, namely passions. In other words, affections are not "acting" but exercising of the will.

In order to develop the well-being of adolescents, SL is therefore a valuable vehicle for adolescents to know about their lives by doing. The cultivation and transformation of life cannot be done by paperwork nor by passing any examination to demonstrate the competence acquired, but through exercising of the will. Throughout facilitating the service trips, I know that SL has not only been beneficial to the service targets and the PolyU students as the service providers, but also to myself. The teaching of this subject enabled me to reflect on my life and the calling every time. The teaching has also driven me to continue my vigorous search from my mind and heart to answer the question of why I still enjoy to serve people around me. The service with Zheng Sheng helped to identify my weaknesses, mostly in terms of my character and my leadership skills. Since my role as a subject teacher was to facilitate my PolyU students to prepare and to conduct the service activities, I was sometimes too "pushy" and rigid with my students and colleagues. Sometimes my ideas may have been too idealistic in that I expected my students to be able to think deeply about the needs of the service targets from multiple perspectives in order to generate their service plans. As such, I think I was a morale killer for my students and sometimes my fellow colleagues, because I put the task over people. The service reminded me that I should take the right balance between the task and people. Once a colleague said to me, "Unlike you, I cannot serve Zheng Sheng stake holders with such effort". At that moment, I thought this was just an excuse. However, as I kept reflecting about the meaning behind it, I found my blind spot that I should have been doing better to inspire my colleague to serve as a subject leader. Since inspiration is essential in service leadership (Chung, 2012), I should now be able to identify this direction for my own leadership development."

5.7 Conclusion

This paper discussed the promotion of service leadership in university students through serving clients in a drug rehabilitation agency. The learning gains of PolyU students were evaluated by means of questionnaire survey and metaphor writing. Both of the quantitative and qualitative results showed the level of reflection of students had increased after completed the services. However, since the sample size was not large enough to represent the learning gains of students in general, the quantitative figures were not significant. Meanwhile, students reflected their learning gains qualitatively through metaphor writing, which came up with four major themes, namely fruitfulness out of hardness, caring disposition, paradigm shift, and reflection of self. The themes supported the development of personal growth to cultivate the well-being of PolyU students.

Appendix 1—Reflection Form

Personal Reflection Form

Student Full Name: ____________ **Student ID:** ____________

Reflective learning is an important element in this subject. After you have completed the subject, we would like to invite you to have some personal reflection about the subject. There are two parts in this reflection. First, use three words or phrases to describe your feelings, perceptions and experiences of this course. Second, think of something that can stand for the course.

I would use the following THREE words or phrases (e.g. interesting, helpful to my development ...etc.) to describe my feeling, perception or experience of this course:

1. ______________________
2. ______________________
3. ______________________

Think about a metaphor (i.e. some object, event or state) which can stand for the subject (e.g., an enjoyable tour, buffet, compass in life ...etc). Give a brief explanation about the meaning of the metaphor.

I would use ________________to stand for the course because:

____

____

____

____

____

Appendix 2—Objectives/Intended Learning Outcomes of the Subject (Excerpt from the Course Outline)

Objectives
This subject is designed to enable students to:

1. Understand the core attributes of service leaders;
2. Apply the core components of service leadership through the engagement of;
3. Community-based service activities;
4. Develop self-awareness of sharing and empathy to others and the community; and
5. Reflect on their service leadership qualities, particularly intrapersonal and interpersonal competencies.

Learning Outcomes
Upon completion of the subject, students will be able to:

1. Address the needs of the service recipients through service delivery;
2. Link their service experiences with academic course materials;
3. Appreciate and respect people from diverse background;
4. Integrate academic learning (e.g., knowledge on service leadership) into the service experience and activities;
5. Demonstrate empathy and care by providing community service;
6. Apply the skills (e.g., active listening) and knowledge (e.g., moral character and competencies) they have acquired in university education to deal with complex issues in the service setting;
7. Reflect on their service leadership qualities through service-learning; and
8. Work effectively with different parties (e.g., students, teachers, family, and community partners) when preparing and delivering service.

References

Barbuto, J. E. Jr., & Wheeler, D. W. (2002). *Becoming a servant leader: Do you have what it takes?*. University of Nebraska-Lincoln Extension. Retrieved from http://extensionpublications.unl.edu/assets/pdf/g1481.pdf.

Biggs, J. B., & Collis, K. F. (1982). *Evaluating the quality of learning: The SOLO taxonomy (Structure of the Observed Learning Outcome)*. New York: Academic Press.

Bringle, R. G., & Hatcher, J. A. (1996). Implementing service learning in higher education. *Journal of High Education, 67,* 211–239.

Chung, P. Y. (2010). *Distinguishing characteristics of service leadership and management education*. Hong Kong: Hong Kong Institute of Service Leadership and Management.

Chung, P. (2011). *Hong Kong Institution of Service Leadership & Management (HKI-SLAM) curriculum framework.* Unpublished document.

Chung, P. (2012). *Service Reborn*. New York: Lexingford Publishing.

Cortina, J. M., Doherty, M. L., Kaufman, G., & Smith, R. G. (1992). The "Big Five" personality factors in the IPI and MMPI: Predictors of police performance. *Personnel Psychology, 45*(1), 119–140.

Crider, C., & Cirillo, L. (1991). Systems of interpretation and the function of metaphor. *Journal for the Theory of Social Behaviour, 21*(2), 171–195.

Kaminsky, A. (2000). Beyond the literal: Metaphors and why they matter. *New Directions for Evaluation, 2000*(86), 69–80.

Lakoff G, Johnson M. (2003). *Metaphors we live by: With a new afterword* (2nd ed.) (p. 256). Chicago, IL: University of Chicago.

Leavy, A. M., McSorley, F. A., & Boté, L. A. (2007). An examination of what metaphor construction reveals about the evolution of preservice teachers' beliefs about teaching and learning. *Teaching and Teacher Education, 23*(7), 1217–1233.

Levin, T., & Wagner, T. (2006). In their own words: Understanding student conceptions of writing through their spontaneous metaphors in the science classrooms. *Instructional Science, 34,* 227–278.

Madaus, G. F., & Kellaghan, T. (2000). Models, metaphors, and definitions of evaluation. In G. F. Madaus, M. Scriven, & D. L. Stufflebeam (Eds.), *Evaluation models: Viewpoints on educational and human services evaluation* (2nd ed.) (pp. 19–32). Boston, MA: Kluwer-Nijhoff Publishing.

Marchant, G. J. (1992). A teacher is like a…: Using simile lists to explore personal metaphors. *Language and Education, 6*(1), 33–45.

Mitchell, T. D. (2008). Traditional vs. critical service-learning: Engaging the literature to differentiate two models. *Michigan Journal of Community Service Learning, 14,* 50–65.

Mohammed, S., Mathieu, J. E., & Bartlett, A. L. (2002). Technical-administrative task performance, leadership task performance, and contextual performance: Considering the influence of team-and task-related composition variables. *Journal of Organizational Behavior, 23*(7), 795–814.

Morgan, G. (1980). Paradigms, metaphors, and puzzle solving in organization theory. *Administrative Science Quarterly, 25*, 605–622.

Morgan, G. (1986). *Images of organization*. Beverley Hills, CA: SAGE Publications.

Munby, H. (1987). Metaphor and teacher's knowledge. *Research in the Teaching of English, 21,* 377–397.

Narcotics Division of Security Bureau (2014). Drug abuse trends for 2004–2013. In *Central registry of drug abuse sixty-third report* (pp.7–18). Hong Kong: Narcotics Division of Security Bureau.

Parlett, M., & Hamilton, D. (1972). *Evaluation as illumitative: A new approach to the study of innovatory programs. University Centre for Research in Educational Science*. UK: University of Edinburgh.

Patton, M. Q. (2002). Teaching and training with metaphors. *American Journal of Evaluation, 23*(1), 93–98.

Shek, D. T. L. (2012). Development of a positive youth development subject in a university context in Hong Kong. *International Journal on Disability and Human Development, 11,* 173–179.

Shek, D. T. L., & Chung P. (Eds.). (2015). *Promoting service leadership qualities in university students: The case of Hong Kong*. Singapore: Springer.

Shek, D. T. L., Yu, L., Ma, C. M. S., Sun, R. C. F., & Liu, T. T. (2013). Development of a credit-bearing service leadership subject for university students in Hong Kong. *International Journal of Adolescent Medicine and Health, 25*(4), 353–361.

SLAM education (2013). *Hong Kong Institute of Service Leadership and Managemen*t. Retrieved from http://hki-slam.org/.

Smith, J. E. (Ed.). (1987). *The works of Jonathan Edwards* (Vol. 2, p. 6). New Haven, CT: Yale University Press.

Smith, N. L. (1988). Mining metaphors for methods of practice. In D. M. Fetterman (Ed). *Qualitative approaches to evaluation in education: The silent scientific revolution*. New York: Praeger.

Spears, L. C. (2010). Character and servant leadership: Ten characteristics of effective, caring leaders. *The Journal of Virtues & Leadership, 1*(1), 25–30.

Starr-Glass, D. (2005). Metaphor and maps in evaluation. *Assessment & Evaluation in Higher Education, 30,* 195–207.

Thomas, L., & Beauchamp, C. (2011). Understanding new teachers' professional identities through metaphor. *Teaching and teacher Education, 27*(4), 762–769.

Warren, J. L. (2012). Does service-learning increase student learning: A meta-analysis. *Michigan Journal of Community Service Learning, 18,* 56–61.

Yusoff, M. S. B., Esa, A. R., Pa, M. N. M., Mey, S. C., Aziz, R. A., & Rahim, A. F. A. (2013). A longitudinal study of relationships between previous academic achievement, emotional intelligence and personality traits with psychological health of medical students during stressful periods. *Education for Health, 26*(1), 39–47.

Chapter 6
Service Leadership Through Serving Socially Deprived Students: Experience Gained from Corporate–Community–University Partnership (Project *WeCan*)

Cecilia M. S. Ma, Daniel T. L. Shek and Pecky P. K. Li

Abstract Service-learning provides an application of academic knowledge in real-life contexts through the process of meeting community needs. It offers university students a chance to collaborate with people from diverse backgrounds and to develop competencies related to leadership, communication skills, and professionalism. With financial support from the Wharf (Holdings) Limited (the Group), a corporate–community partnership program "Project *WeCan*" has been launched to help secondary school students from the underserved community. In this chapter, we evaluated the effectiveness of this project through credit-bearing service-learning courses. Using multiple evaluation methods, different stakeholders provided their feedback on service-learning experiences. Service recipients (secondary school students) and service partners (secondary school teachers) perceived the service experience positively and satisfied with the community–university partnership. University students reported favorable changes in their academic and personal growth after participating in the service-learning activities. Findings suggest the positive impact of the service-learning experiences in corporate–community–university partnership in promoting students' academic, psychosocial, and leadership development.

Keywords Service-learning · Secondary school students · Corporate–community partnership · University students · Low socioeconomic status · Hong Kong

---

C. M. S. Ma (✉) · D. T. L. Shek · P. P. K. Li
Department of Applied Social Sciences, The Hong Kong Polytechnic University, Hunghom, Hong Kong
e-mail: cecilia.ma@polyu.edu.hk

D. T. L. Shek
e-mail: daniel.shek@polyu.edu.hk

P. P. K. Li
e-mail: pecky.li@polyu.edu.hk

D. T. L. Shek et al. (eds.), *Service-Learning for Youth Leadership*,
Quality of Life in Asia 12, https://doi.org/10.1007/978-981-13-0448-4_6

6.1 Introduction

Service-learning is an educational experience that provides experiential learning opportunities for students to enhance their competencies, to strengthen their civic responsibility, and to develop a greater sense of social consciousness (Benson, Harkavy, & Puckett, 2007; Bringle & Hatcher, 1995; Groh, Stallwood, & Daniels, 2011). It bridges educational goals with service designed to satisfy the needs of the community (Schmidt & Brown, 2016). Through active participation in structured service-learning activities, students' professional and personal development are promoted (Felten & Clayton, 2011; Jacoby, 1996). Different from internships, vocational training, or voluntary service, it integrates the components of academic learning in the services that aim to meet the needs of the recipients and community (Deeley, 2004; Pritchard, 2001). This chapter describes the experiences of Chinese university students, who participated in a service-learning subject providing service to socially deprived secondary school students in a corporate–community–university partnership project.

6.1.1 Adolescents with Low Socioeconomic Status in Hong Kong

With over seven million people, Hong Kong is one of the world's most densely populated cities (behind New York and London). Despite the achievement in economic growth, nearly one million people live in poverty in Hong Kong (less than HK$3800) (Hong Kong Census and Statistic Department, 2016). The Gini coefficient reached a record high of 0.539 in 2016 (compared with 0.537 in 2011), reflecting the increased economic disparity and urban poverty in Hong Kong (Hong Kong Census and Statistic Department, 2017). In particular, around 180,000 adolescents (below 18 years) suffered from financial hardship and poverty (Hong Kong Census and Statistic Department, 2016).

Adolescents from low socioeconomic status (SES) were associated with more frequent substance use (Yen et al., 2007), poorer school adjustment (Shek, 2002), unhealthier diet (Sooman, Macintyre, & Anderson, 1993), higher emotional and psychosocial problems (Becker & Luthar, 2002), and larger likelihood of smoking (Wills, Sandy, & Yaeger, 2002) than those from high SES peers. Although they are vulnerable to psychological distress and risk problems, programs focusing on the prevention and promotion of health and well-being of the youth are critical to the development of this population. Previous studies have shown the benefits of organized after-school activities and community-based programs on general (Durlak, Weissberg, & Pachan, 2010), African American (Belgrave, Chase-Vaughn, Gray, Addison, & Cherry, 2000; Tucker & Herman, 2002), Chinese (Sun & Shek, 2012), and disadvantaged (O'Donnell et al., 1999) youths.

Similar findings exist in the field of service-learning research. For example, d'Arlach et al. (2009) examined the impact of a service-learning program and showed the reciprocal benefits between Latino immigrants and university students. This was also supported in a recent study by Cupelli (2016) who found the positive impacts on recipients and undergraduate nursing students. Service-learning is considered as a platform that allows the linkage between community and university (Felten & Clayton, 2011). Unlike other subjects which focus on factual knowledge, service-learning has been considered as an empowering tool of civic learning and personal growth through critical reflection (Felten & Clayton, 2011; Mendel-Reyes, 1998). Kagawa (2007) argued that the role of a university to nurture students to be a change agent by developing their skills and abilities is paramount. Given the importance of this subject, there is a need for more research in this area, especially in Chinese contexts.

6.2 Project *WeCan*

In 2011, the Wharf (Holdings) Limited (the Group) launched a business-in-community "Project *WeCan*" that aims at providing learning opportunities for the less privileged secondary school students. This project serves an open platform by involving local universities and offering various service activities to the target population. To date, more than 50 secondary schools with 50,000 students have benefited from this project. In this chapter, we look at the effectiveness of the project with reference to credit-bearing service-learning courses.

6.2.1 Subject Background

Two credit-bearing service-learning courses (APSS2S05 "*Promotion of Children and Adolescent Development*" and APSS2S09 "*Service Leadership through Serving Children and Families with Special Needs*") were introduced at the Department of Applied Social Sciences at The Hong Kong Polytechnic University. The overall aims of the courses were to apply academic knowledge and satisfy the community's needs through students' tailor-made service activities. The former focused on developing one's potential and strengths utilizing the positive youth development (PYD) approach (Catalano, Berglund, Ryan, Lonczak, & Hawkins, 2004; Damon, 2004). The subject was awarded the Excellence Award from the Communist Youth League in 2016. The latter aimed at integrating the Service Leadership and Management (SLAM) model in service delivery (Chung, 2012). This subject was awarded the Bronze Award in the QS Reimagine Education Awards 2016 under the category of "Social Enterprise." Details are shown in Table 6.1.

Table 6.1 Intended learning outcomes of the courses

	APSS2S05 "Promotion of Children and Adolescent Development"	APSS2S09 "Service Leadership through Serving Children and Families with Special Needs"
Theoretical framework	Positive youth development	Service leadership and management model
Objectives	1. To give a brief overview of different perspectives on child and adolescent development, needs and challenges of children and adolescents living in disadvantaged circumstances to students through design and implementation of a service project 2. To enhance students' competencies of problem-solving, decision-making, communication, and teamwork 3. To cultivate the positive values and strengths orientation among students 4. To nurture students' sense of social responsibility, social awareness and promote prosocial behaviors 5. To nurture students' sense of care and compassion toward other people in the community, especially toward underprivileged children and adolescents	1. To understand the core attributes of service leaders 2. To apply the core components of service leadership through the engagement of community-based service activities 3. To develop the self-awareness of sharing to and empathy with others and the community 4. To reflect on their service leadership qualities, particularly intrapersonal and interpersonal competencies
Intended learning outcomes	Upon the completion of the subject, students will be able to 1. Understand different perspectives of child and adolescent development and apply the concepts to understanding the needs and potential of underprivileged children and adolescents in the community 2. Integrate knowledge on child and adolescent development into real-life situations through service delivery 3. Apply the knowledge and skills they have acquired in university education to deal with complex issues in the service setting 4. Reflect on their roles and responsibilities both as a professional in their chosen disciplines and as a responsible citizen 5. Develop a sense of care and compassion toward other people, especially the underprivileged children and adolescents in the community 6. Enhance psychosocial competencies such as self-confidence, problem-solving, decision-making capabilities, and interpersonal skills	Upon the completion of the subject, students will be able to 1. Address the needs of the service recipients through service delivery 2. Link their service experiences with academic course materials 3. Appreciate and respect people from diverse backgrounds 4. Integrate academic learning (e.g., knowledge of service leadership) into the service experience and activities; 5. Demonstrate empathy and care by providing community service 6. Apply the skills (e.g., active listening) and knowledge (e.g., moral character and competencies) they have acquired in university education to deal with complex issues in the service setting 7. Reflect on their service leadership qualities through service-learning 8. Work effectively with different parties (e.g., students, teachers, families, and community partners) when preparing and delivering service

Table 6.2 Descriptions of courses

	APSS2S05 "Promotion of Children and Adolescent Development"	APSS2S09 "Service Leadership through Serving Children and Families with Special Needs"
Course structure	• 10-h e-learning module • Three 3-h lectures • Six 3-h seminars • 40 direct service hours	• 10-h e-learning module • Three 3-h lectures • Six 2-h seminars • 40 direct service hours
No. of university students	• 78	• 66
Semester	• Fall and Spring semesters	• Spring and Summer semesters
No. of service partners	• Catholic Ming Yuen Secondary School • TWGHs C. Y. Ma Memorial College • TWGHs Kwok Yat Wai College	• Semple Memorial Secondary School • CCC Fung Leung Kit Memorial Secondary School • Lions College • The Yuen Yuen Institute MFBM Nei Ming Chan Lui Chung Tak Memorial College • Caritas Fanling Chan Chun Ha Secondary School • Ju Ching Chu Secondary School (Tuen Mun)
No. of service recipients	• 1991	• 1819
Characteristics of the service recipients	Adolescents with special needs or vulnerable to psychosocial and emotional problems New immigrants from Mainland China Youth from low-income households	

In both subjects, university students were asked to design service activities for students in nine secondary schools. Service recipients (secondary school students) were mainly from low-income or new immigrant families (see Table 6.2). In the first semester, students were required to complete 10-h e-learning to understand the concepts and practices of service-learning, to attend three 3-h lectures, followed by a series of six seminars. University students had the opportunity to work with secondary school staff, students (seven graders to twelve graders), and their parents. Throughout the two semesters, students were asked to complete 40 direct service hours. Prior to the service delivery, they worked with the school staff and proposed the service activities that met the interest and needs of the secondary school students. Examples of the service activities included: conducting after-school interest classes, such as arts, science and cookery classes, academic and life skills preparation, developing leadership or team building workshops and providing on-campus tours/visits (Table 6.3).

Table 6.3 Descriptions of service-learning activities

	Objectives	Description of the activity	Number of activity	Number of participants
After-school activities/ workshop	• To enhance their interest in other subjects • To improve communication skills	• DIY tote bag • Science experiments • Junior Chief: Cooking classes • Health talk • Leadership and team building workshops	85	1166
Language proficiency class	• To increase their language proficiency • To improve written and verbal communication in English	• Watching English-spoken movie • Art jam through English	26	780
Campus/ community visit	• To provide insights into the secondary school students about campus facilities	• Guided talk on museums, athletics facilities, residential halls, and academic buildings	15	456
Life skills training (Academic and Career planning)	• To teach the secondary students essential study and job skills	• Job interview • Preparation of public examination	31	601
		Total	157	3003

6.3 Methodology

A total of 144 university students were enrolled in two courses in the 2016–2017 academic year. To explore the impacts of service-learning courses on secondary school (service recipients) and university (service providers) students, the following methods were used (Fig. 6.1). These included:

(1) Method 1: To evaluate the secondary school students' perceptions of the subject, subjective outcome evaluation was conducted at the end of the courses.
(2) Method 2: To evaluate the university students' perceptions of the subject, subjective outcome evaluation was conducted at the end of the courses.
(3) Method 3: To evaluate the impact on university students' learning and personal growth, objective outcome evaluation was employed at the beginning and the end of the semester.

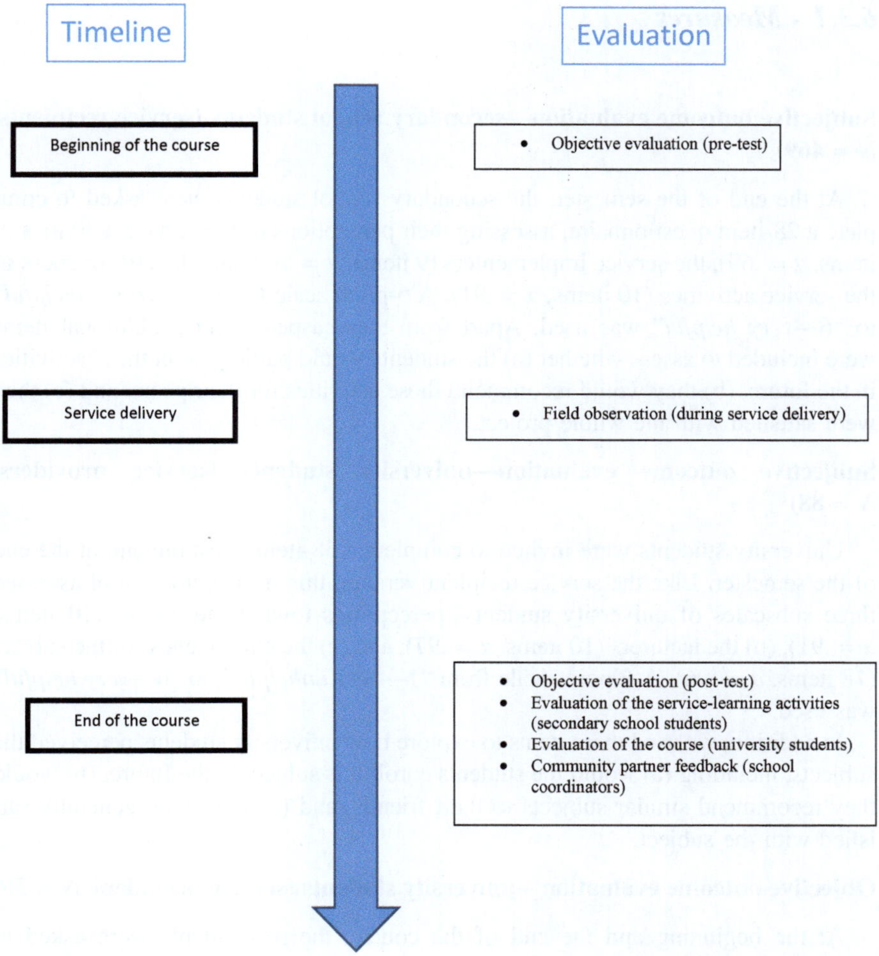

Fig. 6.1 Evaluation process

(4) Method 4: To evaluate the service partners' perceptions of the performance of the university students, field observation was conducted after each service activity.
(5) Method 5: To evaluate the service partners' perceptions of the overall university–community collaboration, partnership evaluation was conducted at the end of the courses.
(6) Method 6: To evaluate the university students' perceptions of the subject, student feedback questionnaire was conducted at the end of the courses.

6.3.1 Measures

Subjective outcome evaluation—secondary school students (service recipients, $N = 469$)

At the end of the semester, the secondary school students were asked to complete a 28-item questionnaire, assessing their perceptions of the service activities (9 items, $\alpha = .69$), the service implementers (9 items, $\alpha = .95$), and the effectiveness of the service activities (10 items, $\alpha = .91$). A 6-point scale from "1—*very unhelpful*" to "6—*very helpful*" was used. Apart from these aspects, three additional items were included to assess whether (a) the students would participate in these activities in the future, (b) they would recommend these activities for their peers, and (c) they were satisfied with the whole project.

Subjective outcome evaluation—university students (service providers, $N = 88$)

University students were invited to complete a 38-item questionnaire at the end of the semester. Like the service recipient version, this measurement tool assessed three subscales of university students' perceptions toward the course (10 items, $\alpha = .91$), (b) the lecturers (10 items, $\alpha = .97$), and (c) the effectiveness of the subject (18 items, $\alpha = .96$). A 6-point scale from "1—*very unhelpful*" to "6—*very helpful*" was used.

In addition, we used three items to explore how university students perceived the subjects, including (a) would the students enroll this subject in the future, (b) would they recommend similar subjects to their friends, and (c) were they generally satisfied with the subject.

Objective outcome evaluation—university students (service providers, $N = 30$)

At the beginning and the end of the course, the respondents were asked to complete a 70-item online questionnaire, assessing (a) positive development constructs, (pretest: $\alpha = .92$; posttest: $\alpha = .96$), where the items were categorized as social competence (3 items), emotional competence (3 items), cognitive competence (4 items), behavioral competence (2 items), moral competence (3 items), self-determination (3 items), clear and positive identity (2 items), belief in future (3 items), spirituality (4 items), and resilience (3 items), b) service leadership (pretest: $\alpha = .94$; posttest: $\alpha = .94$), where the items were categorized as caring disposition (8 items), self-leadership (5 items), character strengths (15 items), and the beliefs and values of service leadership (6 items), and c) other psychosocial variables, such as life satisfaction [5 items, (pretest: $\alpha = .90$; posttest: $\alpha = .97$)]. A 6-point scale from "1—*strongly disagree*" to "6—*strongly agree*" was used.

Field observation form—service partners (secondary school teachers, $N = 69$)

Service partners were invited to complete a field observation form when university students conducted the service activities. A total of 13 items were used to assess the quality (e.g., the sense of responsibility, problem-solving skills, communication skills) and overall satisfaction with the service activities. A 5-point scale from "1—*very good*" to "5—*very poor*" was used.

Community partner feedback form (secondary school teachers, $N = 11$)

At the end of the course, the coordinators of the nine schools were invited to assess their perceptions about the subjects (e.g., suitability for the community's needs), university students' service performance (attitude, caring), and university staff (collaboration process). A 5-point scale "1—*very good*" to "5—*very poor*" was used.

Student feedback questionnaire—university students (service providers, $N = 114$)

At the end of the course, university students were invited to complete an online survey assessing their perceptions of the subject (4 items) and achievements of intended learning outcomes (5 items). A 5-point scale "1—*strongly disagree*" to "5—*strongly agree*" was used.

6.4 Results

Subjective outcome evaluation—secondary school students (service recipients)

There were four parts in the subjective evaluation form: a) the students' evaluation of the contents of the activities, b) the evaluations of the service implementers, c) the evaluation of the effectiveness of the service activities, and d) a summary of the views of the students on all service activities. The descriptive statistics of each aspect is shown in Tables 6.4, 6.5, 6.6 and 6.7.

In general, the secondary school students perceived the service activities positively. The percentage of the rating of "4" or above on a 6-point Likert scale ranged from 82.1% to 97.2% (Tables 6.4, 6.5 and 6.6). Regarding the findings of students' evaluations of the contents of the activities, 93.9% of the students perceived the content design of the activities prepared by the university students as very good, 94.9% of the students felt that the format of the activities was appropriate, and 94.9% of the students found that the atmosphere of the activities was pleasant (Table 6.4). Of the secondary school students, 96.2% found that the university students showed professional attitudes, 97.2% thought that the university students were actively involved in the services, and 96.2% reported that the university students showed readiness to offer help to them when needed (Table 6.5). About the secondary school students' evaluations of the effectiveness of the service activities, 88.1% of the students found that the service activities had enhanced their self-confidence, 90.5% thought that they had broadened their horizons, 89.9% thought that the activities were very useful to them, and 87.9% of them reported that

Table 6.4 Descriptive statistics of the secondary school students' evaluation of the contents of activities

		M	*SD*	Respondents with positive responses (Options 4–6) *n*	%
1.	The content design of the activity is very good	5.01	.98	442	93.9
2.	The format of the activity is appropriate	5.02	.94	447	94.9
3.	The atmosphere of the activity was pleasant	5.14	.98	446	94.9
4.	There was much peer interaction among the students	5.04	1.02	436	92.9
5.	I participated in the activity actively	5.00	1.08	435	92.8
6.	I was encouraged to do my best	4.80	1.11	422	90.3
7.	The learning experience enhanced my interests toward the service	4.93	1.14	427	91.0
8.	Overall speaking, I have a very positive evaluation on the activity	5.07	1.05	437	93.3
9.	On the whole, I like this activity very much	5.04	1.09	426	91.8

Note All items are on a 6-point Likert scale with 1 = strongly disagree, 2 = disagree, 3 = slightly disagree, 4 = slightly agree, 5 = agree, 6 = strongly agree. Only respondents with positive responses (Options 4–6) are shown in the table

it had promoted their holistic development (Table 6.6). About the summary of the views of the secondary school students after completing all service activities, 93.2% of the students reported that they would participate in the activities again in the future and 96.9% of them were satisfied with the service activities (Table 6.7).

Subjective outcome evaluation—university students (service providers)

Table 6.8 shows the descriptive statistics of the impacts of the subject. In general, the university students perceived the course positively. About their impression of the content, 87.5% of the students thought that the objectives of the curriculum were very clear, 87.5% of them reported that they participated in the class activities, including discussions, sharing, and games actively, and 88.6% of them felt that they were encouraged to do their best in the course. Regarding the students' impressions on the lecturers, 89.8% of the students thought that the lecturers had a good mastery of the course, 90.9% of them felt that the lecturers were very involved in the course, 92% of them reported that the lecturers were ready to offer help to them when needed, and 90.9% of them agreed that the lecturers had a lot of interaction with them. About the benefits from the course, the students expressed that this course was able to improve their leadership and interpersonal skills, such as social competence (88.6%), the importance of situational task competencies, character strength, and caring disposition in successful leadership (86.4%). In addition, 84.1% of the students reported that the theories, research, and concepts covered in

Table 6.5 Descriptive statistics of the secondary school students' evaluation of service implementers

				Respondents with positive responses (Options 4–6)	
		M	*SD*	*n*	%
1.	Service implementer(s) was (were) well prepared for the activity	5.21	.93	450	95.9
2.	Service implementer(s) showed professional attitude	5.29	.90	451	96.2
3.	Service implementer(s) understood my needs and potential	4.98	1.02	441	94.0
4.	Service implementer(s) was (were) actively involved	5.32	.88	456	97.2
5.	Service implementer(s) encouraged me to participate in the activity	5.21	.96	446	95.9
6.	Service implementer(s) cared about me	5.17	.99	444	94.9
7.	Service implementer(s) showed readiness to offer help to me when needed	5.27	.97	451	96.2
8.	Service implementer(s) had much interaction with us	5.19	1.04	438	93.6
9.	Overall speaking, I have a very positive evaluation on the university students	5.29	1.01	443	95.3

Note All items are on a 6-point Likert scale with 1 = strongly disagree, 2 = disagree, 3 = slightly disagree, 4 = slightly agree, 5 = agree, 6 = strongly agree. Only respondents with positive responses (Options 4–6) are shown in the table

the course had helped them synthesize the characteristics of successful service leaders. However, the findings demonstrated a relatively neutral impact on students' spirituality, love for life (51.1%), and meaning of life (59.1%). Overall speaking, 68.2% of the students were satisfied with this course (68.2%, Table 6.9).

Objective outcome evaluation—university students (service providers)

The university students were asked to complete the object outcome evaluation forms at the beginning and the end of the course. Some students undertook a work placement and internship after the service delivery and did not complete the posttest. Therefore, only those, who completed both pre- and posttests, were included in data analysis. Table 6.10 shows the descriptive statistics of the impacts of the subject on the university students. A paired samples t-test was conducted to assess the mean differences of the learning outcomes before and after the service delivery. The results are shown in Table 6.11. Positive changes were found in clear and positive identity (pretest: $M = 3.28$, $SD = .85$, posttest: $M = 4.17$, $SD = .62$, $t(29) = -2.72$, $p < .05$), caring disposition (pretest: $M = 3.88$, $SD = .51$, posttest: $M = 4.12$, $SD = .56$, $t(29) = -2.08$, $p < .05$), character strength (pretest: $M = 3.60$,

Table 6.6 Descriptive statistics of the secondary school students' evaluation of the effectiveness of service activities

				Respondents with positive responses (Options 4–6)	
		M	*SD*	*n*	%
1.	It has strengthened my resilience in adverse conditions	4.71	1.22	384	85.9
2.	It has helped me to face the future with a positive attitude	4.72	1.24	389	85.9
3.	It has enhanced my self-confidence	4.80	1.21	401	88.1
4.	It has broadened my horizons	4.96	1.19	402	90.5
5.	It has enhanced my interests toward my studies	4.82	1.20	387	86.6
6.	It has enhanced my ability to care	4.76	1.23	384	86.9
7.	It has helped me to develop a good relationship with adults (for example, teachers and parents)	4.65	1.38	357	82.1
8.	It has promoted my aspiration	4.73	1.34	368	84.8
9.	It has promoted my holistic development	4.82	1.23	386	87.9
10.	On the whole, I think the activity is very useful to me	4.91	1.22	393	89.9

Note All items are on a 6-point Likert scale with 1 = very unhelpful, 2 = unhelpful, 3 = slightly unhelpful, 4 = slightly helpful, 5 = helpful, 6 = very helpful. Only respondents with positive responses (Options 4–6) are shown in the table

$SD = .48$, posttest: $M = 3.85$, $SD = .57$, $t(29) = -2.37$, $p < .05$), and beliefs in service leadership (pretest: $M = 3.88$, $SD = .58$, posttest: $M = 4.20$, $SD = .62$, $t(29) = -2.94$, $p < .01$).

Field observation form—service partners (secondary school teachers)

To evaluate the performance of the service implementers (university students), the teachers from the secondary schools were invited to fill in the field observation form. In general, teachers perceived the performance of the service implementers positively. The percentage of a rating of 3 or above on a 5-point Likert scale ranged from 95.2 to 100% for the various items measured (Table 6.12). The majority of the teachers rated the university students' performance positively in terms of their service attitude, the sense of responsibility, cultural sensitivity, problem-solving skills, application of discipline-related knowledge, reflective attitude, punctuality, and overall performance. These positive perceptions were also reflected from the qualitative comments. For instance, *"A group of energetic and helpful youngsters. Well-organized. Well done!"*, *"During the provision of services, (service implementers) were full of enthusiasm and put a lot of effort."* and *"The helpers (service implementers) get along well with the students. Well done!"* In general, they

Table 6.7 Summary of the views of the students after the completion of service activities

Will you participate in the activities that are designed by university students again in the future? (N = 469)

1		2		3		4		Participants with positive responses (Options 3–4)	
Definitely will not		Will not		Will		Definitely will			
n	%	n	%	n	%	n	%	n	%
6	1.3	26	5.5	284	60.6	153	32.6	437	93.2

Will you suggest your friends participate in the activities that are designed by university students? (N = 469)

1		2		3		4		Participants with positive responses (Options 3–4)	
Definitely will not suggest		Will not suggest		Will suggest		Definitely will suggest			
n	%	n	%	n	%	n	%	n	%
5	1.1	36	7.7	291	62.0	137	29.2	428	91.3

On the whole, are you satisfied with the activity? (N = 452)

1		2		3		4		5		Participants with positive responses (Options 3–5)	
Very dissatisfied		Moderately dissatisfied		Slightly satisfied		Moderately satisfied		Very satisfied			
n	%	n	%	n	%	n	%	n	%	n	%
5	1.1	9	2.0	110	24.3	158	35.0	170	37.6	438	96.9

Table 6.8 Descriptive statistics of the university students' evaluation of the service-learning course

				Respondents with positive responses (Options 4–5)	
		M	*SD*	*n*	%
Impressions concerning the curriculum content					
1.1	The objectives of the curriculum are very clear	4.05	.64	77	87.5
1.2	The content design of the curriculum is very good	3.67	.81	59	67.0
1.3	The activities were carefully arranged	3.86	.71	65	73.9
1.4	The classroom atmosphere was very pleasant	4.06	.72	72	81.8
1.5	There was a lot of peer interaction among the students	4.16	.71	72	81.8
1.6	I actively participated in the class activities (including discussions, sharing, games)	4.20	.68	77	87.5
1.7	I was encouraged to do my best	4.22	.67	78	88.6
1.8	The learning experience enhanced my interests toward the course	3.85	.81	62	70.5
1.9	Overall speaking, I have a very positive evaluation of the course	3.86	.73	66	75.0
1.10	On the whole, I like this course very much	3.80	.82	60	68.2
Impressions concerning the lecturer(s)					
2.1	The lecturer(s) had a good mastery of the course	4.26	.63	79	89.8
2.2	The lecturer(s) was (were) well prepared for the lessons	4.32	.69	77	87.5
2.3	The teaching skills of the lecturer(s) were good	4.18	.78	72	81.8
2.4	The lecturer(s) showed good professional attitudes	4.25	.81	74	84.1
2.5	The lecturer(s) was (were) very involved	4.34	.64	80	90.9
2.6	The lecturer(s) encouraged students to participate in the activities	4.33	.67	78	88.6
2.7	The lecturer(s) cared for the students.	4.34	.68	78	88.6
2.8	The lecturer(s) was (were) ready to offer help to students when needed	4.43	.67	81	92.0

(continued)

Table 6.8 (continued)

				Respondents with positive responses (Options 4–5)	
		M	*SD*	*n*	%
2.9	The lecturer(s) had much interaction with the students	4.33	.64	80	90.9
2.10	Overall speaking, I have a very positive evaluation on the lecturer(s)	4.28	.74	77	87.5
Benefits from the course					
3.1	It has enhanced my social competence	4.08	.66	78	88.6
3.2	It has improved my ability in expressing and handling my emotions	4.00	.79	69	78.4
3.3	It has enhanced my critical thinking	4.00	.77	70	79.5
3.4	It has increased my competence in making sensible and wise choices	4.11	.69	74	84.1
3.5	It has helped me make ethical decisions	4.08	.78	72	81.8
3.6	It has strengthened my resilience to adverse conditions	4.10	.76	71	80.7
3.7	It has strengthened my self-confidence	4.10	.77	72	81.8
3.8	It has helped me face the future with a positive attitude	3.97	.81	68	77.3
3.9	It has enhanced my love for life	3.45	.97	45	51.1
3.10	It has helped me explore the meaning of life	3.63	.95	52	59.1
3.11	It has enhanced my self-leadership ability	4.07	.85	71	80.7
3.12	It has helped me cultivate compassion and care for others	4.11	.75	74	84.1
3.13	It has helped me enhance my character strengths comprehensively	3.91	.74	68	77.3
3.14	It has enabled me to understand the importance of situational task competencies, character strength, and caring disposition in successful leadership	4.10	.71	76	86.4
3.15	It has promoted my sense of responsibility in serving the society	3.99	.69	73	83.0
3.16	It has promoted my overall development	3.99	.75	72	82.8

(continued)

Table 6.8 (continued)

				Respondents with positive responses (Options 4–5)	
		M	*SD*	*n*	%
3.17	The theories, research, and concepts covered in the course have enabled me to understand the characteristics of successful service leaders	3.99	.70	72	81.8
3.18	The theories, research, and concepts covered in the course have helped me synthesize the characteristics of successful service leaders	3.99	.72	74	84.1

Note All items are on a 5-point Likert scale with 1 = strongly disagree, 2 = disagree, 3 = neutral, 4 = agree, 5 = strongly agree. For Part 3, all items are on a 5-point Likert scale with 1 = unhelpful, 2 = not very helpful, 3 = not sure, 4 = helpful, 5 = very helpful

integrated the knowledge (e.g., caring) and skills in their service activities and interacted positively with the secondary school students (service recipients).

Community partner feedback form—service partners (secondary school teachers)

The coordinators (secondary school teachers) from the various secondary schools were also invited to fill in the community partner feedback form to understand more on their perceptions of the collaboration between their secondary schools and the university. They perceived the collaboration positively. The percentages of ratings of 3 or above on a 5-point Likert scale for all items were hundred percent (100%), such as the relevance of service to the needs of their schools, interactions with university staff and students, the performance of students in service delivery, the ability of students to apply subject-related knowledge, and skills to solve problems (Table 6.13). Based on the open-ended comments, coordinators generally perceived the collaboration positively. For example, "*the collaboration process was generally smooth*", "*Good communication… the university students showed passion…look forward to continued collaboration with the university.*" They also gave us some suggestions "*Provide more diversified service activities in order to motivate secondary school students' interest*", "*To avoid scheduling conflicts with our school activities, we can plan a discuss the service schedule earlier next year.*"

Student feedback questionnaire—university students (service providers)

To understand the impact of the course comprehensively, university students were asked to fill in the Electronic Student Feedback Questionnaire (ESFQ) via an online platform. Overall speaking, the students evaluated the course positively (Table 6.14). For example, 84.2% of the students thought that they had a clear

Table 6.9 Summary of students' views after the completion of service activities

Will you suggest your friends take this course? (N = 88)											
1		2		3		4		5		Participants with positive responses (Options 4–5)	
Definitely will not suggest		Will not suggest		Not sure		Will suggest		Definitely will suggest			
n	%	n	%	n	%	n	%	n	%	n	%
4	4.5	10	11.4	24	27.3	36	40.9	14	15.9	50	56.8
Will you participate in similar courses again in the future? (N = 88)											
1		2		3		4		5		Participants with positive responses (Options 4–5)	
Definitely will not suggest		Will not suggest		Not sure		Will suggest		Definitely will suggest			
n	%	n	%	n	%	n	%	n	%	n	%
7	8.0	18	20.5	36	40.9	21	23.9	6	6.8	27	30.7
On the whole, are you satisfied with this course? (N = 88)											
1		2		3		4		5		Participants with positive responses (Options 4–5)	
Very dissatisfied		Moderately dissatisfied		Neutral		Satisfied		Very satisfied			
n	%	n	%	n	%	n	%	n	%	n	%
0	0	5	5.7	23	26.1	48	54.5	12	13.6	60	68.2

Table 6.10 Summary of the impacts of the course and students' developmental characteristics

		Pretest		Posttest	
		Respondents with positive responses (Options 4–6)		Respondents with positive responses (Options 4–6)	
		n	%	*n*	%
1.	I know how to communicate with others	26	86.7	25	86.2
2.	I understand the rules and expectations in interacting with others	25	83.3	26	89.7
3.	I can get along well with others	27	90.0	28	96.6
4.	When I am unhappy, I can appropriately express my emotions	14	46.7	19	67.9
5.	When I have a conflict with others, I can usually manage my emotions	23	76.7	24	82.8
6.	I can stand in the shoes of others	23	76.7	24	82.8
7.	I know how to see things from different angles	24	80.0	27	93.1
8.	I try new ways to solve my problems	16	53.3	22	75.9
9.	I know how to find the causes of and solutions to a problem	23	79.3	27	93.1
10.	I can differentiate between the good and the bad aspects of things	26	89.7	25	86.2
11.	I can face criticisms with an open mind	20	66.7	26	89.7
12.	I can express views that are different from others'	20	66.7	24	82.8
13.	I have high moral standards about my behaviors	25	86.2	24	82.8
14.	I fulfill my promises	25	83.3	28	96.6
15.	It is no big deal to give up some of our moral principles in exchange for money	2	8.0	4	17.4

(continued)

Table 6.10 (continued)

		Pretest		Posttest	
		Respondents with positive responses (Options 4–6)		Respondents with positive responses (Options 4–6)	
		n	%	*n*	%
16.	I have a habit of self-reflection	19	63.3	20	69.0
17.	I am capable of making wise choices	20	66.7	25	86.2
18.	I am confident about my decisions	19	63.3	21	72.4
19.	I believe things that will happen in my life are mostly determined by myself	21	70.2	23	79.3
20.	I am a person with self-confidence	12	40.0	15	50.0
21.	I believe I have the qualities and abilities of a leader	13	43.3	18	60.0
22.	I have the confidence to solve my future problems	20	66.7	25	83.3
23.	I have the confidence to graduate from university	28	93.3	28	96.6
24.	I have confidence that I will be a useful person after I graduate	23	76.7	23	76.7
25.	In most ways, my life is close to my ideal	13	43.3	14	48.3
26.	The conditions of my life are excellent	15	50.0	17	58.6
27.	I am satisfied with my life	15	51.7	16	55.2
28.	So far, I have gotten the important things I want in life	12	40.0	13	44.8
29.	If I could live my life over, I would still choose the life I have now	14	46.7	18	62.1
30.	My life is meaningful	16	55.2	19	65.5
31.	I have found my purpose in life	12	41.4	15	51.7
32.	I have considered committing suicide before	5	25.0	7	31.8

(continued)

Table 6.10 (continued)

		Pretest		Posttest	
		Respondents with positive responses (Options 4–6)		Respondents with positive responses (Options 4–6)	
		n	%	*n*	%
33.	I believe spiritual riches are more important than material prosperity	25	83.3	22	73.3
34.	When I face difficulties, I do not give up easily	19	63.3	21	70.0
35.	My belief is that even though tomorrow becomes worse, I will still live in a good manner	15	50.0	20	66.7
36.	I believe problems in life can be solved	22	73.3	21	72.4
37.	I understand the importance of self-development	25	83.3	25	83.3
38.	I know my strengths and weaknesses	23	76.7	23	76.7
39.	I am capable of managing my own life	21	70.0	26	86.7
40.	I have planned my life well	17	56.7	18	60.0
41.	I control my own behavior to avoid stepping out of line	27	90.0	24	80.0
42.	I am sensitive to others' needs	15	50.0	21	70.0
43.	I pay attention to others when they are talking to me	27	93.1	26	86.7
44.	I offer advice to others when there is a need	23	76.7	26	86.7
45.	I am always ready to lend a hand to those in need	19	63.3	25	83.3
46.	I know how to appreciate others, even those who are completely different from me	22	73.3	24	80.0
47.	I treat others with dignity and respect	25	83.3	29	96.7
48.	I care about others	23	76.7	29	96.7
49.	I am kind and friendly to others	24	82.8	29	96.7

(continued)

Table 6.10 (continued)

		Pretest		Posttest	
		Respondents with positive responses (Options 4–6)		Respondents with positive responses (Options 4–6)	
		n	%	*n*	%
50.	I open my mind to embrace new knowledge	23	79.3	27	90.0
51.	I am grateful for many things in my life	21	70.0	22	73.3
52.	Lying or cheating is not my way	21	70.0	23	76.7
53.	I persist in pursuing my goals even though I encounter setbacks	16	53.3	22	73.3
54.	I do not like to show off good things happening to me	14	46.7	21	70.0
55.	I do not hesitate to fight against what I think is wrong despite opposition	11	36.7	13	44.8
56.	I place my interests after the interests of others	7	23.3	14	48.3
57.	I regard integrity as the most important aspect of life	18	60.0	23	79.3
58.	It is my pleasure to obey rules and regulations	20	66.7	21	70.0
59.	I would feel ashamed if I did something wrong	23	76.7	24	80.0
60.	I try to maintain harmony in interpersonal relationships	26	86.7	27	90.0
61.	I will fight against injustice	10	33.3	16	53.3
62.	I do not attempt to possess anything undeserved	15	50.0	18	60.0
63.	I live my life in the way I have claimed	12	40.0	23	76.7
64.	Most of the time, I can keep my mind peaceful when facing gains or losses	17	56.7	20	69.0
65.	Leadership is a service for oneself, others, groups, and the society	23	76.7	25	86.2

(continued)

Table 6.10 (continued)

		Pretest		Posttest	
		Respondents with positive responses (Options 4–6)		Respondents with positive responses (Options 4–6)	
		n	%	*n*	%
66.	Everyone has opportunities to practice leadership every day	23	76.7	23	76.7
67.	Leadership effectiveness is determined by situational task competencies, character strength, and caring ability	23	76.7	27	90.0
68.	A successful leader should try his/her best to improve his/her competencies and satisfy others' needs	23	76.7	27	90.0
69.	A service leader needs to provide high-quality service to the people he/she is in contacts with, regardless of their position and capacity	22	75.9	27	90.0
70.	A service leader needs to improve his/her character strength and caring ability continuously	24	80.0	28	93.3

Note All items are on a 6-point Likert scale with 1 = strongly disagree, 2 = disagree, 3 = slightly disagree, 4 = slightly agree, 5 = agree, 6 = strongly agree. Only respondents with positive responses (Options 4–6) are shown in the table

Table 6.11 Differences in the impacts of the course and students' developmental characteristics before and after conducting service activities using paired samples t-test

	Pretest	Posttest	Paired sample t test	
	M (*SD*)	*M* (*SD*)	Mean difference	*t*
Social competence	4.04 (.50)	4.06 (.93)	−.01	−.07
Emotional competence	3.74 (.60)	3.84 (1.03)	−.10	−.51
Cognitive competence	3.78 (.63)	4.03 (.95)	−.26	−1.34
Behavioral competence	3.87 (.58)	4.01 (.92)	−.14	−.94
Moral competence	4.39 (.47)	4.44 (.50)	−.05	−.41
Self-determination	3.71 (.53)	3.93 (.96)	−.22	−1.40
Clear and positive identity	3.28 (.85)	4.17 (.62)	−.38	−2.72*
Belief in the future	4.04 (.59)	4.17 (.62)	−.12	−1.17
Life satisfaction	3.22 (.90)	3.35 (1.23)	−.13	−1.07
Spirituality	3.05 (.57)	3.16 (.72)	−.11	−1.2
Resilience	3.69 (.70)	3.83 (.69)	−.14	−1.45
Self-leadership	3.83 (.69)	3.96 (.68)	−.13	−1.16
Caring disposition	3.88 (.51)	4.12 (.56)	−.23	−2.08*
Character strength	3.60 (.48)	3.85 (.57)	−.25	−2.37*
The beliefs and values of service leadership	3.88 (.58)	4.20 (.62)	−.32	−2.94**

Note $^{*}p < .05$; $^{**}p < .01$

understanding of what they were expected to learn from this course and 84.2% of them reported the teaching and learning activities such as lectures, discussions, case studies, projects had helped them to achieve the course learning outcomes. 84.2% of them thought they could apply their knowledge and skills in this course, and 83.2% of them responded they clearly understood the course criteria.

Table 6.12 Summary of teachers' perceptions of the performance of service implementers

			Respondents with positive responses (Options 3–5)	
	M	*SD*	*n*	%
1. Service attitude	4.43	.56	69	100.0
2. Sense of responsibility	4.48	.61	69	100.0
3. Awareness of needs	4.00	.82	67	98.5
4. Sense of care	4.07	1.30	63	98.4
5. Cultural sensitivity	3.64	1.63	59	100.0
6. Teamwork	4.23	.60	68	98.6
7. Problem-solving skills	4.07	1.04	65	100.0
8. Communication skills with service targets	4.23	.79	67	98.5
9. Teaching skills	3.64	1.37	60	95.2
10. Application of discipline-related knowledge	3.84	1.26	64	100.0
11. Reflective attitude	3.03	2.00	47	100.0
12. Punctuality	4.57	.79	68	100.0
13. Overall performance	4.28	.54	68	100.0

Note All items are on a 5-point Likert scale with 1 = very poor, 2 = poor, 3 = fair, 4 = good, 5 = very good. Only respondents with positive responses (Options 3–5) are shown in the table

Table 6.13 A summary of service partners' perceptions of the collaboration between the secondary schools and the university

			Respondents with positive responses (Options 3–5)	
	M	*SD*	*n*	%
1. The relevance of the service to the needs of your organization/clients/the community	3.91	.70	11	100.0
2. Interactions and communication with university staff (teachers, tutors, or other support staff)	4.64	.50	11	100.0
3. Interactions and communication with university students	4.09	.70	11	100.0
4. Responsiveness to suggestions, inputs, and feedback from your organization	4.09	.30	11	100.0
5. Students' attitude and commitment to service	4.09	.70	11	100.0
6. Students' preparedness for delivering the service	4.27	.79	11	100.0
7. The performance of students in service delivery	4.09	.70	11	100.0

(continued)

Table 6.13 (continued)

			Respondents with positive responses (Options 3–5)	
	M	*SD*	*n*	%
8. The ability of students to apply subject-related knowledge and skills to solve problems in the service setting	3.73	.79	11	100.0
9. The overall effectiveness of the service-learning project in addressing the important need(s) of your organization/clients/ the community	4.27	.47	11	100.0

Note All items are on a 5-point Likert scale with 1 = very poor, 2 = poor, 3 = fair, 4 = good, 5 = very good. Only respondents with positive responses (Options 3–5) are shown in the table

Table 6.14 A summary of university students' feedback for the service-learning courses

				Respondents with positive responses (Options 4–5)	
		M	*SD*	*n*	%
Your learning experience of the subject					
1.	I have a clear understanding of what I am expected to learn from this subject	4.02	.74	96	84.2
2.	The teaching and learning activities (e.g. lectures, discussions, case studies, projects) have helped me to achieve the subject learning outcomes	4.00	.79	96	84.2
3.	The assessments require me to demonstrate my knowledge, skills, and understanding about the subject	4.00	.79	96	84.2
4.	I understand the criteria according to which I will be graded	3.97	.77	94	83.2
Feedback on achievement of learning objectives/outcomes					
1.	I can link the service-learning activities and experiences with the academic content of the subject	3.95	.79	91	80.5
2.	I have learned to apply the knowledge and skills I have acquired at the university to deal with complex issues in the service setting	4.02	.76	98	86.0
3.	This subject has enabled me to reflect on my role and responsibilities both as a professional and as a responsible citizen	4.00	.78	94	82.5

(continued)

Table 6.14 (continued)

				Respondents with positive responses (Options 4–5)	
		M	*SD*	*n*	%
4.	I have felt more empathy toward people in need as a result of studying this subject	3.99	.78	95	83.3
5.	I have developed a stronger sense of civic responsibility	3.99	.81	91	81.3

Note All items are on a 5-point Likert scale with 1 = strongly disagree, 2 = disagree, 3 = no strong view, 4 = agree, 5 = strongly agree. Only respondents with positive responses (Options 4–5) are shown in the table

6.5 Discussion

The purpose of the present study was to explore the effectiveness of service-learning for serving secondary school students by adopting several evaluation methods. Results indicate that service recipients (secondary school students) generally reported positive service-learning experiences. Through the subjects, they interacted with university students from different disciplines and cultural backgrounds and were satisfied with the service activities. They reported that the service activities were well organized and promoted their self-esteem and awareness of oneself.

The secondary school students reported that the university students showed care and were actively involved in service delivery. Their horizon was broadened after they participated in a service activity. This is perhaps related to the small age gap between the secondary school and university students. This is in line with the study of Bialka and Havlik (2016) who found that the secondary school students viewed the university students as peers and helped them understand university experiences better. The individualized and small group service-learning activities allowed the university students to build a closer connection with the secondary school students who might not have prior exposure to university contexts. Through personal interaction and sharing, the secondary school students found the university students more relatable, felt more comfortable to build a reciprocal relationship, and showed more interest in the university that their service partners were attending (Bialka & Havlik, 2016, p. 222). In addition, service partners shared similar views. The findings shed light on the importance of building reciprocal relationships between service recipients and service patterns.

The present study was significant also because it explored the voices of service recipients. The majority of the research in this area focuses on service-learning providers or faculty members (academic providers) while a little is known how the service recipients perceive their service experience (d'Arlach, Sánchez,

& Feuer, 2009). Feedback from service recipients is imperative as "poorly implemented service-learning programs can actually do more harm than good" by reinforcing the stereotypes and prejudices of social issues (Bialka & Havlik, 2016). Researchers have noted the importance of including the service recipients' voices when evaluating the impact of a service-learning program (d'Arlach, Sánchez, & Feuer, 2009; Sperling, 2007). The present study suggests that service-learning offers an opportunity to disadvantage students for interaction with university students.

The benefits of service-learning for the university students were demonstrated in the present study. Consistent with past studies (Barnes, 2016; Brown & Bright, 2017; Groh et al., 2011, Leung et al., 2014), the students experienced positive changes in their leadership abilities in teamwork, problem-solving, communication skills, and caring. This is further supported by Brail (2016), who found out that those university students who enrolled in service-learning subjects showed better academic outcomes (i.e., grade achievement) than those who did not enroll. Both the formative (field observation) and summative (subjective outcome evaluation) results supported the positive impact of service-learning participation on enhancing student learning through the connection between community service and academic coursework. Using the pre- and posttest design, positive changes were shown in clear and positive identity, caring, character strength, and the beliefs and values of service leadership.

"Service-learning, in combining academic theory with experiential learning, is a powerful learning tool, through which the process of consciousness-raising can be nurtured" (Deeley, 2010, p. 50). Where the promotion of personal and professional development is an integral part of university education, service-learning presents an excellent real-world context for students to foster transferable and practical skills in workplace (e.g., interpersonal and team building skills) and to facilitate the behavioral attributes, such as the ability to collaborate with people from diverse backgrounds (McCarthy & Tucker, 2002). The students in the courses formed small groups and conducted service activities that met the recipients' needs. The student engagement in designing service activities is beneficial for fostering students' commitment to learning (Popkess & McDaniel, 2011). The students reported a favorable attitude toward working with people from diverse backgrounds. Providing to learn outside the classroom seems to be more effective in promoting learning for professional and personal development (Bringle & Hatcher, 1996). This indicates the importance of transforming students' attitudes toward deprived groups in enriched care environments.

6.6 Future Directions

The present study suggests that service-learning can deepen students' leadership competencies and learning and offers an opportunity to solve community problems by building a connection with the community (Bates, 2010). Service-learning integrates academic instruction and meaning experiences and critical reflection to facilitate the development of personal growth, the sense of civic responsibility, community building, and educational success (Ryan, 2012). This approach allows university students to enhance their communication, real-life problem-solving, and teamwork skills. Through service-learning programs, university students build a relationship with the secondary school students and are able to experience the socioeconomic differences in real-world settings. More research is needed to complement the quantitative findings. This could be done, for example, by using in-depth or focus group interviews. Also, a post-graduation follow-up study would be helpful to illuminate the long-term effects of service-learning experiences on students' professional learning. In addition, the degree to which student characteristics (e.g., year, gender, major) play a role in the impact of service-learning participation should be investigated.

6.7 Conclusion

Service-learning serves as a teaching method that plays an additional role in deepening student learning, embracing people from diverse backgrounds and cultures, and promoting civic engagement (Felten & Clayton, 2011). The present study highlights the reciprocal benefits of service-learning among university students when working with the disadvantaged population in a corporate–community–university partnership project. Providing university students with real-world opportunities to collaborate with community partners facilitates their awareness and understanding about social disadvantage and commitment to work with people with diverse backgrounds.

References

Barnes, M. E. (2016). The student as teacher educator in service-learning. *Journal of Experiential Education, 39*(3), 238–253.

Bates, L. M. (2010). *Service-learning as strategy of aging and environment: Developing generations of socially responsible interior designers*. Retrieved from http://proquest.umi.com/pqdweb?did=2063853551&Fmt=7&clientId=29550&RQT=309&VName=PQD.

Becker, B. E., & Luthar, S. S. (2002). Social-emotional factors affecting achievement outcomes among disadvantaged students: Closing the achievement gap. *Educational Psychologist, 37*(4), 197–214.

Belgrave, F. Z., Chase-Vaughn, G., Gray, F., Addison, J. D., & Cherry, V. R. (2000). The effectiveness of a culture- and gender-specific intervention for increasing resiliency among African American preadolescent females. *Journal of Black Psychology, 26*(2), 133–147.

Benson, L., Harkavy, I. R., & Puckett, J. L. (2007). *Dewey's dream: Universities and democracies in an age of education reform*. Philadelphia: Temple University Press.

Bialka, C. S., & Havlik, S. A. (2016). Partners in learning: Exploring two transformative university and high school service-learning partnerships. *Journal of Experiential Education, 39*(3), 220–237.

Brail, S. (2016). Quantifying the value of service-learning: A comparison of grade achievement between service-learning and non-service-learning students. *International Journal of Teaching and Learning in Higher Education, 28*(2), 148–157.

Bringle, R. G., & Hatcher, J. A. (1995). A service-learning curriculum for faculty. *Michigan Journal of Community Service Learning, 2*(1), 112–122.

Bringle, R. G., & Hatcher, J. A. (1996). Implementing service learning in higher education. *Journal of Higher Education, 67*(2), 221–238.

Brown, K. M., & Bright, L. M. (2017). Teaching caring and competence: Student transformation during an older adult focused service-learning course. *Nurse Education in Practice, 27,* 29–35.

Catalano, R. F., Berglund, M. L., Ryan, J. A. M., Lonczak, H. S., & Hawkins, J. D. (2004). Positive youth development in the United States: Research findings on evaluation of positive youth development programs. *The Annals of the American Academy of Political and Social Science, 591,* 98–124.

Chung, P. (2012). Service: The business reality of the 21st century. In *Service Reborn* (pp. 1–25). New York, NY: Lexingford Publishing.

Cupelli, L. (2016). An innovative service-learning project to develop cultural competency in undergraduate nursing students. *Teaching and Learning in Nursing, 11,* 113–117.

D'Arlach, L., Sánchez, B., & Feuer, R. (2009). Voices from the community: A case for reciprocity in service-learning. *Michigan Journal of Community Service Learning, 16*(1), 5–16.

Damon, W. (2004). What is positive youth development? *Annals of the American Academy of Political and Social Science, 591*(1), 13–24.

Deeley, S. J. (2004). The impact of experience: A comparative study of the effects of international partnership for service-learning students within welfare agencies in Scotland and Jamaica. In H. Tonkin (Ed.), *Service-learning across cultures: Promise and achievement* (pp. 197–232). New York, NY: International Partnership for Service-Learning and Leadership.

Deeley, S. J. (2010). Service-learning: Thinking outside the box. *Active Learning in Higher Education, 11*(1), 43–53.

Durlak, J. A., Weissberg, R. P., & Pachan, M. (2010). A meta-analysis of after-school programs that seek to promote personal and social skills in children and adolescents. *American Journal of Community Psychology, 45*(3–4), 294–309.

Felten, P., & Clayton, P. H. (2011). Service-learning. *New Directions for Teaching and Learning, 128,* 75–84.

Groh, C. J., Stallwood, L. G., & Daniels, J. J. (2011). Service learning in nursing education: Its impact on leadership and social justice. *Nursing Education Perspectives, 32*(6), 400–405.

Hong Kong Census and Statistic Department. (2016). *Hong Kong Poverty Situation Report 2015*. Retrieved from http://www.povertyrelief.gov.hk/pdf/poverty_report_2015_e.pdf.

Hong Kong Census and Statistic Department. (2017). *Census and Statistics Department announces results of study on household income distribution in Hong Kong*. Retrieved from http://www.censtatd.gov.hk/press_release/pressReleaseDetail.jsp?pressRID=4180&charsetID=1.

Jacoby, B. (1996). Service-learning in today's higher education. In B. Jacoby (Ed.), *Service learning in higher education: Concepts and practices* (pp. 3–25). CA: Jossey-Bass.

Kagawa, F. (2007). Dissonance in students' perceptions of sustainable development and sustainability: Implications for curriculum change. *International Journal of Sustainability in Higher Education, 8*(3), 317–338.

Leung, H., Ma, C. M. S., Shek, D. T. L., & Law, M. Y. M. (2014). *Nurturing service leaders through service learning for university students*. Paper will be presented at the 2nd Summit on University Social Responsibility cum Inaugural International Conference on Service-Learning. The Hong Kong Polytechnic University, Hong Kong (Oral presentation).

McCarthy, A. M., & Tucker, M. L. (2002). Encouraging community service through service learning. *Journal of Management Education, 26*(6), 629–647.

Mendel-Reyes, M. (1998). A pedagogy for citizenship: Service learning and democratic education. *New Directions for Teaching and Learning, 73,* 31–38.

O'Donnell, L., Stueve, A., Doval, A. S., Duran, R., Haber, D., Atnafou, R., … Piessens, P. (1999). The effectiveness of the reach for health community youth service learning program in reducing early and unprotected sex among urban middle school students. *American Journal of Public Health, 89*(2), 176–181.

Popkess, A. M., & McDaniel, A. (2011). Are nursing students engaged in learning? A secondary analysis of data from the National Survey of Student Engagement. *Nursing Education Perspective, 32*(2), 89–94.

Pritchard, I. A. (2001). Community service and service-learning in America: The state of the art. In A. Furco & S. H. Billig (Eds.), *Service-Learning: The essence of the pedagogy* (pp. 3–21). Greenwich, CT: Information Age.

Ryan, M. (2012). Service-learning after learn and serve America: How five states are moving forward. Retrieved from www.ecs.org/clearinghouse/01/02/87/10287.pdf.

Schmidt, N. A., & Brown, J. M. (2016). Service learning in undergraduate nursing education: Strategies to facilitate meaningful reflection. *Journal of Professional Nursing, 32*(2), 100–106.

Shek, D. T. L. (2002). Family functioning and psychological well-being, school adjustment, and problem behavior in Chinese adolescents with and without economic disadvantage. *The Journal of Genetic Psychology, 163*(4), 497–502.

Sooman, A., Macintyre, S., & Anderson, A. (1993). Scotland's health–a more difficult challenge for some? The price and availability of healthy foods in socially contrasting localities in the West of Scotland. *Health Bulletin, 51*(5), 276–284.

Sperling, R. (2007). Service-learning as a method of teaching multiculturalism to white college students. *Journal of Latinos and Education, 6*(4), 309–322.

Sun, R. C. F., & Shek, D. T. L. (2012). Positive youth development, life satisfaction and problem behavior among Chinese adolescents in Hong Kong: A replication. *Social Indicators Research, 105*(3), 541–559.

Tucker, C. M., & Herman, K. C. (2002). Using culturally sensitive theories and research to meet the academic needs of low-income African American children. *American Psychologist, 57*(10), 762–773.

Wills, T. A., Sandy, J. M., & Yaeger, A. M. (2002). Stress and smoking in adolescence: A test of directional hypotheses. *Health Psychology, 21*(2), 122–130.

Yen, J. Y., Yen, C. F., Chen, C. C., Chen, S. H., & Ko, C. H. (2007). Family factors of internet addiction and substance use experience in Taiwanese adolescents. *CyberPsychology & Behavior, 10*(3), 323–329.

Chapter 7
Nurturing Service Leadership Qualities in University Students Through Corporate-Community-University Partnership

Daniel T. L. Shek, Mabel N. S. Cheng and Cecilia M. S. Ma

Abstract The Hong Kong Polytechnic University (PolyU) started its collaboration with the Project WeCan since 2014 to implement a Service Learning course to serve disadvantaged secondary schools. A qualitative study based on in-depth interviews with four teachers was conducted to evaluate this collaborative venture. Results revealed that the greatest challenges were conflict of time and communication problems between university and secondary schools. Despite the challenges encountered, university students showed enhanced self-reflection ability, broadened horizon, development of moral character, and growth in civic engagement. PolyU teachers also reported having increased reflection on teaching and improved relationship with colleagues and students. The service also had positive influence on secondary school students. The factors contributing to successful collaboration and suggestions for improvement are highlighted.

Keywords Service-Learning · Project WeCan · The Hong Kong Polytechnic University · Corporate-community partnership · Leadership

7.1 Introduction

Different from typical classroom teaching, Service Learning is "a form of experiential education" that engages students with the community through enhancing their understanding about the needs of the community and providing opportunities for them to practice and apply their knowledge by serving other members in the community (Werder & Strand, 2011). Unlike volunteering and other service programs, Service Learning seeks to make a good balance in fulfilling the learning

D. T. L. Shek (✉) · M. N. S. Cheng · C. M. S. Ma
Department of Applied Social Sciences, The Hong Kong Polytechnic University, Hunghom, Hong Kong
e-mail: daniel.shek@polyu.edu.hk

D. T. L. Shek et al. (eds.), *Service-Learning for Youth Leadership*, Quality of Life in Asia 12, https://doi.org/10.1007/978-981-13-0448-4_7

needs of students and the service needs of the community (Furco, 2002; Tam, 2014). According to Bringle, Hatcher, and McIntosh (2006):

> Service Learning is a course-based, credit-bearing educational experience in which students a) participate in an organized service activity that meets identified community needs, and b) encourage/provide opportunities for students to reflect on the service activity in such a way as to gain further understanding of course content, a broader appreciation of the discipline, and enhanced sense of personal values and civic responsibility.

Based on a meta-analysis of 11 empirical studies involving 2129 students, Warren (2010) concluded that Service Learning has an overall positive impact on students' learning outcomes. Previous studies also showed that Service Learning effectively promoted students' social responsibilities, including civic responsibility and civic engagement (Weder & Strand, 2011; Ngee, 2011; Niehaus & Crain, 2013; Newman, Dantzler, & Coleman, 2015; Seider, Gillmor, & Rabinowicz, 2012), multicultural awareness (Gross & Maloney, 2012; Cupelli, 2016; Holsapple, 2012), interpersonal skills (Weder & Strand, 2011; Conner, 2010; Cupelli, 2016), academic performance (Lockeman & Pelco, 2013; Newman et al., 2015), as well as knowledge and practical skills (Weisee, Haijar, & Joseph, 2016; Ngee, 2011; Kazemi, Behan, & Boniauto, 2011; Conner, 2010; Jarrell et al., 2014). Lin, Wu, We, Pan, and Liao (2013) also showed that Taiwanese students put greater value on teamwork after completion of Service Learning.

Service Learning promotes empathy in students. Conner (2010) suggested that Service Learning provides opportunities for students to interact with diverse populations. Throughout the experience, they did not only learn more about other groups of people, but also have the chance to change their personal biases. Jarrell et al. (2014) also found that the service learning experience increased the level of empathy among a group of nursing students after they gained awareness of the difficulties faced by their patients.

Besides, with sufficient self-reflection and guidance provided by the supervisor, personal growth can be facilitated (Chang, Anagnostopoulos, & Omae, 2011). Sanders, Oss, and McGeary (2016) reported that students who wrote structured reflection throughout the Service Learning period had significantly higher personal growth and self-efficacy compared with those who did not. Service Learning also promoted service providers' professional skills and competence in their own expertise (Gross & Maloney, 2012; Weder & Strand, 2011). In addition, self-efficacy, intrinsic motivation, and positive emotions such as pride in students were also noted (Ho & Lee, 2012; Newman et al., 2015).

Many Service Learning programs require the involvement of the community and business sector to ensure students' exposure and learning are enriched. Partnerships involving schools, business sectors, and universities have been developing rapidly in the USA since 1990s (Beyerbach, Weber, Swift, & Gooding, 1996). The goals of most of these triangle coalitions included enhancing mutual understanding between business and education sectors, increasing students' exposure to the workforce, and helping students to see the linkage between education and employment. This kind of program has been seen as innovative and effective, as community resources are well utilized to improve students' learning.

In Australia, the School-Business-Community-Partnership Brokers Program, also known as Partnership Brokers, has been implemented, involving over 2300 schools, 1800 business companies, and 6400 community organizations. These involved parties aim to harness community resources and share the responsibilities to improve education and the development of all young people (The Smith Family Research Report, 2014). Their report published in the year of 2014 documented the collaboration of 11 partnerships, which showed that the Partnership Brokers has been able to facilitate mutual benefits in all parties. The Australian Council for Education Research also published a report in 2011 investigating the school-business connection in general (ACER, 2011). It showed that such relationships can bring benefits to all involved parties, including students, teachers, business employees, and schools as a whole. Overall, students' and teachers' understanding about the world of business was improved significantly, schools as a whole were benefited from the human and financial resources provided by the business sectors, while the business employees gained mentoring experiences as well as personal satisfaction experienced when witnessing the growth of the students.

In this chapter, a Service Learning project conducted within the context of a multi-sectoral collaboration involving a business corporation, a university, and some secondary schools was evaluated to provide input on this tripartite mode of collaboration with particular reference to Service Learning provided by the university students.

7.1.1 Service Learning Project Related to Project WeCan

Initiated by The Wharf (Holdings) Limited, the Project WeCan (PWC) is a multi-dimensional program that aims to provide financial and volunteer support to disadvantaged secondary schools in Hong Kong. The project adopts the Business-in-Community model, which means every participating school is coupled with a business company under Wharf. Project WeCan strives to enhance secondary school students' basic competencies, such as enhancing communication skills and exposure, cultivating characters, developing common sense, and fostering innovativeness and creativity. Staffs in corresponding business companies are invited to sign up for volunteering. In general, these employees serve as a mentor to the collaborating school, where they initiate and hold activities for the students throughout the academic year. Internship and company visit opportunities are also provided. Currently, 53 secondary schools are benefited by the project, with 34 business companies signed up for volunteering and five universities involved (Project WeCan, 2017).

The Hong Kong Polytechnic University has been collaborating with Project WeCan since 2014. The Service Learning project has been implemented in ten

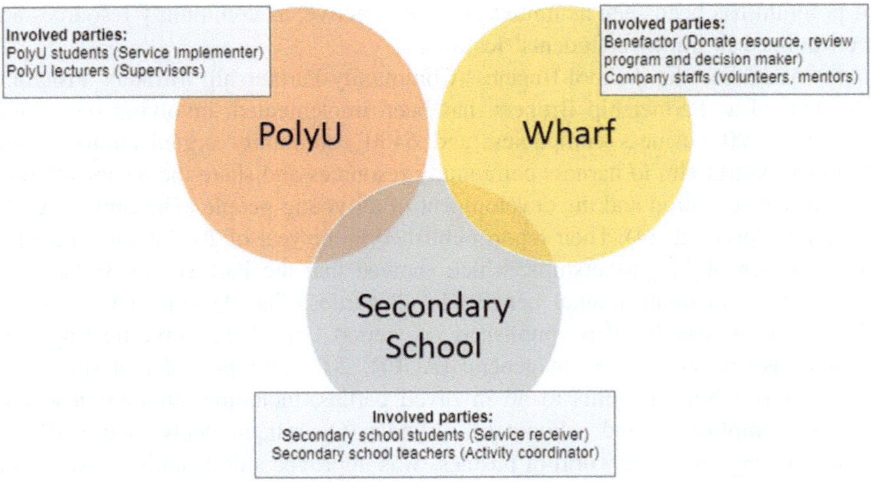

Fig. 7.1 Overview of the Service Learning project in PolyU in collaboration with Project WeCan

Project WeCan schools. Employees from Wharf, secondary school teachers, and PolyU teachers have been working together in the past three years. In every year, around 270 PolyU students sign up for the Service Learning courses and provide services to over 600 students from the participating schools. Figure 7.1 shows an overview of the collaboration, including the involved parties and their role in the Service Learning project. In general, the collaboration has three stages: program planning, program implementation, and program evaluation (see Fig. 7.2). The program planning stage takes place before the academic year begins, with the teachers from PolyU meeting with Wharf and the coordinators of the secondary schools to understand their needs and expectations. A wish-list is prepared by the secondary school. The teachers will then share the wish-lists with PolyU students, brief them about the basic background of the corresponding school, and assign the students in designing activity plans accordingly.

Currently, two departments are offering Service Learning course in the Project WeCan, including the Department of Applied Social Sciences (APSS) and the Department of Biomedical Engineering (BME). For APSS, the length of the course lasts for two semesters, while the course offered by BME only lasts for one semester. Details of the courses are presented in Table 7.1. Generally speaking, students spend the first six weeks acquiring the new knowledge about Service Learning, the corresponding schools, STEM (Science, Technology, Engineering, and Mathematics) subjects or youth development. APSS students are required to design service activities based on the school wish-list. For some schools, the program implementation period takes place in the seventh week of the semester, while some start in the second semester, depending on the school's schedule. Different from APSS, the Service Learning course under BME has a fixed curriculum and core activity. Hence, BME students do not need to write a proposal or create new

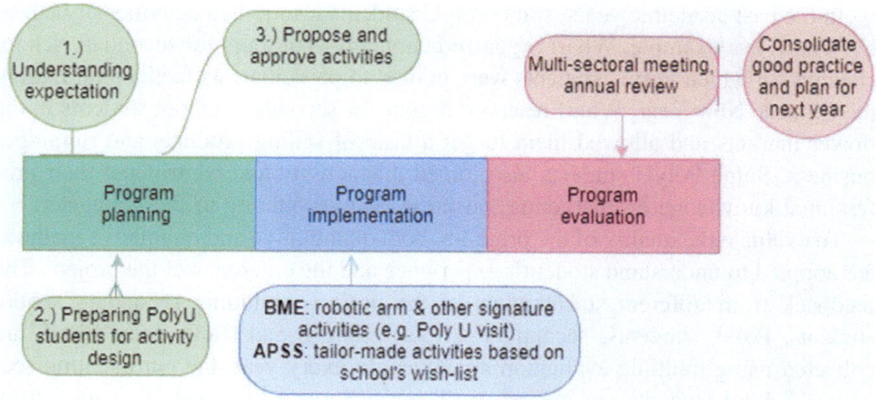

Fig. 7.2 Stages of Service Learning course implementation with Project WeCan schools

activities for their service. Instead, students spend the first six weeks to acquire knowledge, then a five-day program in secondary schools will be held to teach the youngster how to make a robotic arm.

Throughout the years, some activities are perceived to be particularly effective and are favored by most secondary schools. These activities include PolyU visit, STEM workshop, overnight camping, career-life development workshop, and career talk. These activities are now known as the "signature activities" and are provided in every academic year. Apart from the fixed activities in their own curriculum, BME students also provide these abovementioned signature activities to corresponding secondary schools.

Table 7.1 Details of the PolyU Service Learning courses in Project WeCan

Department	Applied social sciences	Biomedical engineering
Course title	1. Promotion of children and adolescent development 2. Service leadership through serving children and families with special needs	Reducing the scientific divide in secondary students through STEM (science, technology, engineering, and mathematics) projects
Course duration	Two semesters	One semester
Enrolled students	From all discipline	Students who major in engineering
Fixed curriculum	No. Students are responsible for designing their own service activities based on the wish-list provided by secondary school	Yes. A 5-day workshop on robotic arm will be taught by PolyU students. Enrolled students are not responsible for creating new activities
Service hour provided	40	40
Number of collaborating school	9	1

In the past academic years, some PolyU students also joined activities organized by Wharf. For example, Wharf organized company visit tours for secondary school students, in which PolyU students were invited to participate as facilitators. During the Chinese New Year, Wharf reserved booths for secondary school students in the flower markets and allowed them to get a taste of selling products and running a business. Some PolyU students also joined this activity and contributed their professional knowledge on marketing, business, and accounting to the youngster.

To evaluate the quality of the program, both quantitative and qualitative methods are adopted to understand student's experience and the outcomes of the project. The feedback from different stakeholders of the project, including secondary school students, PolyU students, secondary school teachers, and staffs from Wharf, are collected using multiple evaluation strategies. In every year, the participating secondary school students are invited to fill out a Service Learning evaluation form upon the completion of the program, where the quality of the activities, performance of PolyU students, and perceived program effectiveness are assessed. Secondary school teachers and Wharf staffs are also invited to fill out an individual evaluation form to rate PolyU students' performance when they participate in the activities as an observer. Additionally, secondary school teachers are invited to fill out the "Community Partner Feedback on Service-Learning Project," which evaluates their collaboration experience with PolyU students. As service implementers, PolyU students fill out a pre-post questionnaire to evaluate their own attitude, competence, and limitation.

For qualitative study, all the PolyU students are required to submit a 1000–1500-word reflection paper upon the completion of the course. Furthermore, focus groups are conducted among secondary school students, secondary school teachers, Wharf staffs, PolyU students, and PolyU teachers. The current study aims to gain a better understanding of the experience of PolyU teachers throughout the collaboration as well as to explore the partnership quality and program effectiveness. This chapter presents the qualitative findings based on the responses of PolyU teachers.

7.2 Method

7.2.1 Participants

Purposive sampling was used to select participants for the current study. A total of four teachers from The Hong Kong Polytechnic University were invited to participate. Three participants have been teaching the Service Learning course and collaborating with Project WeCan since 2014, while one participant joined the team in Fall 2016. Table 7.2 presents a brief summary of the participants.

Table 7.2 Teachers' year of participation in the Project WeCan and number of schools in-charge

Participant	Period of participation	Department	Number of schools in-charge
Participant 1	2014–current	Applied social sciences	4
Participant 2	2014–current	Biomedical engineering	1
Participant 3	2014–2017	Applied social sciences	3
Participant 4	2017–current	Applied social sciences	2

7.2.2 Data Collection and Analysis

The current study employed a general qualitative research method with the use of one-on-one in-depth interview. Each interview lasted for approximately 60–90 min. A semi-structured interview guide (see Appendix 1) was designed and used to explore the followings: (1) participants' view on Service Learning, (2) their experiences in program implementation, (3) their perceived program effectiveness on university students, service beneficiaries, and the PolyU teaching team, and (4) the quality of multi-sectoral partnership (PolyU, Wharf, and secondary schools). The questions related to partnership evaluation was designed and modified based on the framework proposed by the Nuffield Institute for Health's Partnership Assessment Tool (PAT) (Hardy, Hudson, & Waddington, 2003), where the key elements of good partnership included recognition of the need for partnership, clear purpose (shared value and goals), commitment, development of trust, clear responsibility and arrangement (communication), and evaluation. The interviews were audio-recorded and transcribed verbatim. Data were analyzed using NVivo 11 Pro (QSR, 2015).

7.3 Results

7.3.1 Views on Service Learning

All participants saw Service Learning to be different from volunteering and other social services, which is a give-and-take relationship, with a main goal to foster the growth of the learner through serving others. Service Learning created numerous opportunities for students to utilize their strengths and creativities, and often allowed them to interact with diverse groups. It was seen as effective in enhancing students' interpersonal skills and team spirit, which they do not get to practice as much in typical classroom learning.

Most importantly, such unique learning experience required students to apply their knowledge and expertise when providing service to the community. Learning to apply the theories and skills learned was regarded by the interviewees to be one of the most important and valuable parts of Service Learning. The serving experiences with supervision encouraged students to reflect more on their own strengths and weaknesses. The early exposure to the workforce allowed students to set a more realistic expectation on their path after the completion of the undergraduate degree. In addition, two participants described Service Learning as a platform that bridged university students and the community. It was believed that providing service to the general public can enhance students' sense of responsibility as a citizen, which is seen as an important part of personal growth among university students. The related narratives are as follows:

- "When we put too much focus on developing our own profession, we forgot our obligation to serve our community. Service Learning guided them to think more about how to use their professional knowledge to contribute to the community."
- "It is not only about fulfilling the service hour required or to teach students about adolescent's development. I think our course aims to enhance student's self-understanding, to help them understand what it means to serve and to contribute. Of course we need to ensure the quality of the service provided, but the most important thing is not for them (university students) to create activities, the most important thing is they learn how to connect with others."

7.3.2 Experience in Program Implementation

7.3.2.1 Obstacles in Undertaking Service Learning

The university and many participating secondary schools experienced tremendous difficulties setting schedules for service activities. Some schools had difficulties providing sufficient hours for students to conduct their planned activities, as the school timetables were often packed. Some secondary schools could only offer one to two hours for the services during weekdays. As most of the school locations were remote, it was rather time-consuming for the university students to travel back and forth. Similarly, as university students tended to have different class schedules than their groupmates, it was a challenge for them to come up with sufficient time slots as a team. In addition, university students finish their academic year in around April or May, and this period is close to the final examination period for secondary school students. Hence, it was quite a challenge for both parties to come up with a schedule that fits everyone.

As mentioned above, most secondary schools tended to have an intense academic schedule for their students. In order to provide 40 hours of service time slots for university students as required by their course, many activities were scheduled on weekend. Such had led to another problem—low attendance of secondary school students in activities. Many secondary school students were not willing to travel a long way to school during the holidays. Hence, the activities held in weekend tended to have low attendance. This challenge was encountered by all PolyU students. It was reported that the low attendance rate was somewhat discouraging to them as they spent a lot of time preparing for the activities.

Furthermore, the teachers reflected that many complaints were made by students regarding the communication problem with secondary school teachers. School teachers tended to have busy schedules and were not able to pick up calls during the day. In some occasions, the teachers were not able to get back to the PolyU students until the last minute before their activities started.

7.3.2.2 Positive Experiences

All the participants shared their positive experiences teaching the Service Learning course. The important themes emerged from the data included enhanced relationships with PolyU students and colleagues, enriched teaching experiences, and increased self-reflection on teaching. As PolyU collaborated with ten secondary schools in Project WeCan, much internal and external communication was required. Throughout the program, they learned to communicate effectively and tackle the obstacles together. As mentioned earlier in the chapter, the schedules of both university students and secondary schools were tight. Hence, there were many sudden changes in plan. To cope with these unexpected changes, the teaching team learned to have communication more frequently to exchange their management strategies in order to provide adequate support to students.

Apart from the remarkable working experience with colleagues, many participants disclosed their positive experiences working with undergraduate students. One interviewee shared a story about student showing gratitude toward their coordination in this program, as students understood the coordination work required a lot of time and energy. When the students learned to appreciate the effort of their teachers, they become more devoted in their coursework. Having the opportunity to witness the growth of students was described as another positive experience in the program. The teachers worked closely with students from activity planning to program termination, with the entire process lasted for the whole academic year for some teachers. One interviewee described the process as "walking alongside them." In Service Learning, the teachers had greater chances to interact with students and to tackle the challenges together, which is different from typical classroom learning, where the teacher–student relationship is mostly hierarchical.

As the course structure and course nature were different from most modules, the Service Learning teaching experience allowed the participants to work with more students from different disciplines. With the realization that students from different disciplines carried different characteristics, some teachers were inspired to use different teaching methods that best suited the students. As shared by one participant, "it is rather important to facilitate the meaning behind providing service, and the responsibility to serve the community" and "that's the shared goal behind all the different kinds of activity in this program."

As reported by one of the teachers, a lot of self-reflection was required when collaborating with the business sector, secondary schools, as well as university students. Since this is a multi-sectoral collaboration which involved different parties, it is essential to stand in everyone's shoes to understand their needs and struggles. As shared by a participant, "it is a matter of making balances for the needs and responsibilities of the three sectors, and also for all of our colleagues involved. We need to keep reflecting on the purpose of our collaboration and our ultimate goals."

7.3.3 Perceived Program Impact

7.3.3.1 Positive Impact on PolyU Students

In terms of program effectiveness, one of the most common themes emerged in the interviews was the widened horizon of students. Not only that PolyU students gained the valuable opportunity to interact with youth, the service experience allowed students to gain a taste of what working is like, as they "learned more about the society," as well as "knowing more about the standard and expectation in the working industries."

The exposure to new people and new environment also provided PolyU students a place to reflect. Most of the university students initially appeared to be unfamiliar with the lives of schoolchildren from disadvantaged backgrounds. From this experience, they gained another new lens to look at the world. Some students reflected on their teenage years while giving advices to the young, while some thought deeper about the meaning of education and the underlying needs of the underprivileged students.

According to the PolyU teachers, personal growth and the development in moral character among university students were remarkable. First of all, it was noted that Service Learning fostered a sense of responsibility among the university students. Seeing themselves as the representatives of the university, students became more self-disciplined. Despite the remote location of secondary schools and the long traveling hours, students monitored themselves to be well prepared and punctual for activities. Although the service experience was filled with obstacles as mentioned in the last section, students were observed to be more persistent when they encountered obstacles. With adequate guidance and support from the teachers, students were able to overcome their fears and tackled the difficulties. Such act had also led to enhanced interpersonal skills, management skills, increased self-efficacy, and increased self-esteem, according to the participants. A teacher shared as follows:

> There was a student, whose major was not fashion design, but he was responsible for sewing clothes. He stayed in the secondary school and worked until 11 p.m. few days in a row. He eventually received the scholarship. Many secondary school teachers remembered him and asked about him in the next two academic years.

Another significant theme emerged was empathy. A few participants addressed that's students become more sensitive to the emotions and the needs of others. As pointed out by a teacher,

> A PolyU student, who graduated from an underprivileged secondary school, was emotional while providing service. In the debriefing, the student expressed feeling disappointed when he saw some of the secondary school teachers have given up on teaching the secondary school students. This student shared with his classmates, 'they (secondary school students) will actually listen to what you teach, you just have to find the right method.'

Two participants described Service Learning as a platform that bridged university students and the community. By providing service in secondary schools, students gained a greater understanding about the underprivileged families in the community, and started to concern about the struggles experienced by these families. Although the curriculum only required students to provide 40 h of direct service, despite their busy schedules with classes and examinations, many students continued their service after the requirement had been fulfilled. Every year, there were at least three students who would come back for volunteering after the completion of the course. According to the participants, students developed a sense of belonging to the community, as well as a good relationship with the service beneficiaries. Many students started to see the needs in the community and wanted to make contributions.

7.3.3.2 Positive Impact on Secondary School Students

All participants stated that the Service Learning program enhanced secondary school students' exposure to the world outside the campus. The Service Learning course provided a unique opportunity for secondary students to interact with university students. Not only that good relationships with university students were established over time, but also the visit to the university campus and sharing about university school life were invaluable. It was believed that these exposures played an important role in their decision making in career development. In some activities, PolyU students shared their struggles in DSE. Their sharing helped the secondary school students to understand that underprivileged students were not destined to fail. One can make changes in his or her path by putting greater effort on their studies.

Most importantly, it was highlighted that secondary school students greatly benefited from the interpersonal relationship, as most of them felt respected and encouraged throughout the process. Many secondary school students expressed appreciation toward PolyU students' effort and patience in holding activities. PolyU students were seen as role models. The care and patience provided by them did not only have a positive impact on the beneficiaries' motivation on learning, but also enhanced their self-value and sense of hope.

The findings suggest that teacher's vision about Service Learning is a basic factor conducive to the positive outcomes in PolyU students. According to one teacher, "Service Learning is not just about guiding students to create interesting activities, the quality of the activities is certainly important, but what's more important is that we shall never forget Service Learning is an education, it is a learning process. The teachers should understand the value of Service Learning, and embed such value in students." As mentioned earlier in the chapter, the expected outcomes of Service Learning are for students to "understand themselves," "understand what it means to contribute," and "understand what serving means." As shared by one teacher, "students would initiate meetings to communicate with us, because they did not only see it as a 40-hour-service, they see the value in their services." As students viewed their work as meaningful, they became more engaged and involved. The value eventually enhanced one's sense of belonging to the community. The identity of citizen became more salient; they started to see the obligation to serve as their empathy level increased.

7.3.4 Factors Contributing to Multi-sectoral Collaboration

From the data, several factors influencing the quality of multi-sectoral collaboration were identified. The first factor is recognition of the need for partnership, shared goals, and shared value. All the collaborating parties have shown mutual understanding about each other's goals, as it was made clear before the program was launched. According to the participants, all the parties understood the benefits of Service Learning and agreed that both university and secondary school students can benefit more from the program, though every collaborating school has their own views and values on education. Schools' views and values appeared to be important elements, as the partnership quality and the involvement were directly affected. For example, some collaborating schools put great emphasis on academic achievement and language proficiency, while others wanted to focus more on enhancing students' career exposure and innovative learning. As most PolyU students were expecting to utilize their professional knowledge and innovative ideas in the course, being overly academic and achievement-oriented on activity design were likely to shape them into a "tutor," which directly affected their motivation to engage to this program. Similarly, if the designed activity did not match the expectation of secondary school, the perceived commitment level tended to be low.

It was concluded that schools without shared value seemed to be more reserved and had a lower level of openness toward innovative activities and experiential learning. Schools which seen the collaboration as a long-term partnership were observed to be more devoted, supportive, with a higher level of openness, and more willing to interact with the service providers. It was emphasized that the lack of shared value is not due to poor communication, though adequate communication can establish mutual understand and respect.

The second factor identified is commitment of different stakeholders. In general, the commitment level of each party was seen as satisfactory. As mentioned in the previous section, it was rather difficult for secondary schools to provide sufficient time slots for PolyU students, especially during the first year of collaboration. However, it seemed that the level of commitment increased over time. All the teachers agreed that such situation was significantly improved throughout the years, as schools understood more about the Service Learning course requirement, they began to reserved open time slots for the services. In the Partnership Assessment Tool, sense of ownership was also considered as a significant element in commitment. According to the teachers, most of the schools seemed to have a low level of ownership, as usually it was PolyU who took the lead in activity design. One teacher suggested that communication and mutual understanding can increase the ownership of both sides.

Most of the discussion about commitment was focused on the partnership between PolyU and secondary schools, as PolyU teachers mostly worked with secondary school teachers directly, while Wharf involved less in the decision making and program planning process. Nevertheless, Wharf's participation in this triangle coalition was seen as very important, as they enhanced both university and secondary school students' exposure to the outside world by involving them in various innovative activities in the business area, which stimulated personal growth and insights. In addition, Wharf also offered generous financial support to secondary schools to encourage positive development of the students. In general, they showed their ownership by monitoring the quality of collaboration and the program progress monthly. It was also noted that Wharf played a significant role in mediation, who served as a bridge for communication when PolyU or secondary schools encountered difficulties in the collaboration.

The third influence is trust. Overall, all the teachers agreed that there was a trusting relationship between Wharf and the secondary schools. Trust was identified as one of the most important elements in establishing a satisfying partnership in this project. The first year of collaboration required lots of adjustments for both university and secondary schools. With little understanding about the university culture, collaboration mode, and the service program, secondary schools were more reserved at the beginning. As stated by one participant, "some secondary school teachers might be worried and were protective toward their students by nature," and "those worries might include not having enough time and resource to coordinate the activities, not getting used to the collaboration, or our students might possibly look down on their secondary school students as they came from a disadvantaged background, and so on." However, as the collaboration went on, these worries were resolved, as the program was proved to be effective. All the participants agreed that they have established stable relationships with the collaborating schools.

It was further pointed out that the level of trust is positively correlated to the commitment and ownership of PolyU students and secondary school teachers' level of openness toward new activities. One participant remarked that "at the beginning, students tended to just work to fulfill the hours. But in the later stage of the program when the trust is gained, they (PolyU students) were so committed that they go beyond the required service hours, and even came back for volunteering in the next year because they found sense of purpose in this relationship." The importance of communication emerged as a significant theme, which is embedded in the process of trust building.

Another factor influencing the quality of collaboration is clarity in responsibility and communication. One participant shared that "school did not have enough trust toward us in the initial stage, however the partnership becomes stronger when we get to understand each other. The best way of enhancing such understanding is to communicate," and "we create opportunities to foster effective communication." Apart from emails and phone calls, the teachers would invite corresponding secondary school teachers to attend the seminar to interact with PolyU students. The participant further elaborated that "in the seminar, we were simply chit-chatting instead of delivering information about the secondary school. We might not understand each other's needs and expectation at the beginning, yet through discussion, and more discussion, we eventually reached a mutual understanding. We learn from each other, and eager to help each other at the same time."

To improve communication with schools, it was suggested to involve all the corresponding teachers in the annual meeting for program planning. Some participants pointed out that most of the time it was the school principal who made the decision and it is rather important to include the program coordinator as well, because they are the executor. "It would be more practical to include the executor in the initial stage, because they know the best about the needs of the school and students. Most importantly, when the executors agreed with the activities planned, they were more committed in the implementation stage."

Even though there were positive ways to foster communication between the two parties, external communication has always been known as a common challenge in most partnerships. As mentioned in the previous section, communication with schools was highlighted as one of the major obstacles in this project. Due to the different working schedule, secondary school teachers were busy most of the time and weren't able to return calls. To eliminate the impacts of such obstacle, the signature activities, such as PolyU visit and overnight camp, were planned ahead.

All the participants agreed that their communication with Wharf has been smooth. Wharf is responsible for providing financial support and monitoring the program progress; hence, no frequent communication is required between Wharf and PolyU. It was pointed out that Wharf was able to provide sufficient support when needed. Although the program has been running progressively smoother throughout the years, it was addressed that the role and the responsibility of each party in this project were never clearly and formally defined. It is believed that a clear definition of such might enhance the sense of responsibility and motivation of each party.

Last but not least, the final element is the review of the program implementation. To constantly monitor the program development and quality, a progress report prepared by PolyU was submitted to Wharf on a monthly basis. Details included the summary of activities conducted, number of beneficiaries, number of service hours, number of participating PolyU students, and a plan for the upcoming month.

In every year, a review meeting was conducted among the three collaborating parties. The review meetings were held right after the end of the academic year, when the secondary schools were making academic plans for the upcoming year. In the meeting, the three parties raised out their concerns in the past year and good practices were consolidated. Activities that were perceived as effective were provided again in the next academic year. Hence, by the end of the review meeting, a brief plan was made based on the evaluation and discussion.

7.4 Direction for Future Refinement

To enrich the program content for both secondary school and PolyU students, collaborating parties are encouraged to look into their scheduled activities in the upcoming year before the review meeting and explore the opportunity for their partner's involvement. For example, the university can invite both business sector and secondary schools to participate in their school festival. It would help the partners to learn more about the university, and foster interaction and enhance exposure among the participating parties.

Another example is that business sector scheduled a Christmas exhibition in December, and they might discuss with the university and secondary school teachers and see if their students would like to get involved in the preparation process. It could be a good opportunity for the beneficiaries to learn about design and event management. In addition, the findings suggested that the collaboration allowed the participating parties to learn from each other. The diverse background led them to exchange insight from different perspectives. The increased involvement of business sector might bring in professional business advice and innovative idea that stimulate both teachers and student's learning.

In the program implementation stage, PolyU students had sufficient interaction with secondary school students, teachers, and PolyU teachers. However, it was found that very few occasions can bring together the business staffs and university students. As the university students are in the process of exploring their career path, it is believed that they can be greatly benefited from enhanced exposure to the business world. For example, activities such as company visit tour and flower market booth were considered as particularly effective in multi-level learning. The setting provided opportunities for university students to learn from the business sector, and to pass on their learning to the secondary school students.

Finally, although review meeting has been conducted on an annual basis, most of the meeting content was focused on program planning. In order to improve the quality of collaboration, it is suggested that partners should be open to each other regarding their opinions toward the collaboration. For example, role and responsibility should be clearly defined, reviewed, and redefined if necessary. Evaluation of partnership should be ongoing instead of one-off. It is believed that the continuous evaluation of the partnership quality will have positive impacts on the level of trust and commitment in the collaboration.

7.5 Conclusion

Service Learning is a partnership that is more "arduous, time-consuming, and pedagogically complex" than typical teaching, and its workload and responsibility can be heavy for students, instructors, as well as the collaborating partners (Kahn, 2011, p. 113). Nevertheless, the impact Service Learning brings to students, teachers, and beneficiaries is undeniable. According to our findings, Service Learning is more than just a credit-bearing module or a learning opportunity, and it is a lesson in life that allows one to learn to communicate and connect with one other in the community. It provides a safe environment for the students to see new things, to get closer to the world of work, and to fully utilize their strengths. Meanwhile, the multi-sectoral collaboration created a platform that fosters professional development and continuous learning opportunity for staffs from both business and education sectors. Such valuable experience does not only enrich both students and staff's experiences but also strengthen their identities as a citizen by endorsing a sense of meaning in their services. Involving business sector in education is still a relatively new concept in Hong Kong. The Project WeCan has proven the positive impacts the collaborative approach brought to our society. It is hoped that a more systematic evaluation can be constructed to measure the business-education partnership in the Hong Kong context. Future studies might continue to document and consolidate good practices and disseminate the findings to interested parties who wish to make contributions in education. It is hoped that such collaborative approach will be promoted and adopted by more stakeholders in the community in order to maximize the positive outcome in education for the new generation.

Acknowledgements The Service-Learning subjects in Project WeCan were financially supported by The Hong Kong Polytechnic University. The coordination and evaluation work as well as the present manuscript are financially supported by Project WeCan.

Appendix 1: In-Depth Interview Guide for PolyU Teachers

Part One: On Promoting Service Learning

1. Please share your view on Service Learning
2. When did you start teaching this subject and work with the Project WeCan?
    a. Who are your collaborating secondary schools?
3. Please share your experience assisting the students to design their activities.
    a. What are the core activities?
    b. What was the most unforgettable activity?

4. In your opinion, what are the key elements that had smoothen the program implementation process?
5. While implementing the program, have you encountered any difficulties? If yes, please share with us of some examples.
   a. How did you deal with these difficulties?
6. Overall, what are the greatest challenges encountered by the students?
   a. How did you help them to overcome these challenges?

Part Two: Evaluation of the Effectiveness of the Program

1. Have you noticed any changes in your students after participating in the Service-Learning program? If yes, what are the changes?
2. If you noticed changes in students, what are the factors you anticipated to cause such changes?
3. If you have not noticed changes in your students, what are the factors that caused your students with least changes?
4. In your opinion, what are the program impacts on
   a. Secondary school students,
   b. Secondary school in general, and
   c. PolyU teachers
5. Are the aforementioned changes comparable to the goals of the program?

Part Three: Overall Evaluation of Service Learning

1. What are the most unforgettable experiences in this program?
2. As the lecturer/coordinator of this program, did you gain any insight or reflection on education?
3. In your opinion, what factors or arrangement can foster the benefits of participating students?

Part Four: Collaboration with Wharf and Corresponding Secondary Schools

1. Please describe your collaboration with corresponding secondary schools in the past three years
   1.1. Please evaluate your collaboration based on the following aspects:
      1.1.1. Shared goals/value
      1.1.2. Communication (understanding each other's expectation/communicate to solve problem when encountering difficulties)
      1.1.3. Level of trust (in regards of program planning, decision making, and program implementation)
      1.1.4. Commitment (participate in activities held by PolyU students/give advice/provide support/supervise students/provide administrative support)
      1.1.5. Program evaluation (review of the quality of program and the collaboration)

2. Please describe your collaboration with corresponding secondary schools in the past three years
   2.1. Please evaluate your collaboration based on the following aspects:
      2.1.1. Shared goals/value
      2.1.2. Communication (understanding each other's expectation/communicate to solve problem when encountering difficulties)
      2.1.3. Level of trust (in regards of program planning, decision making, and program implementation)
      2.1.4. Commitment (participate in activities held by PolyU students/give advice/ provide support/supervise students/provide administrative support)
      2.1.5. Program evaluation (review of the quality of program and the collaboration)
3. Please share your view on multi-sectoral collaboration.
4. In your opinion, what changes can be made within the multi-sectoral relationship in order to smoothen the program implementation?
5. In your opinion, what changes can be made within the multi-sectoral relationship in order to expand the benefits of participating PolyU students and secondary school students?

Part Five: Other Opinion

1. Are you satisfied with the program? What are the satisfied or dissatisfied areas?
2. From your perspective, in what areas can the program be improved?
3. Do you have any other comments or feelings?

References

Australian Council for Educational Research. (2011). *ACER final report on the benefits of school-business relationships*. Retrieved from Department of Education, Employment and Workplace Relations website. https://docs.education.gov.au/system/files/doc/other/benefits_sbr_acer_report.pdf.

Beyerbach, B. A., Weber, S., Swift, J. N., & Gooding, C. T. (1996). A school/business/university partnership for professional development. *The School Community Journal, 6*(1), 101–112.

Bringle, R. G., Hatcher, J. A., & McIntosh, R. E. (2006). Analyzing morton's typology of service paradigms and integrity. *Michigan Journal of Community Service Learning, 13*(1), 5–15.

Chang, S. P., Anagnostopoulos, D., & Omae, H. (2011). The multidimensionality of multicultural service learning: The variable effects of social identity, context and pedagogy on pre-service teachers' learning. *Teaching and Teacher Education, 27,* 1078–1089.

Conner, J. O. (2010). Learning to unlearn: How a service-learning project can help teacher candidates to reframe urban students. *Teaching and Teacher Education, 26,* 1170–1177.

Cupelli, L. (2016). An innovative service-learning project to develop cultural competency in undergraduate nursing students. *Teaching and Learning in Nursing, 11,* 113–117.

Furco, A. (2002). Is service-learning really better than community service? In A. Furco & S. H. Billig (Eds.), *Service-learning: The essence of the pedagogy* (pp. 23–50). Greenwish, CT: Information Age.

Gross, P. A., & Maloney, V. A. (2012). Embracing diversity through service learning the clearing house: A. *Journal of Educational Strategies, Issues and Ideas, 85*(5), 192–196.

Hardy, B., Hudson, B., & Waddington, E. (2003). *Assessing strategic partnership: The partnership assessment tool* (Nuffield Institute for Health).

Ho, S. Y., & Lee, V. M. W. (2012). Toward integration of reading and service learning through an interdisciplinary program. *Asia Pacific Education Review, 13*(2), 251–262. https://doi.org/10.1007/s12564-011-9188-3

Holsapple, M. A. (2012). Service-learning and student diversity outcomes: existing evidence and directions of future research. *Michigan Journal of Community Service Learning, 18,* 5–18.

Jarrell, K., et al. (2014). Constructing the foundations for compassionate care: How service-learning affects nursing students' attitude towards the poor. *Nurse Education in Practice, 14,* 299–303.

Kahn, H. E. (2011). Overcoming the challenges of International service learning: A visual approach to sharing, authority, community development, and global learning. In *International service learning conceptual frameworks and research* (pp. 113–124). Sterling, Virginia: Stylus.

Kazemi, D., Behan, J., & Boniauto, M. (2011). Improving teaching strategies in an undergraduate community health nursing program: Implementation of a service-learning preceptor program. *Nurse Education Today, 31,* 547–552.

Lin, C. Y., Wu, S. W., We, S. F., Pan, B. S., & Liao, H. C. (2013). Effects of service-learning in a university in Taiwan. *Procedia—Social and Behavioral Sciences, 116,* 902–906.

Lockeman, K. S., & Pelco, L. E. (2013). The relationship between service-learning and degree completion. *Michigan Journal of Community Service Learning, 20,* 18–30.

Newman, J. L., Dantzler, J., & Coleman, A. N. (2015). Science in action: How middle school students are changing their world through STEM service-learning projects. *Theory into Practice, 54*(1), 47–54.

Ngee, L. M. (2011). Youth-led initiative in community service-learning projects and their learning experience. *US-China Education Review, 2,* 281–288.

Niehaus, E., & Crain, L. K. (2013). Act local or global? Comparing student experiences in domestic and international service-learning programs. *Michigan Journal of Community Service Learning, 20,* 31–40.

NVivo for Windows version 11 Pro. (2015). (QSR International Pty ltd, Melbourne, Australia).

Project WeCan overview. (2017). Retrieved from http://www.projectwecan.com/about-us/overview/.

Sanders, M. J., Van Oss, T., & McGeary, S. (2016). Analyzing reflections in service learning to promote personal growth and community self-efficacy. *Journal of Experiential Education, 39*(1), 73–88. https://doi.org/10.1177/1053825915608872

Seider, S. C., Gillmor, S., & Rabinowicz, S. (2012). The impact of community service learning upon the expected political voice of participating college students. *Journal of Adolescent Research, 27*(1), 44–77.

Tam, M. (2014). Intergenerational service learning between the old and young: What, why and how. *Educational Gerontology, 40*(6), 401–413.

The Smith Family's Partnership Brokers. (2014). *Improving young people's educational outcomes through school business community partnerships*. Retrieved from https://www.thesmithfamily.com.au/~/media/files/research-advocacy/research/Partnership_Brokers_Report_2014.ashx?la=en.

Warren, J. L. (2010). Does service learning increase student learning? A meta-analysis. *Michigan Journal of Community Service Learning, 18,* 56–61.

Weder, K. P., & Strand, K. (2011). Measuring student outcomes: An assessment of service-learning in the public relations campaigns course. *Public Relations Review, 37,* 478–484.

Weisee, D., Hajjar, E. R., & Joseph, A. S. (2016). Student perception of academic and professional development during an introductory service-learning experience. *Currents in Pharmacy Teaching and Learning, 8,* 833–839.

Chapter 8
Science for Healthy and Sustainable Living Environments

Kwok Wai Mui and Ling Tim Wong

Abstract This service learning project focuses on organizing learning activities for school students in which schools and teachers can ensure that education for sustainable development is integrated into the other learning activity (OLE) in the school curriculum. The objectives can be achieved by (i) exposing school students to situations of poor families, they will be encouraged to look at the ways how the sustainability can be integrated into everyday living; (ii) introducing them to interesting ways of learning scientific topics and exposing them to activities related to higher education, and spending extended periods of time with university students, they may be better motivated to spend more time pursuing their studies, and (iii) working in teams to complete a project; they will build up their communication skills, teamwork and self-confidence.

Keywords Integrated school curriculum · Sustainable environment education
Other learning experience · Service learning project · Learning reflection
Student development

8.1 How It Benefits to Community?

The focus of this subject is on cultivating an ethic of environmental sustainability through teaching and learning of engineering science-related concepts and theories (Barth, Adomßent, Fischer, Richter, & Rieckmann, 2014). Students will require to experience the situation of poor families to learn about their living situation, especially with respect to energy efficiency and sustainability in everyday life in Hong Kong. They may have to conduct investigations, interviews and surveys to

K. W. Mui · L. T. Wong (✉)
Department of Building Services Engineering, The Hong Kong Polytechnic University, Hunghom, Hong Kong
e-mail: beltw@polyu.edu.hk

K. W. Mui
e-mail: behorace@polyu.edu.hk

D. T. L. Shek et al. (eds.), *Service-Learning for Youth Leadership*,
Quality of Life in Asia 12, https://doi.org/10.1007/978-981-13-0448-4_8

get a sense of issues such as energy usage, water usage. They will then use this experience to design learning activities for primary or secondary school students. Students will be required to integrate issues of sustainability into their activities and use interactive and learner-centered activities (Lehmann, Christensen, Du, & Thrane, 2008).

The target of this subject is to work with primary and secondary schools that serve mostly underprivileged children, so the issues that the students encounter in their preparatory site visit should be familiar to the primary and secondary students. We intend our service to fit into the other learning activities (OLE) component in the primary and secondary school curriculum frameworks (Ramos et al., 2015). The schools that we will work with lack the extra resources required to support such activities.

Examples of project topics include: water and energy efficiency, trash reduction and waste audit. Examples of service project topics include: benchmarking utility consumption in home consumption (water, fuel gas, and electricity), willingness in adopting energy efficient/water conservation appliances, home waste quantification, trend of air pollution, measurement of indoor temperature and energy impacts. Students will have to integrate examples from built environment sustainability, organize relevant and meaningful learning activities, demonstrate engineering experiments, design teaching materials and worksheets. The activities for the primary and secondary students will end with a project presentation, in which our students will act as instructors and mentors to the schoolchildren.

8.2 Academic Focus of the Subject

This subject looks at the following issues:

(a) The impacts of sustainability and living environments, especially pertaining to underprivileged people in Hong Kong.
(b) The link between basic scientific thinking principles and applying these to teach and demonstrate concepts relating to sustainability and healthy living environments;
(c) The challenges facing underprivileged primary and secondary schoolchildren in Hong Kong.

The service project supports the academic focus on the following ways:

(a) Through the visit to underprivileged families and conducting the associated investigations, interviews and surveys, our students will get a better sense of the hardships faced by underprivileged people in Hong Kong society.
(b) Through investigating the related issues and preparing the teaching plans and project proposals for the primary and secondary schoolchildren, students will better understand the impact of sustainability, energy efficiency and other issues on living environments

(c) Through integrating these concepts into scientific teaching activities and participating in projects with the schoolchildren, students will understand more about the challenges facing primary and secondary schoolchildren in learning about scientific concepts.

8.3 Service Programme and Implementation

The subject works with two partner secondary schools; with presented philosophy of the subject and the subject academic requirement and operation timeframe; collaboration is confirmed and the programme gains support of school teachers.

PolyU students offered two service programmes, (a) one for senior form schoolchildren (Form 4) and another one for selected junior form schoolchildren (Form 1 & Form 2). Students teamed up as service teams, each team consisted of 3–4 students and worked as facilitators. Each team proposed a project related to science for healthy and sustainable living environments, designed project details and scheduled activity plan for the recipients in a timeframe of four days. Activities covered the project theme, key concept of science and technology involved in the project, schoolchildren-based project work and training on presentation.

The e-learning module, which is developed and delivered by the Office of Service Learning at PolyU, consists of readings, exercises and assessments that are designed to introduce students to the basic concepts and practices of service learning. They are designed to assess students' ability to link service learning with the academic content of the subject and their understanding of their roles and responsibilities in society. Students are required to successfully complete the module within the first four weeks of the semester in which they are taking the subject.

Discipline/Project-specific lectures, seminars, tutorials (including reflection and review tutorials), and/or workshop were scheduled on week basis. The focus of the projects is on cultivating an ethic of environmental sustainability through teaching and learning of engineering science-related concepts and theories. Students worked in groups with participating primary and secondary school students.

8.3.1 Briefing Session with PolyU Team

The students are briefed in the first lecture for the expected subject outcomes. The teaching and learning (T&L) methods adopted to achieve the expected outcomes include interactive lectures, supplemented by worked examples, tutorials, seminars and workshops. Lecture notes, worked examples and feedback were issued to students at the appropriate time to enhance learning.

In the service project preparatory stage, students are required to write project proposals and plans to substantiate their understanding of relevant engineering science concepts in relation to sustainable built environment and their ability to apply their knowledge in living environment for poor families. These proposals and plans include activity designs, case study and visit, sample deliverables, lesson plans, worksheets, suggested answers. As sustainable building involves making choices that take resource use and energy efficiency into account, students should plan ways that are environmentally responsible.

The schools that students worked with mostly serve children from underprivileged backgrounds. Students shall propose the project theme related to sustainable built environment for the described environment. Some examples are:

(a) Collecting data to highlight issues of sustainability and related issues at home, e.g. benchmarking utility consumption in home (water, fuel gas and electricity), home waste quantification.
(b) Identifying challenges to healthy and sustainable living, e.g. trend of air pollution, measurement indoor temperature and energy impacts.
(c) Developing ideas and proposals to improve sustainability and living environment.

Examples of tasks that students can undertake are organizing environmental awareness workshops, competitions, exhibitions and other activities for primary and secondary students, etc.

8.3.2 Briefing Session with Recipients

Project titles are made available for school teachers to team-up suitable schoolchildren. A briefing session to schoolchildren is to be arranged, so that the PolyU team can meet up and can make known to recipients. Each PolyU team will prepare a one-page project summary showing schoolchildren about the content of works and schedule during the briefing session. Schoolchildren team will share with PolyU about their backgrounds, introduced their school and facilities and arranged a campus tour. After the session, a debriefing session is arranged for the PolyU student team; then they can review their project plan and prepare the first reflection journal.

8.3.3 Student Reflections

For students to learn through reflection, review and reflective sessions are held to supervise and guide students during and after the service learning project (Turns, Sattler, Yasuhara, Borgford-Parnell, & Atman, 2014). Experts and facilitators from outside the subject-offering department (e.g. Office of Service Learning, local schools) are invited to contribute to some of these sessions as appropriate. Moreover, group discussions are conducted to encourage students to review, refine and continuously improve service delivery. Service delivery performance will be evaluated.

During the project, students will be required to write two reflective journals, one after the briefing session and another one at the end of the entire project. The journals are to (a) document their works; (b) reflect upon their service learning experiences; (c) identify their learning gains and weaknesses; and (d) propose changes for future sessions. They will be asked to keep a bi-weekly progress log and/or an activity log as appropriate (Cowan, 2014). Moreover, regular peer sharing sessions will be arranged for students to exchange their service learning experiences. These sessions will not form part of assessment but will encourage interactions among different groups.

8.3.4 Rendering Service

Student team delivered service as planned. They are required to review their performance after the schedule service time everyday and fine-tune their service plan for remaining days. During the project execution, students are exposed to issues and challenges facing the schoolchildren with whom they are going to work. In addition to applying basic scientific thinking principles to demonstrate issues of sustainability in a service setting, students need to be able to communicate effectively with the schoolchildren.

For students to learn through reflection, review and reflective sessions will be held to supervise and guide students during and after the service learning project. Students will be supervised throughout the service component either by members of the teaching team. Students' performance will be evaluated based on their attitudes and performance in the rendering of service, their degrees of engagement and interaction with the service recipients, and their collaboration with other students.

8.3.5 Presentation and Final Summative Report

PolyU students acted as the organizer for an end-subject one-day symposium; each student–schoolchildren team would present their project in front of participants in the symposium. It acts as a demonstration outcome of the service project. The presentation day also serves as a ceremony of the whole activity. The best presentation teams will be determined by the assessing team formed by school principals and science subject leaders and the team will be awarded in the ceremony.

Students are also required to write a final summative report. Through the report and presentation, students should demonstrate their ability to: (a) link their service learning experiences with the academic focus/discipline-specific content of the subject; (b) reflect on their service learning experiences to recognize their learning gains as well as areas for future improvements; and (c) reflect on their roles and social responsibilities.

All journals, reports, presentations and discussions are used to assess students' abilities to link service learning with the academic content of the subject, to reflect upon the challenges related to sustainability and living environment faced by the underprivileged community, reflect upon the challenges facing the schoolchildren from underprivileged backgrounds and to reflect on their roles and responsibilities in society (Waterman, 1997).

8.4 Changes in University Students

8.4.1 Student Reflection

Changes of the first cohort students were measured by assessment of their two reflection journals, one made after the briefing session and another one submitted at the end of the project (Han, Capraro, & Capraro, 2015).

Major changes ($\geq 10\%$) of the marked issues of (i) the problems encountered by the PolyU students; (ii) changes, modifications, revisions to project, and (iii) student reflection in the reflection journals are highlighted in Tables 8.1, 8.2 and 8.3.

Table 8.1 shows some University students overestimated difficulties on English language proficiency but underestimated the difficulties on their presentation skill and time management. Indeed, some of them thought school and schoolchildren expectations were high and finally they found that they had delivered too difficult projects for the schoolchildren; the difficulty was mainly on the experimental works. It was confirmed that a high and increased schoolchildren number who felt the content uninterested/not attractive. The university students also found difficulties in dealing with passive schoolchildren, of inactive/passive characters and their questions. A number of them expected difficulties in dealing with schoolchildren group of individual variations of capability, but finally they could manage well.

Table 8.2 shows a significant number of University students made changes, modifications and revisions to their plan of projects, in the aspects of activities, content, interactive components. Many changes were made after the first briefing session and further changes were made during the project delivery; changes were on the aspects of more interactive teaching, re-distribute assigned works, better communications and more clarification, explanation and monitoring for problems handled by school students. They also learnt to seek help from others.

Table 8.3 summarizes university student reflection, focuses on their changes at the end of this subject, most changes that they found after the service delivered

Table 8.1 Problems encountered mentioned (*N* = 76)

Items	Reflection journal 1 * >40%	Reflection journal 2 * >40%	Changes * >10%
1. Insufficient basic technical knowledge	23	21	−2
2. English language			
(i) Underestimated	4	0	−4
(ii) Not proficient	22	13	−9*
3. Personal limitation			
(i) Communication	18	15	−3
(ii) Knowledge to the project	8	9	+1
(iii) Personal character e.g. worry, embarrassing	24	31	+7
(iv) Preparation	5	11	+6
(v) Language barrier	1	8	+7
(vi) Presentation skill	8	33*	+25*
(vii) Leadership skill and experience	0	1	+1
4. Design of the project			
(i) Too difficult	11	22	+11*
(ii) Too simple	4	1	−3
(iii) Language used	2	0	−2
(iv) Schedule	2	13	+7
(v) Idea of the topic	6	5	−1
(vi) Applicability	6	3	−3
5. Service delivery			
(i) Location	6	1	−5
(ii) Time management	10	38*	+28*
6. Logistic	3	10	+7
7. School student group members			
(i) Gender combination	6	0	−6
(ii) Number of people/identify	10	10	0
(iii) Character (inactive, shy)	34*	6	−28*
(iv) Variation in ability and interest	30	6	−24*
(v) Learning style	6	5	−1
(vi) Harmony among members	2	9	+7
(vii) Doubt about own ability	1	6	+5
(viii) Experimental skills	1	11	+10*
(ix) With special education needs	0	3	+3
(x) Team cohesion	0	3	+3
8. School students towards project			
(i) Uninterested, not attractive	20	37*	+17*
(ii) With expectation/interested in	33*	2	−31*
(iii) Disappointment	3	4	+1

(continued)

Table 8.1 (continued)

Items	Reflection journal 1 * >40%	Reflection journal 2 * >40%	Changes * >10%
(iv) Misunderstanding	2	0	−2
(v) With questions	0	9	+9*
(vi) Passive/not initiative	0	13	+13*
(vii) Not serious/dependent	0	3	+3
9. University/school arrangement			
(i) As a marker/teacher	5	7	+2
(ii) High expectation from school	14	1	−13*
(iii) Without prior notice	1	1	0
(iv) room arrangement/facilities	0	1	+1
(v) involuntary participation/grouping	0	3	
10. Teamwork			
(i) Claimed other's problem/difficulty	2	9	+7
(ii) Work division	3	4	+1
(iii) Number of member changed	3	4	+1
(iv) Lack of communication/ disagreement	1	11	+10*
11. Connection			
(i) Generation gap	2	2	0
(ii) Individual member	0	7	+7
(iii) Different background	0	5	+5
12. Conduct service work			
(i) Fail experimental results	0	4	+4
(ii) Other problems	0	22	+22*
(iii) No/not comprehensive backup plan	0	2	+2

except they reported project-related knowledge gained at the first briefing session to school students (Keshwani & Adams, 2017). Over 40% of university students developed a better interpersonal relationship and got a higher sense of contribution to the society. Over 20% students reported skill improved in communication, social, problem-solving, decision-making, teaching, organizing and planning. Over 20% students reported personal growth in enhancement of self-understanding, self-confidence, sense of achievement and satisfaction. Over 20% students thought their work was applicable to daily life.

Table 8.2 Changes, modifications, revisions to project (*N* = 76)

Items	Reflection journal 1 * >40%	Reflection journal 2 * >40%	Changes * >10%
1. Attitude			
(i) Towards the project	8	0	−8*
(ii) Towards the school students	20	13	−7
2. Revise plan			
(i) Activities	55*	71*	+16*
(ii) Materials/equipment	40*	41*	+1
(iii) Content	67*	24	−43*
(iv) Medium of instruction	14	4	−10
(v) Teaching style (e.g. more interactive)	0	40*	+40*
(vi) Materials with Chinese interpretation	0	3	+3
3. Preparation			
(i) Research	24	12	−12*
(ii) Rehearsal	10	9	−1
(iii) Demonstration	5	7	−2
4. Interaction with students			
(i) Clarification and explanation	18	29	+11*
(ii) Discussion	27	18	−9*
(iii) Communication	44*	25	−19*
(iv) Monitor for problem handle	0	15	+16*
5. Development of positive relationship	17	9	−8*
6. Team			
(i) Communication	2	27	+25*
(ii) Seek help from others	10	23	+13*
(iii) Work distribution	12	32*	+19*
7. Student			
(i) Grouping, seating arrangement	3	4	+1
(ii) Handle conflicts	1	4	+3
(iii) Work distribution	0	7	+7

Table 8.3 University student reflection (*N* = 76)

Items	Reflection journal 1 * >20% ** >40%	Reflection journal 2 * >20% ** >40%	Changes * >10%
1. Gain			
(i) Project-related knowledge	49**	18*	−31*
(ii) Experimental skills	4	3	−1
(iii) Meaning of service learning	7	6	−1
2. Skills improved			
(i) Communication and social skills	22*	27*	+5
(ii) Problem-solving skills and decision-making	3	25*	+22*
(iii) Listening skills	2	2	0
(iv) Presentation (expressing) skills	7	11	+4
(v) Critical and multiple thinking	2	8	+6
(vi) Teaching skills	6	17*	+11*
(vii) leadership skills	4	7	+3
(viii) Organizing and planning	1	19*	+18*
(ix) Explanation skills	0	3	+3
(x) Observation and interpretation skills	0	4	+4
3. Importance of team work and cooperation	15	15	0
4. Interpersonal			
(i) Developed better relationship	14	36**	+22*
(ii) Understanding on others	2	12	+10*
5. Personal growth			
(i) Enhance self-understanding	4	27*	+23*
(ii) Self-confidence	7	18*	+11*
(iii) Not particularly specified and others	3	8	+5
(iv) Responsibility	7	6	−1
(v) Flexibility	4	15	+11*
(vi) Sense of achievement and satisfaction	1	26*	+25*
(vii) Time management	1	6	+5
(viii) Working efficiency	1	4	+3
(ix) Patience	0	4	+4
(x) Emotion	0	2	+2
(xi) Persistent and resilience	0	2	+2
6. Sense of contribution			
(i) To the society	0	39**	+39*
(ii) Suggestions made to government, organization and school	0	5	+5
7. Future career	0	12	+12*
8. Applications			

(continued)

Table 8.3 (continued)

Items	Reflection journal 1 * >20% ** >40%	Reflection journal 2 * >20% ** >40%	Changes * >10%
(i) Applicable to daily life	0	16*	+16*
(ii) Increase interest	0	4	+4

8.5 Conclusions

This service learning project consists of organizing learning activities for school students in which schools and teachers can ensure that education for sustainable development is integrated into the other learning activity (OLE) in the school curriculum through the components of briefing session with recipients, student reflections, rendering service, presentation and final summative report. Over 40% of university students developed better interpersonal relationship and got a higher sense of contribution to the society. Over 20% students reported skill improvement in communication, social, problem-solving, decision-making, teaching, organizing and planning.

References

Barth, M., Adomßent, M., Fischer, D., Richter, S., & Rieckmann, M. (2014). Learning to change universities from within: A service-learning perspective on promoting sustainable consumption in higher education. *Journal of Cleaner Production, 62,* 72–81.

Cowan, J. (2014). Noteworthy matters for attention in reflective journal writing. *Active Learning in Higher Education, 15*(1), 53–64.

Han, S., Capraro, R., & Capraro, M. M. (2015). How science, technology, engineering, and mathematics (STEM) project-based learning (PBL) affects high, middle, and low achievers differently: The impact of student factors on achievement. *International Journal of Science and Mathematics Education, 13*(5), 1089–1113.

Keshwani, J., & Adams, K. (2017). Cross-disciplinary service-learning to enhance engineering identity and improve communication skills. *International Journal for Service Learning in Engineering, 12*(1), 41–61.

Lehmann, M., Christensen, P., Du, X., & Thrane, M. (2008). Problem-oriented and project-based learning (POPBL) as an innovative learning strategy for sustainable development in engineering education. *European Journal of Engineering Education, 33*(3), 283–295.

Ramos, T. B., Caeiro, S., Hoof, B., Lozano, R., Huisingh, D., & Ceulemans, K. (2015). Experiences from the implementation of sustainable development in higher education institutions: Environmental management for sustainable universities. *Journal of Cleaner Production, 106,* 3–10.

Turns, J., Sattler, B., Yasuhara, K., Borgford-Parnell, J., & Atman, C. J. (2014). Integrating reflection into engineering education. In *Proceedings of 121st ASEE Annual Conference & Exposition, American Society for Engineering Education, Paper 9230.*

Waterman, A. S. (1997). *Service-learning: Applications from the research.* London: Lawrence Erlbaum Association.

Chapter 9
Integrating Majors and Non-majors in an International Engineering Service-Learning Programme: Course Design, Student Assessments and Learning Outcomes

Kenneth W. K. Lo, Alison K. Y. Ip, Chi Kin Lau, Wing S. Wong, Grace Ngai and Stephen C. F. Chan

Abstract The trend towards a globalized and knowledge-based society is one of the development hallmarks of the twenty-first century, and there have been numerous education reforms in response to this trend. Engineering education is no exception. Traditionally, engineering education places heavy emphasis on technical aspects, such as mathematical and scientific fundamentals. This heavy focus on the theory and technical aspects often hinders other professions from understanding the world of engineering. As a result, the general public often views engineering as a field that is isolated and difficult to comprehend, which also limits the development of engineering (Morris et al. in Eur J Eng Educ 32(2):135–142, 2007). However, it has become increasingly difficult to perform professionally in this evolving global environment within traditional curricular (National Academy of Engineering in The engineer of 2020: Visions of engineering in the new century. National Academies

K. W. K. Lo (✉) · A. K. Y. Ip · C. K. Lau · W. S. Wong · S. C. F. Chan
Office of Service-Learning, The Hong Kong Polytechnic University,
Hunghom, Hong Kong
e-mail: kenneth.wk.lo@polyu.edu.hk

A. K. Y. Ip
e-mail: alison.ip@polyu.edu.hk

C. K. Lau
e-mail: chi-kin.lau@polyu.edu.hk

W. S. Wong
e-mail: wing.ww.wong@polyu.edu.hk

S. C. F. Chan
e-mail: stephen.c.chan@polyu.edu.hk

G. Ngai
Department of Computing, The Hong Kong Polytechnic University,
Hunghom, Hong Kong
e-mail: grace.ngai@polyu.edu.hk

D. T. L. Shek et al. (eds.), *Service-Learning for Youth Leadership*,
Quality of Life in Asia 12, https://doi.org/10.1007/978-981-13-0448-4_9

Press, Washington, DC, 2004). The National Academy of Engineering forecasts that, in 2020, engineers not only need to be technically competent, but also be trained in other 'soft skills', such as civic responsibility, intercultural competence, leadership, communication and management, for them to be able to contribute to society (Galloway in Civ Eng Mag Arch 77(11):46–104, 2007). In this chapter, we present an engineering service-learning subject that was designed to incorporate major and non-major students. This multidisciplinary subject, which incorporates an international service-learning project, aims to provide a holistic learning experience that raises the problem-solving skills and general knowledge for all students, in particular, to teach students about the impact of engineering on society, and human and societal factors in engineering. Course design, challenges that we encountered, impacts on major and non-major students, and the limitations of this multidisciplinary approach will be discussed.

Keywords International Service-Learning · Engineering · Multidisciplinary Course design

9.1 Literature Review

9.1.1 International Service-Learning

International service-learning is a structured academic experience outside the host country in which students apply theoretical knowledge and utilize hands-on field experience in an organized service activity that addresses identified community needs (Jacoby, 1996). These service projects require students to leave their communities and be immersed in a different culture and environment (Ngai & Chan, 2015). During the service project, students have ample opportunities to interact and cooperate with people from different cultural backgrounds. The project also includes structured reflections to maximize student's learning. Through these learning experience, students can not only understand the course content and appreciate their discipline, but also further understand the related social and intercultural issues behind (Bringle & Hatcher, 2009). As such, international service-learning has been shown to have a high educational impact across the spectrum of disciplines (Bringle, Hatcher, & Jones, 2011).

Apart from the benefit to the students, an effective and structured service-learning programme can also benefit the community. The international service activities are often designed to address the identified human and community needs. With careful design, the services can increase the resources for the community and empower the beneficiaries. These international service projects have been shown to bring positive impacts to both the community partners and the community (Chupp & Joseph, 2010).

Engineering service-learning projects, in particular, may be especially impactful in benefiting the community, especially in developing countries where engineering expertise is often not readily available. By integrating engineering expertise and appropriate technology and with the help of community assessment, these engineering service-learning programmes can introduce different engineering solutions in these communities (Bielefeldt & Pearce, 2012), thereby enhancing the living environment and quality of life.

9.1.2 Service-Learning in Engineering

Since the 1990s, universities and engineering organizations have organized engineering-related service-learning projects that bring students from First World countries to serve in developing regions, often as part of first-year design courses (Duffy, Tsang, & Lord, 2000; Hobson, 2000; Knizley & Coleman, 2014; Lin & Vernaza, 2016), capstone projects (Bielefeldt, Dewoolkar, Caves, Berdanier, & Paterson, 2011; Dewoolkar, George, Hayden, & Rizzo, 2009; Duffy et al., 2008), extracurricular student teams (Kaunonen, 2010; Ramírez, Bengo, Mereu, Bejarano, & Silva, 2011) or other learning and teaching activities (Coyle, Jamieson, & Oakes, 2005; Ropers-Huilman, Carwile, & Lima, 2005).

We illustrate with some examples. Mississippi State University integrated service-learning projects into the freshman-level mechanical engineering course in 2013 to allow first-year students to utilize basic engineering principles (Knizley & Coleman, 2014). One hundred forty-five students participated in one of the five engineering projects. These projects included serving as mentors for high school students participating in a robotics competition or teaching STEM-related lessons for elementary schools. Gannon University introduced service-learning projects into a required first-year seminar in engineering (Lin & Vernaza, 2016). Engineering students worked in a group and collaborated with different community partners. The first half of the course was dedicated to drafting design proposals, and students would implement the selected proposals during the second half. Through these community-based design projects, students can understand the engineering design process and employ their problem-solving skill in a real-world setting.

Bielefeldt et al. (2011) examined different models for incorporating service-learning projects into capstone projects. At Duke University, service projects are required in a biomedical engineering course. Their collaborating partners include individuals with disabilities, their families and the clinical professionals. Students are required to have eight to twelve face-to-face meetings with their service targets and submit two structured reflective essays.

The Engineering Projects in Community Service (EPICS) programme, which was created at Purdue University, allowed undergraduates to earn academic credit for their contributions to solving problems identified by non-profit organizations in the community. The EPICS framework matches the ABET EC 2000 criteria, which emphasizes multidisciplinary and customer-driven design in projects. The EPICS model has been subsequently adopted by 14 other institutions in the USA (Coyle et al., 2005). The College of Engineering at the University of Massachusetts Lowell successfully integrated service-learning into 35 various undergraduate core programmes (Duffy et al., 2008).

These successful examples show that this pedagogy has a positive impact on students. It not only strengthens their academic learning but also develops non-technical attributes, such as civic responsibility, critical thinking and moral development.

9.1.3 Interdisciplinary Approach

Studies have shown that interdisciplinary service-learning experiences are an effective strategy for maximizing student learning outcomes (Stebleton, Jensen, & Peter, 2010; Zeidmane & Cernajeva, 2011). A multidisciplinary team allows each discipline to independently contribute its expertise to solve a common set of problems. Students can enhance teamwork skills, communication skills, conflict resolution skills and leadership skills through working with students from other disciplines. For example, in 2000, the College of St. Catherine initiated a community–campus partnership-building process. Students and faculty from five professional disciplines developed and implemented a service-learning course (Gupta, 2006). Positive feedback was received from the students and faculty, in which they appreciated the diversity of professional and personal identities. The interdisciplinary approach exposed them to expertise, experience and perspectives from different disciplines and, therefore, enhanced skills and knowledge in diverse curricula.

It would be ideal if engineering service-learning projects could adopt an interdisciplinary approach that optimally incorporates an interdisciplinary team that extends beyond engineering. The interdisciplinary approach can enrich engineering projects with complementary skills such as community assessment. Students from non-engineering backgrounds can also gain a better understanding of infrastructural and industrial development through working on these projects. However, such a true collaboration is often difficult to achieve due to differences in structure and intended learning outcomes between different disciplines. As a result, most interdisciplinary engineering service-learning projects integrate different engineering majors, instead of other disciplines.

9.2 Course Description

The Hong Kong Polytechnic University has a long tradition of organizing engineering-related service-learning projects that bring students to serve underprivileged communities. Since 2005, the Department of Computing has been organizing various projects in local and overseas communities. In the beginning, most projects were instructional-type projects, in which our students delivered STEM and digital storytelling workshops to under-served schools or communities.

The last few years have seen a change in project nature. The projects have become more technical and infrastructural. These include building a computer laboratory, wireless networking and library system in 2007 to a renewable energy project in 2015 where students constructed solar-powered charging stations and installed a community learning centre. Since 2007, students have contributed over 17,000 man-hours of service in over 20 engineering-related projects to communities in rural China, Cambodia, Rwanda and Myanmar. With the launch of the new four-year university curriculum in 2012, this community service project was formalized as a credit-bearing service-learning subject.

The target of study in this paper is this two-semester service-learning subject, offered by the Department of Computing, titled 'Technology Beyond Borders: Service-Learning across Cultural, Ethnic and Community Lines'. Unlike many other engineering subjects, this subject was designed to be accessible to all undergraduate students, regardless of discipline. Through this subject, students learn about the impact of technology, how proper use of technology can benefit people in many different ways and how one can harness technology for the benefit of the underprivileged, even for those who are not from engineering disciplines. The formal intended learning outcomes of this course are as follows:

1. To increase our students' awareness and knowledge of communities that are culturally, ethnically or socially distinct from their own.
2. To acquaint students with significant issues of social need, justice and ethics related to the information age, such as the concept of the information divide and how technology may be used to meet needs.
3. To cultivate an awareness of information ethics and professional responsibility in our students.
4. To nurture a sense of civic responsibility and engagement in our students.

From 2014/15 to 2016/17, 347 students enrolled in this subject. Projects ranged STEM-related teaching projects in primary or secondary schools to infrastructure improvement projects in rural villages. In this paper, we consider only the infrastructure programmes implemented in our two most mature overseas sites: Cambodia and Rwanda. In total, 134 students were involved in these projects.

9.2.1 Subject Components

As an academic service-learning subject, we adopt a blended-learning approach, combining e-learning, classroom discipline-specific lectures, project-specific laboratory tutorial sessions, experiential learning and reflective learning.

The concepts and theories are covered through e-learning and lectures. The e-learning module is designed as an induction to help students understand what service-learning is and why they need to do it. It covers the concept and practices of service-learning, the benefits of service-learning, some general guidelines about serving and learning through reflection. Four to six discipline-specific lectures then introduce students to the relevant academic topics and issues, such as digital divide, appropriate technology, information literacy and energy poverty.

To enable students to gain an understanding of the target community and equip them with the skills necessary for delivering the services, hands-on project-specific tutorial and laboratory sessions are used. For example, students who will be building a learning centre in Cambodia might get lessons in setting up solar systems, computer networks, models of maintaining computer centres, along with cultural training that educates them about the culture and history of the country in which they will be serving. This ensures that students can understand the social aspects of the project, connect the academic dimension to the services and identify the community impacts. They will also learn technical skills such as basic electronic circuitry, use of power and mechanical tools, laser cutting, soldering, installation of a solar system, or setting up computer networks and content hosting servers.

The execution of the service project is arguably the most important component of an SL subject. Hence, students are intensively supervised and assessed during the service delivery. Their contribution to the team and project, their attitude, performance, the degree of engagement with service recipients, collaboration with other students and relationship with collaborating organizations are observed.

Our projects usually last for 2–3 weeks and involve three main components:

1. *Understand the local culture and community*: These activities are designed to help students to understand cultural norms, prepare them to deal with cultural differences and serve sensitively, and enable them to build up the linkage between the service projects and the social issues or historical factors. Activities may include sharing and activities organized by local non-government organizations (NGOs) or universities, visiting historical museums and a generally immersive experience to acclimate them to the local context. For example, in Cambodia, students participate in a training workshop to learn about Khmer, traditional dancing, the living style in rural villages, etc. They also visit the genocide museum and the killing fields, a community centre and a slum school.
2. *Training and preparation with local peers*: Our students are necessarily handicapped by the fact that they are serving in a community that they are not a part of. For this reason, and for sustainability purposes, our projects are designed such that our students will serve with local peers—young people or university students. Hence, a second component of the project involves building up the rapport and teamwork between our students and their local peers. This process may involve working together to finalize the design, construct, and test the deliverables.
3. *Project implementation*: During the service delivery, students work in groups with their local peers to install the solar system or set up the learning centre.

This requires students to work in close proximity and collaboration with others who may be very different from them in language, culture or appearance. It teaches our students global competencies and communication. The local young people also practise and master the technical skills, some of them to an extent that they are able to help our local collaborating NGO partner to maintain the equipment in the long run.

Throughout the project, students are expected and guided to make observations about how their experiences link with the academic concepts taught in class. When students are on-site, they will generally have a reflection session every one or two service sessions. The reflection sessions are designed to clarify and make sense of their observations, helping them to understand the background and causes behind the phenomenon observed, guide them to reflect more deeply on their experiences and give them support if they encounter difficulties. To help them to clarify and solidify their learning, students are required to submit reflective journals and reports both during and after the projects.

Since 2015, our projects have followed two main themes: renewable energy and education infrastructure, both in the context of rural communities:

1. *Solar energy system for rural communities*: These projects involve building solar power solutions for rural communities off the electrical grid. Following the principle of appropriate technology, the solar power solutions took the form of a public charging station shared by a group of nearby households. Our students assembled the solar panels and wired up homes with low-powered electrical appliances.
2. *Community learning centre*: These projects involve building informal learning spaces for children and youths. They are meant to supplement the regular school education and to serve as a resource for continued education and self-guided study. The centres are powered with solar energy, and offline educational resources are used in lieu of Internet access. Students were responsible for designing and installing the electrical support for the centre, and identifying and deploying a customized computer library with electronic learning resources.

9.2.2 Evaluation Methods

Students' attainment of the intended learning outcomes was evaluated using three approaches: (1) grading by the teaching team according to the subject rubrics, (2) a self-reported post-experience survey and (3) reflective journals submitted after the completion of the projects.

1. *Teaching team assessment*: The students' performance was accessed according to a set of rubrics in three phases, preparation, execution and reflection. Each student was evaluated independently by at least four teachers and tutors, and a

meeting was organized to finalize the result. The grading is ranged from 0 to 4.5 (0 = inadequate; 1 = barely satisfactory; 2 = satisfactory; 3 = good; 4 = outstanding; 4.5 = extraordinary).

2. *Post-experience survey*: A standard post-experience survey was administered at the end of the course. This survey comprised a set of questions asking students to rate, on a seven-point scale (1 = very little; 4 = a fair amount; 7 = very much), their attainment of the intended learning outcomes relating to their intellectual (4 items), social (2 items), civic (5 items) and personal (1 item) development as a result of attending the service-learning subject.
3. *Student's reflective journal*: Students were required to submit a reflective report that summarized their experience, observations and analyses under three dimensions: social, personal and academic. For the social impact, they are required to support their observations and their arguments regarding the project's community impact with data and concrete examples. For the personal dimension, students need to reflect on their personal, social and professional changes. In the academic dimension, they reflected on the linkage between their observations from the service project and the academic topic covered in the first half of the course (digital divide or appropriate technology).

9.3 Findings and Observation

9.3.1 Grading and Intended Learning Outcomes

A total of 134 students participated in the engineering-based service projects studied in this paper. Of these, 63 students (47%) were studying engineering; the others were from a variety of disciplines including health sciences, social sciences and the humanities. This diversity poses extra challenges to the running of such projects but also makes additional learning gains available to the students. The majority of students were in year 1 (n = 80, 60%), 46 (34%) were in year 2, and the remaining 8 (5%) were in years 3 and 4 (final year).

The descriptive statistics for the learning outcome are summarized in Table 9.1. Among the four learning outcomes, the personal aspect had the highest mean for both engineering students (6.03 on a seven-point scale) and non-engineering students (6.34), whereas intellectual had the lowest: 5.81 for engineering students and 5.99 for non-engineering students. However, the rating was still significantly higher than the mid-point of 4. The standard deviations of the scores ranged from 0.74 to 0.97 for the engineering group and 0.65–0.70 for the non-engineering group. Also, non-engineering students rated themselves higher on all four learning outcomes, though the differences were small, ranging from 0.18 to 0.31.

This result shows the non-engineering students perceived themselves as learning more in all four dimensions, i.e. intellectual, social, civic and personal, than the engineering students. The intellectual learning gain covers the understanding of the

Table 9.1 Descriptive statistics of the learning outcomes

Variables included in the study	Group[a]	Min	Max	Mean	Std. dev.
Learning outcomes (scale from 1 to 7)					
Intellectual	E	3.00	7.00	5.81	0.85
	NE	4.00	7.00	5.99	0.70
Social	E	2.50	7.00	5.94	0.94
	NE	5.00	7.00	6.24	0.66
Civic	E	3.00	7.00	5.89	0.74
	NE	4.25	7.00	6.13	0.68
Personal	E	3.00	7.00	6.03	0.97
	NE	5.00	7.00	6.34	0.65

[a]*E* Engineering; *NE* non-engineering

linkage between service-learning and the academic content of the subject, application of knowledge to deal with complex issues, real-life problem solving and critical thinking. The non-engineering students have a relatively lower level of engineering knowledge and skills, and many did not have any related learning experience before taking this interdisciplinary service-learning subject. This project challenged the non-engineering students to apply and polish their hard and soft skills in order to catch up with the engineering students and achieve the project goal, which may account for the higher self-perceived learning gains.

In most of the student groups, the non-engineering students took up tasks which mainly involved interacting with the service recipients and the community, such as conducting community assessments, while the engineering students chose to take up the engineering tasks, such as electrical wiring and solar panel installation. This may explain the reason why the non-engineering students perceived that they gained a deeper understanding of the social issues, as they had more opportunities to interact directly with the community members.

In terms of personal awareness, the non-engineering students would understandably find the service project more challenging. As such, they were forced to leave their comfort zone and learn new knowledge and skills. Facing and overcoming these challenges helps students to know their own strengths and be more aware of their weaknesses, which is more conducive to facilitating personal growth.

Figure 9.1 shows the grade differences between the engineering and non-engineering students. Compared to the non-engineering students, the engineering students received slightly higher grades for their performance during the preparation, execution, and reflection stages, with the difference ranging from 0.14 to 0.19. As project preparation and execution require a certain level of discipline knowledge and skill, it is not surprising that the engineering students perform better than the non-engineering students, especially during the initial preparation stage.

The reflection grade is more surprising. Upon examination of the reflective reports, it appears that engineering students are more aware of the connection between the service project, the academic topic covered in the course, the impact on

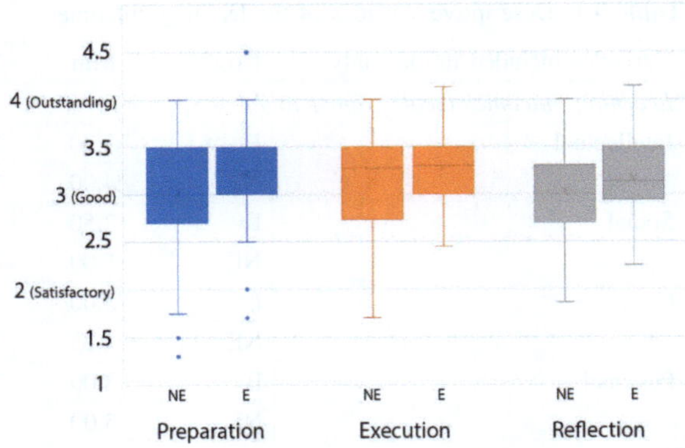

Fig. 9.1 Comparison between engineering and non-engineering students: assessment results

the target community and on society in general. The non-engineering students, in contrast, put more emphasis on their personal development and their interaction with their engineering peers. They are in general able to articulate the immediate impact of their service project, but find it more difficult to demonstrate high-level critique.

To examine differences in the grading and learning outcomes, an independent t-test was conducted. The results, depicted in Table 9.2, show that engineering students received a higher grading in preparation (M = 3.21) than non-engineering students (M = 3.02). This difference is statistically significant, but it only represents a small-sized effect ($d < 0.5$). There was also a significant difference in the self-perceived social and personal learning outcome dimensions between engineering and non-engineering students. Non-engineering students rated themselves 0.29 and 0.31 higher than engineering students in the social and personal dimension representatively.

Table 9.2 Assessment results and self-reported learning outcomes: statistical comparison between engineering and non-engineering students

Variables included in the study	*T*	df	Sig. (two-tailed)	Mean diff.	Std. err. diff.	Effect size
Grading (scale from 1 to 4)						
Preparation	2.00	132	0.05	0.19	0.10	0.35
Execution	1.76	132	0.08	0.14	0.08	0.31
Reflection	1.70	132	0.09	0.14	0.081	0.29
Learning outcomes (scale from 1 to 7)						
Intellectual	1.34	132	0.18	0.18	0.13	0.23
Social	2.12	132	0.04	0.29	0.14	0.37
Civic	1.90	132	0.06	0.23	0.12	0.33
Personal	2.17	132	0.03	0.31	0.14	0.38

9.3.2 Benefit to Students

Based on the teaching team's observations and students' reflections, we identify four benefits to students' learning through our application of the multidisciplinary approach to an international engineering service-learning programme.

A. *Appreciation for One's Own Discipline*

The National Academy of Engineering's 'The Engineer of 2020' reports that the engineer of 2020 will need strong analytical skills combined with interdisciplinary competence; ability to synthesize information from a broad range of disciplines and contextual competence; and ability to understand the constraints and impacts of engineering solutions on social, cultural, political and environmental contexts (National Academy of Engineering, 2004).

We observed that working on a tangible project that impacted real people helped engineering students to understand the value of their discipline. Most of our students are accustomed to living in a highly developed city, where much of the engineering infrastructure is taken for granted. The Hong Kong economy is also strongly dependent upon the service industry and the service sector. As a result, engineering students often feel underappreciated compared to their peers in, for example, the health sciences or business, where the impact is more visible and the profession tends to be more highly valued by society.

> Most people think that economists and politicians are the people who run countries, and engineers are the ones who simply invent technology and drive the human race forward.—Student 62c, Mechanical Engineering

Working on a project in a developing region gives students the opportunity to experience, in a very vivid way, the value and impact of the engineering discipline. These service projects require students to put their classroom learning into practice and observe the immediate impact on the service recipients, in a way which is not possible in Hong Kong because of the multiple layers of existing infrastructure. Working with and for communities that are not as familiar with the constant availability of high technology also teaches them a better understanding on the role of human factor in engineering.

> I learnt a lot about the principles, the benefits, drawbacks and its impact on the environment of renewable energy from my studies. However, I also wanted to know how renewable energy impacts the society. After conducting the service project, I learnt that it could help people undoubtedly. Before the advancement of the technology in producing solar panels, it was difficult to provide electricity to these remote areas as building a grid in these areas is always too costly for a developing country. With the advancement in energy engineering, we could install solar panels in their village. The panels are lighter and safer to use. I totally understand that engineering can change a lot through this service project, from no electricity to lighting up the house with the solar power. To conclude, I learnt that humans as the promoters and beneficiaries of engineering enhances the development of the community, the country and the world in different aspect of life. It definitely deepens my knowledge on my major.—Student 87c, Environmental Engineering

In many schools, engineering is a relatively isolated field. Due to the packed programme structure, engineering students often only take engineering classes, interact only with their engineering peers and have not much spare time to venture into the other academic fields during their undergraduate study. Although most universities now require all students to study some broadening courses, i.e. courses that are not from their own disciplines, these courses are often lecture-based and do not require a deep collaboration among students from different backgrounds. Students also often have the conception that these broadening courses are less important compared to their discipline-related subjects, and these subjects do not require their full devotion. As a result, their interaction is mainly with people from a similar background, who share the same thinking style, language and culture.

In contrast, the design of the current international service-learning project forces engineering students to truly cooperate with students from other disciplines for a considerable amount of time. Engineering students had opportunities to explain their technical logic to non-engineering students in an understandable way and to work to come up with a compromise.

> During the preparation, we had so many arguments. On every little problem, we always had a fight and mostly I won the arguments. Even though I was wrong I would not say that I was wrong. However, I realised that debating was not the best solution to solve a problem. It was not about who wins the arguments, it should be a discussion among the group members to come up with the best idea. Discussions are always better than arguments, because an argument is to find out who is right, and a discussion is to find what is right. It was also not good if all the idea came from me, as we work as a team and need all their minds.—Student 89c, Electronic and Information Engineering

Meanwhile, they learn how non-engineering groupmates perceive their discipline. Non-major students are also often able to observe different facets of the societal and global issues, especially to those related to their own disciplines. This sharing of views and opinions helps to develop students' understanding of the human side of engineering, including the role of engineering in promoting sustainable development.

> Now the human aspect in engineering itself is an important element often forgotten by a lot of—even professional engineers. Humans are basically both the start line and the finish line of the whole engineering process itself. Engineering is done from and for humans. It's a beautiful and most of the time unseen form of loving each other.—Student 5c, Mechanical Engineering

During the reflection sessions, some engineering students reflected that the engagement in serving the communities could inspire them to consider what they could do for the society after the attainment of the engineering degree. The project helped them to acquire better understanding of the actual needs of people in developing countries, which changed their mindset about engineering changed through an insight into the contribution of engineering to development.

> Engineering can bring an affordable technology to a developing country. Basic utilities, infrastructure, and communication are essential for a development of a country. It is not only about providing the latest affordable technology for the people, but also about the need

to be concerned about the sustainable development of the country. … This kind of activities can help me understand more about the global issue. I should use my knowledge to work on more international projects and start to think of working in overseas developing countries. —Student 53r, Electrical Engineering

B. *Building Appreciation for other Disciplines*

Students also learnt through collaborating with students whose thinking styles and cultures are very different. For instance, students in the business fields are trained to be more attuned and observant of body language and non-verbal communication, something that the engineering students felt they lacked:

I did learn a lot from my teammate, and I wish I can learn more from him. He taught me what empathetic communication means. For example, he taught me to think "Do I need the answer for this question? Or I can already get the answer from my observations?" every time before I ask. He shared with me about how to be more conscious about others' feelings.—Student 89r, Aviation Engineering

Most non-engineering students expressed concerns about the technical demands of these engineering projects at the beginning of the subject. They often feared that it would be impossible for them to acquire these knowledge and skills which seem alien to them. For them, it is especially rewarding when they overcome these hurdles and see how the end product immediately improves the service recipient's daily life. The experience of overcoming these challenges also ignites their 'can-do' attitude and sense of achievement.

Through this project I learnt that no matter which major of study you are—you can do anything as long as you are willing to learn. I had to make an extra effort to understand all the unfamiliar words and equipment; I got cut by a knife and blacked out during the service. But all this experience is worth the time because this is an experience I would never will learn in any other subject in my major.—Student 45c, Business Management.

Being a non-engineering student, I cannot imagine being involved in an engineering project before, especially the wiring parts. Our group completed the indoor wiring in nine houses successfully and built one solar panel station. It is surely our biggest success in this service trip. We can influence the community in a more long-lasting and sustainable way. We can actually make the world a better place to live in. We can help the villagers with real needs, saving their money for charging their phones and commuting time. We have gained a sense of satisfaction in the service.—Student 82c, Building Surveying.

Some students reflected that though they were not engineering majors, their skill sets could contribute to the project even in a very technical way:

I used to doubt what I could contribute to the team. Being a Design student, I did not have any technical or science background. I relied on my teammate and tried my best to work on the design of the solar station. Following the instructions from the engineering students, I drew the three-dimensional diagram with precise measurements. During the execution, I was the only one who understood the whole setting and measurement; therefore, I stepped beyond my comfort zone and took the role of leader to build the solar station. My teammates appreciated what I did and felt grateful that I was part of the team. Engineering to me

> is an auxiliary to other dimensions and an important way to make a difference, both to the rural villagers and to me.—Student 26c, Design

Some non-engineering students reflected that the engineer's mindset enhanced the working attitude in their own profession. The service-learning project provides a good platform for students to learn and demonstrate consideration for the community and individuals under the constraints of resources and time. Some students drew a parallel from this engineering working process to their own discipline:

> The villagers are like the patients. When I was interviewing them, it was like diagnosing patients. I need to fully understand their situation and problems so that I can provide the best treatment and help. The building of solar station and the indoor wiring are like the treatments we provide. Therefore, the service is just like a whole treatment process. With different limitations at the site, our group needed to change our design of the station… patients may have different symptoms and I need to use those as the basis to provide the best way to help them. In the medical field, there is a term called "patient-centered care". It means that health professionals need to put the patients and their families at the center of decisions so as to get the best outcome. In this service, we were villager-centered so that we could provide the best for them. To conclude, some of the attitudes of a physiotherapist is like an engineer's attitudes and I also learnt the ways of thinking and dealing things and people, which will help me to become a better physiotherapist in the future.—Student 66c, Physiotherapy

Many students also shared how working with people with differing strengths helped them to gain respect for others:

> In the past, I hated to work in a team. I think that we have to discuss and debate in every team effort. However, I learnt that the strength of everyone are different. We are actually the leaders of different parts of the work. For example, engineering students are the leader of thinking about the whole wiring system, design students are the leader of construction of solar panels, surveying students are the leader of checking the detail, etc. I learnt to appreciate everyone and be patient to explain to others, as others may not be as professional as you in certain aspects. We need different people to make things better. This is the first time I see that importance of teamwork. I believe that this is a good practice of the real workplace.—Student 23c, Design

C. *Breaking Traditional Stereotypes and Learning Respect*

We observed the breaking of traditional stereotypes during the process. At the beginning of the project, for instance, some male students would not let their female groupmates work on the more physically demanding tasks. Instead, they relegated the female teammates to the less demanding (and often less consequential) parts of the project:

> I could feel that the male groupmates want to be gentlemen, they deny me and other female groupmates to do 'physically demanding jobs', such as carry heavy things and drill holes. In their perspective, they think that girls should do 'clean jobs', such as adjusting screws and doing measurements.—Student 88c, Optometry

Some engineering students did not think their non-engineering peers had the abilities to carry out the project. They insisted on checking every step these non-engineering students have completed.

> Reflecting back on the first week of our trip, I felt really disappointed with myself. Being the only person in my group with a passion and background of engineering, I often felt prideful and arrogant for having the skills that I possessed. One small moment I remember was in the first few days, when each group started building their solar panel modules. It was the first time our group worked together after a few months and we immediately had our hands down working on the solar panels. I remember how I didn't trust anyone else but me to drill or solder, and how I had to recheck all of the measurements any of my teammates had made. Although I was sure that all of what I did was important, I now realize that I was being prideful and not trusting my teammates enough.—Student 62c, Mechanical Engineering

On the flip side, the engineering students too suffered from the stereotype that non-engineering students had of them—that engineers were great technical people but poor communicators. Some non-engineering students unilaterally decided to take charge of tasks such as community and needs assessment without consulting with their engineering peers. As expected, those who were denied the opportunities were frustrated about being victims of these stereotypes.

The teaching team deliberately reassigned tasks so that students who were not comfortable with these activities would still need to practise them, and encouraged the students who were denied the chances to work extra hard to earn their teammates' trust. This process helped students to realize that stereotypes were often not accurate, and led them to question their own way of dealing with people:

> With just four hits, the nail went through in front of everyone… my Cambodia female group mate nails the wood better and quicker than all my Hong Kong male group mates… I was so amazed by her and ashamed of myself at the same time… I realized that I've made too many false assumptions and interpretations … that have made me totally underestimated the things they can do… I sometime judge people by how they look, where they come from and what their gender is. From that, treat them in certain ways, like how I often just let her do some simple work for me.—Student 39c, Industrial and Systems Engineering

D. *Building Students' Self-efficacy*

The experience of building a tangible construction and overcoming challenging tasks boosted the self-efficacy of the students, engineering and non-engineering alike. Self-efficacy is defined as 'beliefs in one's capabilities to organize and execute the courses of action required to produce given attainments' (Edwin, 1997). This self-belief or the personal judgment about one's competencies significantly affects students' learning motivation and performance (Pajares, 1996; Schunk, 2003). It was found that students' self-efficacy can be boosted with careful design of an educational programme (Van Dinther, Dochy, & Segers, 2011).

The project required non-engineering students to overcome the technical tasks that they had have very low confidence in at the beginning and engineering students to use their skills for something that would be of real consequence to a real person.

During the course, the teaching team repeatedly reassured students that these skills, though new to them, were achievable with learning and practice. At the same time, they were working under the pressure that their works affect the daily lives of the real people. The demanding situation together with abundant opportunities forced them to rethink their perceptions and overcome their reservations:

> I remember feeling pessimistic and afraid of being a burden to my group as I have no clear idea on what to do and have not much knowledge about engineering concepts. I continue feeling this way and without my realization, I truly labelled myself as a 'burden', and did nothing much to help my group as I feel ashamed of sharing my 'invalid' opinions. This feeling soon come to an end once we arrived in Cambodia … I realized that the more I label myself as a burden, the more likely that would become a reality.—Student 33c, Global Supply Chain Management

Many students found the whole experience rewarding, especially when they first finished wiring up a house and observed the house owner's satisfaction when he/she turned on the light or when they saw the finished solar charging station:

> I, personally, did not expect that we would do all the tasks and even more than what was assigned to us. Especially, when it came to build the solar station. It was so beautiful that even I was amazed by our work.—Student 89c, Electronic and Information Engineering

Working on tangible solutions brings the issue home to the students and makes it more realistic to them. The challenges appear to be bigger, and the sense of reward is much higher when they succeed in overcoming the challenges. It is true that most non-engineering students would not need to use their learnt technical skills after the project. However, we believe that the process of overcoming the challenges in the mastery of these technical skills helps to build up their resilience and self-efficacy in facing future challenges.

9.4 Conclusion and Future Work

The students' work in multidisciplinary teams and integration into an engineering project was found to impact positively not only the project but also both engineering and non-engineering students. This mixed group approach can offer other learning experiences to the teams, including tolerance for diversity, break the traditional stereotypes, stimulate the students to think differently about engineering, build up their self-efficacy and enhance the interpersonal development.

Having said that, the key to building up these experiences rests with the teachers. Left to themselves, it is natural for students to divide up the tasks according to their own expertise—this would result in students simply staying in their comfort zone, either out of convenience or efficiency. Quality assurance is also an issue—when executing real projects that impact real people, it is only natural to assign the best, most skilled workers to the task—who usually are the engineering major students. It is up to the teacher, then, to properly prepare and train the students, educate them to listen and consult with each other, show them the benefits of a multifaceted view, and even to intervene and force students to switch roles when necessary.

A proper project design and holistic assessment are also important for parity and fairness. If the project were solely about technical installation and the assessment purely based on the quality of the technical implementation, it would be inevitable for engineering students to have the upper hand, simply because of their increased exposure and practice during their own discipline major. However, this would not only be unfair to the non-engineering students, it would also neglect the human and societal factor, which is critical to service-learning and the success of appropriate technology solutions in developing communities.

As teachers, designing and organizing this course has been a challenge, albeit a rewarding one. Taking the step to admit students from other disciplines into our course, and by extension, committing to giving them as good a learning experience as we would offer to our own students, has taught us to think out of the box, communicate differently, manage expectations, but also raise hopes and standards. We believe that we have grown as teachers as a result of this initiative. In the future, we will investigate designing and offering multidisciplinary courses with teachers from other disciplines.

References

Bielefeldt, A. R., & Pearce, J. M. (2012). *Service learning in engineering. Convergence: Philosophies and pedagogies for developing the next generation of humanitarian engineers and social entrepreneurs.* Retrieved from http://digitalcommons.mtu.edu/materials_fp/54/.

Bielefeldt, A. R., Dewoolkar, M. M., Caves, K. M., Berdanier, B. W., & Paterson, K. G. (2011). Diverse models for incorporating service projects into engineering capstone design courses. *International Journal of Engineering Education*, 1206–1220. Retrieved from http://www.scopus.com/inward/record.url?eid=2-s2.0-81155137230&partnerID=40&md5=64ed58246995c00b802766617d710206.

Bringle, R. G., Hatcher, J., & Jones, S. G. (2011). *International service learning: Conceptual frameworks and research.* VA, USA: Stylus.

Bringle, R., & Hatcher, J. (2009). Innovative practices in service learning and curricular engagement. *New Directions for Higher Education*. Retrieved from http://onlinelibrary.wiley.com/doi/10.1002/he.356/full.

Chupp, M. G., & Joseph, M. L. (2010). Getting the most out of service learning: Maximizing student, university and community impact. *Journal of Community Practice, 18*(2–3), 190–212. https://doi.org/10.1080/10705422.2010.487045.

Coyle, E. J., Jamieson, L. H., & Oakes, W. C. (2005). EPICS: Engineering projects in community service. *International Journal of Engineering Education, 21*. Retrieved from http://staging.community-wealth.org/sites/clone.community-wealth.org/files/downloads/article-coyle-et-al.pdf.

Dewoolkar, M. M., George, L. A., Hayden, N. J., & Rizzo, D. M. (2009). Vertical integration of service-learning into civil and environmental engineering curricula. *International Journal of Engineering Education, 56*(6), 1257–1269.

Duffy, J., Barington, L., Moeller, W., Barry, C., Kazmer, D., West, C., & Crespo, V. (2008). Service-learning projects in core undergraduate engineering courses. *International Journal for*

Service Learning in Engineering, Humanitarian Engineering and Social Entrepreneurship, 3 (2). http://doi.org/10.24908/ijsle.v3i2.2103.

Duffy, J., Tsang, E., & Lord, S. (2000). Service-learning in engineering: What, why, and how? *American Society for Engineering Education (ASEE) Annual Conference.*

Edwin, A. (1997). Self-efficacy: The exercise of control. *Choice Reviews Online, 35*(3), 35–1826. https://doi.org/10.5860/CHOICE.35-1826.

Galloway, P. D. (2007). The 21st-century engineer: A proposal for engineering education reform. *Civil Engineering Magazine Archive, 77*(11), 46–104. https://doi.org/10.1061/ciegag.0000147.

Gupta, J. (2006). A model for interdisciplinary service-learning experience for social change. *Journal of Physical Therapy Education, 20*(3), 55–60. Retrieved from https://login.proxy.bib.uottawa.ca/login?url=http://search.ebscohost.com/login.aspx?direct=true&db=cin20&AN=2009521318&site=ehost-live.

Hobson, R. S. (2000). Service-Learning as an educational tool in an introduction to engineering course. In *American Society for Engineering Education (ASEE) Annual Conference* (p. 3253).

Jacoby, B. (1996). Service-learning in today's higher education. In *Service-learning in higher education: Concepts and practices.* San Francisco, CA: Jossey-Bass.

Kaunonen, G. (2010). Engineering world health. *IEEE Pulse, 1*(2), 28–33. https://doi.org/10.1109/MPUL.2010.938710.

Knizley, A., & Coleman, T. (2014). Implementing service-learning into an introductory mechanical engineering course. In *American Society for Engineering Education.* Retrieved from http://asee.cs.southern.edu/proceedings/ASEE2014/Papers2014/4/54.pdf.

Lin, Z., & Vernaza, K. (2016). Teaching first year engineering students engineering design process and problem solving through service learning projects. In *2016 IEEE Frontiers in Education Conference (FIE)* (pp. 1–7). http://doi.org/10.1109/FIE.2016.7757495.

Morris, R., Childs, P. R., & Hamilton, T. (2007). Sustainability by design: A reflection on the suitability of pedagogic practice in design and engineering courses in the teaching of sustainable design. *European Journal of Engineering Education, 32*(2), 135–142. https://doi.org/10.1080/03043790601118549.

National Academy of Engineering. (2004). *The engineer of 2020: Visions of engineering in the new century.* Washington, D.C.: National Academies Press. http://doi.org/10.17226/10999.

Ngai, G., & Chan, S. C. (2015). How much impact can be made in a week? In *Proceedings of the 46th ACM Technical Symposium on Computer Science Education—SIGCSE '15* (pp. 645–650). New York, USA: ACM Press. http://doi.org/10.1145/2676723.2677267.

Pajares, F. (1996). Self-efficacy beliefs in academic settings. *Review of Educational Research, 66* (4), 543–578. https://doi.org/10.3102/00346543066004543.

Ramírez, M. C., Bengo, I., Mereu, R., Bejarano R., A. X., & Silva, J. C. (2011). Participative methodology for local development: The contribution of engineers without borders from Italy and Colombia: Towards the improvement of water quality in vulnerable communities. *Systemic Practice and Action Research, 24*(1), 45–66. https://doi.org/10.1007/s11213-010-9175-3.

Ropers-Huilman, B., Carwile, L., & Lima, M. (2005). Service-learning in engineering : A valuable pedagogy for meeting learning objectives. *European Journal of Engineering Education, 30*, 155–165. https://doi.org/10.1080/03043790410001664363.

Schunk, D. H. (2003). Self-efficacy for reading and writing: Influence of modeling, goal setting, and self-evaluation. *Reading and Writing Quarterly: Overcoming Learning Difficulties, 19*(2), 159–172. Retrieved from https://eric.ed.gov/?id=EJ672802.

Stebleton, M., Jensen, M., & Peter, G. (2010). Enhancing student engagement in a multidisciplinary, first-year experience course. *College Teaching Methods & Styles Journal, 6*, 1–6. Retrieved from http://libaccess.mcmaster.ca/login?url=http://search.proquest.com/docview/964182470?accountid=12347%5Cnhttp://sfx.scholarsportal.info/mcmaster?url_ver=Z39.88-2004&rft_val_fmt=info:ofi/fmt:kev:mtx:journal&genre=article&sid=ProQ:ProQ%3Aericshell&atitle=Enha.

Van Dinther, M., Dochy, F., & Segers, M. (2011). Factors affecting students' self-efficacy in higher education. *Educational Research Review, 6*(2), 95–108. https://doi.org/10.1016/j.edurev.2010.10.003.

Zeidmane, A., & Cernajeva, S. (2011). Interdisciplinary approach in engineering education. In *2011 IEEE Global Engineering Education Conference, EDUCON 2011* (pp. 1096–1101). http://doi.org/10.1109/EDUCON.2011.5773284.

Chapter 10
Where Programming Skills Meet the Social Needs

Peter H. F. Ng and Memory W. H. Chiu

Abstract This chapter describes *Technology Beyond Borders*, a service-learning course offered by the Department of Computing. The course, which is open to all students, focuses on using programming skills to meet social needs. In 2016 and 2017, the project centered on the development of computer-aided edutainment products for special education needs children. The projects and the collaborating partners were carefully chosen so as to achieve maximal learning impact for our students while at the same time fulfilling a needed service that is not currently met by the commercial sector. Analyses of our students' products show that even though all of these are undergraduate students and many of them are not from computer science or engineering, they are able to develop a product that works well and can be deployed in situ for real use and that the design of the course and project helped to address many of the issues with motivation and engagement that were witnessed in previous similar courses.

Keywords Assistive technology · Special education needs · Computer-aided learning · Non-major students · Computational thinking

10.1 Overview of Technology Beyond Borders

Our subject is named, "Technology Beyond Borders: Service Learning across Cultural, Ethnic and Community Lines." (Technology Beyond Borders). The design of this subject emphasizes hands-on tasks, involving team as well as individual work. Students are encouraged to research on specific problems and challenged to design and implement a solution, applying their knowledge in information technology to solving social problems. The development and infrastructure projects

P. H. F. Ng (✉) · M. W. H. Chiu
Department of Computing, The Hong Kong Polytechnic University, Hunghom, Hong Kong
e-mail: cshfng@comp.polyu.edu.hk

M. W. H. Chiu
e-mail: cswhchiu@comp.polyu.edu.hk

D. T. L. Shek et al. (eds.), *Service-Learning for Youth Leadership*,
Quality of Life in Asia 12, https://doi.org/10.1007/978-981-13-0448-4_10

allow students to design and develop IT solutions for underprivileged communities or non-governmental organizations (NGOs).

In 2016 and 2017, the theme of this subject was interactive and educational computer games. In this chapter, we will share the experience of teaching game programming skills to achieve this objective.

Teaching game programming is not an easy task in computer science. It is hard to transfer the knowledge of game design, such as reinforcement model, reward system, and gamification. It is also hard to set up studio-based learning and create some meaningful game for the society in the space of just one course. It is made even more difficult by the fact that this subject is not restricted to computer science students, but is also made available to students from other disciplines as a general education course.

The setting of a service learning subject allows us to create an intentionality environment and subject setting to teach programming concepts and to motivate our students through constructivist teaching. By creating meaningful interactive products, we show computer science students with concrete examples and experience that programming skills are meaningful to our society. By learning the computing and programming skills necessary to create a workable computer game that can be deployed to the community partner, we demonstrate to non-computer science students that computational thinking is not something that is so difficult as to be unlearnable, and we also demonstrate how even introductory computational skills can be used to serve niche populations in the community. The teaching team and the students have also interacted at length and formed strong relationships.

10.1.1 Objectives of Technology Beyond Borders

The focus of this subject is the digital divide, the impact of technology on the community, and how responsible use of technology can contribute to the betterment of needy individuals and communities. The formal objectives of this subject are:

1. To introduce the concept and practice of learning through community service to our students.
2. To increase our students' awareness and knowledge of communities that are cultural, ethnically, or socially distinct from their own.
3. To acquaint students with significant issues of social needs, justice, and ethics related to the information age, such as the concept of the information divide and how technology may be used to meet these needs.
4. To cultivate an awareness of information ethics and professional responsibility in our students.
5. To nurture a sense of civic responsibility and engagement in our students.

Similarly, the intended learning outcomes state that upon completion of the subject, students should be able to:

1. Demonstrate an awareness of the impact of the information/digital divide, and the linkage between social disadvantages and the availability of appropriate technology.
2. Demonstrate an awareness of the impact of culture and ethnicity, and empathy for the preconceptions, concerns, and needs faced by disadvantaged individuals or community groups.
3. Articulate the needs of the underprivileged in society, analyze complex issues in the service setting and design, implement or deploy appropriate and ethical technological solutions to meet the needs of the target recipients.
4. Work effectively in teams to solve problems encountered in planning and delivering the service.
5. Communicate effectively with clients and/or other stakeholders.
6. Reflect on the relationship between their service learning activities and experiences with the academic content of the subject, in particular, the needs of the underprivileged in society and their discipline and sense of civic responsibility, especially about use and deployment of technological solutions.

10.1.2 Subject Setting of Technology Beyond Borders

The core concept of Technology Beyond Borders can be summarized in Fig. 10.1. We have created an intentionality environment and subject setting to motivate our students. First, lectures were provided to introduce the concept of service learning, digital divide, usability, and human–computer interaction (HCI), the latter two in the context of developing products for mentally and physically impaired children. By increasing the awareness of the empathy for the preconceptions, and needs faced by disadvantaged groups, the objectives of our subjects can be delivered to our students. The real-life setting of our course also motivates students to be responsible and active learners.

After the academic concepts were delivered, workshops were provided to teach necessary skills, such as the basic concept of game programming, game logic and mechanism, computer graphics, and animation. Since our subject is not intended as a computer science subject, we focus on the skills and skip the theory of these topics. Only task-based materials and examples of Unity3D were created and provided to students, who were then facilitated to practice these skills in laboratory and through exercises. The objective was to equip students with the basic technical skill to integrate the task-based example into their prototypes.

After that, we apply the constructivist teaching approach as shown in the cycle of Fig. 10.1. A preparatory visit was organized to bring students to meet the people

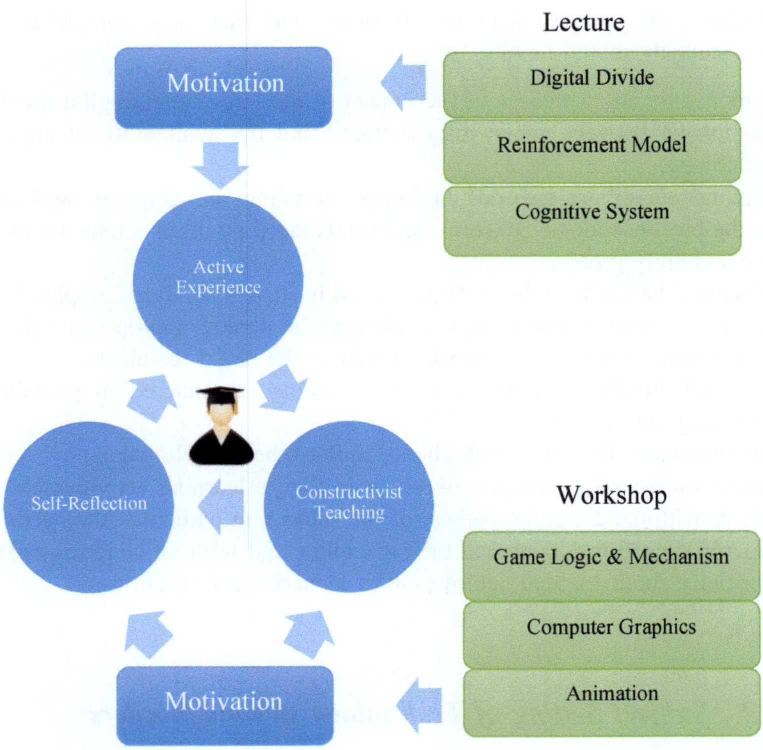

Fig. 10.1 Core concept of Technology Beyond Borders

who would ultimately be using their games, through which they could observe and learn their needs and constraints which would inform their design. These findings were then used to construct the prototype. Follow-on visits allowed students to test their prototype in situ. To encourage and facilitate learning from these experiential activities, students were asked to write a self-reflective journal for each cycle, in which they were required to expand on their experience and link it to the academic concepts taught in class. This journal is assessed for student learning, along with their performance and attitude during each visit. Therefore, their knowledge can be actively constructed.

The students' work in the quality of the prototype and product is also assessed. Unlike traditional assignments in computer science, we do not provide concrete requirements, as identifying the constraints and needs of the users is part of the assignment. Students took the lead in proposing a design, and, once accepted, created the user requirements by themselves. We acted as a facilitator to teach and provide support for the technical content for development in each regular meeting. In this sense, the concept is similar to a flipped classroom (Anderson-Patton & Bass, 2000; Bergmann & Sams, 2012).

10.1.3 Assessment of Technology Beyond Borders

The core concept of our assessment is to allow failure and refinement. Unlike traditional undergraduate projects that are assessed once only, the prototypes, reflective journals, and the conduct of service will be assessed multiple times throughout our subject. This also means that even if we judge the design and the user requirements of our students as not perfect, we would not reject their ideas and would encourage them to try and explore further. To support the students, we provided consultation sessions where students could get suggestions and technical help. In the spirit of iterative design and refinement, students were encouraged to create the prototype first, test, observe, and reflect on the effectiveness and usability, and from this feedback, refine the prototype.

To reinforce the importance of this iterative process, the course assessment is designed to be continuous, reflecting improvement and learning over the entire process, unlike many computer science project courses where the assessment grade is based on the final product only.

1. Preparation phase (30%)

   The first assessment component reflects the extent to which students are able to learn and practice the skills to design and build the first prototype after the classroom lectures and workshops. The evaluation will be based on the following criteria.

- Quality of proposal/design (team evaluation)
- Teamwork, participation, performance in the lessons (individual evaluation)
- Quality of their first prototype (team evaluation)

2. Execution (40%)

   The second-stage evaluation reflects students' ability to conduct on-site evaluations of their prototypes, and their ability to realize these observations into refinement of their product. The evaluation will be based on the following criteria.

- Quality of service provided during the testing of prototype (individual evaluation)
- Responsibility, contribution, teamwork, adaptability/flexibility, empathy, attitude, etc.
- Quality of their final product (team evaluation)

3. Reflections (30%)

   Reflections provide an intentional and structured means for students to learn from their experiences. After each visit to the community, the students were required to submit a short reflective journal. At the end of the whole course, the students were required to submit a full reflective report (around 2500 words). The evaluation was based on:

- Quality and organization of final report (individual evaluation)
- Demonstration of learning gains (individual evaluation)

10.2 Service Project

10.2.1 Criteria for Selecting Service Project

In our experiences, the service site and project have a strong relationship with the student learning experience. Therefore, it is very important that the collaborating partners be selected carefully. We wish to prepare a fruitful environment for our students to learn an awareness of the impact of culture and empathy for the preconceptions, concerns, and the needs faced by disadvantaged individuals or community groups. At the same time, we wish for them to be able to actually be in a position to contribute something tangible and beneficial in return.

We follow three criteria when we select a service site:

1. The collaborating partner should be an underprivileged community. Examples are mentally or physically impaired children, children from low-income families, or elderly. Our students need to be able to relate to the members of this community and thus develop empathy for them.
2. The service site should take students outside of their familiar comfort zone. As one of our teaching objectives is observing the need of the underprivileged community, the requirement of the client should be unique and hard to imagine from students' daily life. Therefore, the students are willing to do the observation.
3. The behavior of the client should be easy to observe and understand. Although we expect our students to be strongly motivated by the subject setting, they are not experts on human–computer interface (HCI) or multiple learning disabilities. If the behavior of the clients consists of multiple actions and complicated hierarchy, this would create too big a challenge for our students to understand and analyze.
4. We are not interested in creating direct competition with the commercial sector or putting other businesses out of work. Therefore, we also need to ensure there is no similar product on the market, and that we are serving a deserving niche community.

10.2.2 Children with Physical and Mental Impairments

Based on these three criteria, we chose to work with physically and mentally impaired children in 2016 and 2017. We collaborated with two special schools in

Hong Kong, with a total of over 200 children aged from 6 to 18. The children resident in these schools suffers from a range of conditions ranging from mild mental and physical handicaps to PMLD, or Profound and Multiple Learning Difficulties, a catch-all term that is usually associated with severe physical and mental impairments.

Working with these children in these settings matches with our requirement in a number of ways. First, many children in these settings suffer from multiple ailments, meaning that the need of each child is unique and, therefore, does not come close to the critical mass needed for the development of commercial products. The setting of these special schools is also unfamiliar to our students, most of whom have never been in close contact with severely physically or mentally impaired people. This takes them outside of the comfort zone and helps them to learn. Due to the children's mental handicaps, the interaction and reinforcement model used by the schools are simple and direct, for example, action–reaction pairs (for severely disabled children), or simple and straightforward rules (for mildly disabled children), which makes it feasible for our undergraduate students to observe and study.

10.2.3 Criteria for Forming Student Teams

Diversity was a concern on the subject. This being a computer science class, we had quite a large number of computer science students enroll. However, we wanted our students to meet and learn to work together with other students in other domains, such as design and social science. Therefore, students from different domains were invited. There were around 50 students in each year. One-third of them were from computer science, and another one-third were engineering students. The remaining were from different disciplines, including finance, design, social science. We wished the students from different disciplines to interact and mix together. Therefore, instead of allowing students to form their own groups, we adopted a hybrid approach. We allowed students to find a pair partner whom they were mutually happy to work with. Each pair was then carefully matched up with two other pairs to ensure that each group would end up with students from computer science, engineering, and a non-CS/engineering discipline.

10.3 Service Products

10.3.1 Students' Products

The service project of our subject was to create an interactive learning computer product for physical and mental impaired students. Quite unexpectedly, the products that our students developed were impressive. In 2016, out of nine interactive products, seven of them were of a high enough quality and could be deployed to the collaborating school for long-term usage.

The therapists or teachers in the special schools proposed some ideas for the games and the target competence that they wished the game to develop. Most of our student groups were happy to pick up on these ideas and develop their products along the same line. However, some students surprised us by coming up with completely unexpected ideas that also worked.

Broadly speaking, the products of our students can be divided into three categories:

Category 1: 2D edutainment

These types of products usually required lower technical skill and could conceivably be constructed using drag-and-drop programming. Most of these products were based on examples that we used for teaching in class, and were modified by the students after the observation sessions at the special schools.

Several of these products were designed to teach the children some basic concepts, such as matching (Fig. 10.2), for severely mentally disabled children, or money counting or public transport (Fig. 10.7). Some of these applications allowed the teacher to customize the game with their own pictures and videos.

Another interesting application was a mini-game that taught the concept of progression and ordering. This application allowed the teacher to input a series of images. The images will be displayed one by one when the player clicked the button. For example, one series of pictures showed the evolution from egg to chicken (Fig. 10.2). As simple as this application was, it was very popular with the severely mentally disabled children and their parents.

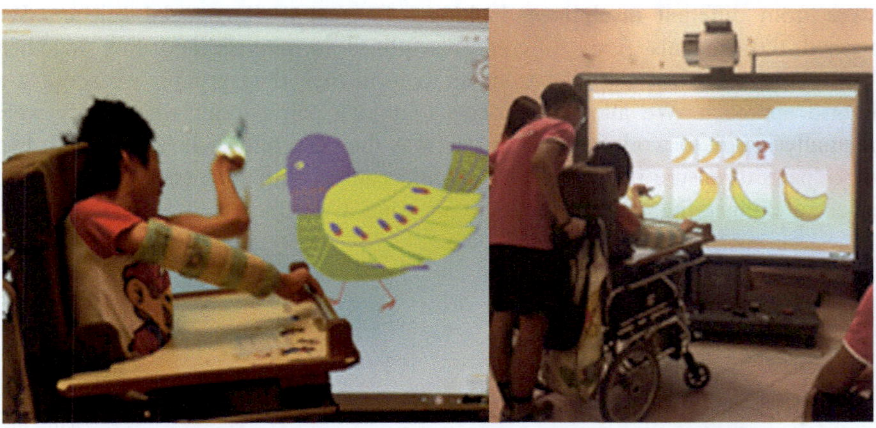

Fig. 10.2 Products in the first category designed for severely disabled children

Category 2: Gesture detection or Tangible Interaction

This category of products attempted to break out of the keyboard-video-mouse means of interaction and, in general, required higher technical skill. Most of these products used the Microsoft Kinect or the Makey Makey as an interactive input device. In general, these products required textual programming, and some of the applications even required learning about 3D graphics, invention tool, and gesture detection devices.

Figure 10.3 shows a motor training game that combines the Kinect with an exercise treadmill. The students in this group observed that part of the treatment regimen for the mentally disabled children was exercise, during which they had to stretch out their arms and move them, so that the muscles would not atrophy. Usually, a physiotherapist gives instructions, which the children follow. However, the children usually did not understand the purpose of this exercise, they felt that they were being forced to move, and their emotions were disturbed as a result. Therefore, our students designed interactive gesture detection game. The player was prompted to perform certain gestures, which were specified by the physiotherapist. If the player performed the gesture correctly, a special particle effect was played as an encouragement. Some other applications used the same paradigm to train social interaction and emotion control (Fig. 10.4). Other applications used the Makey Makey input device as a mnemonic to replace the keyboard and mouse (Fig. 10.8).

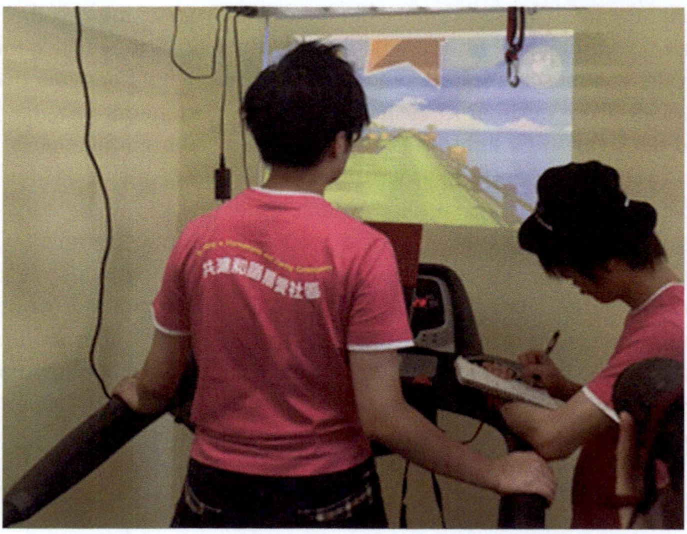

Fig. 10.3 A motor training game for mentally impaired people

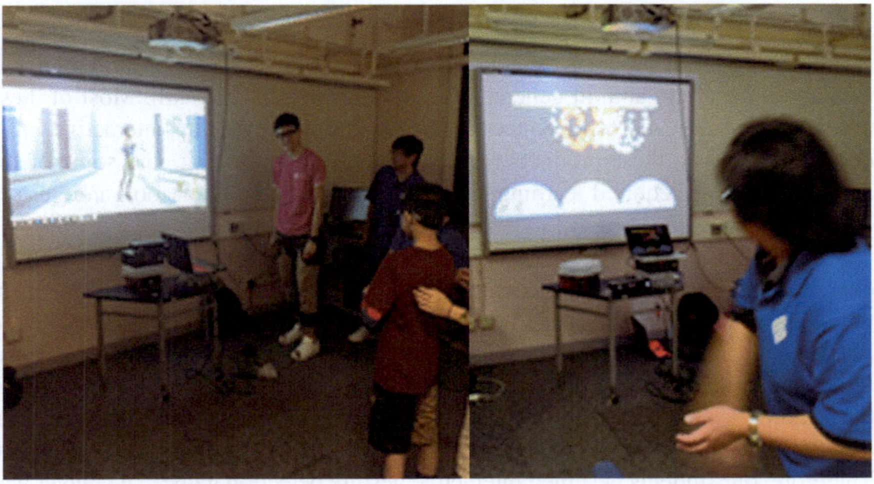

Fig. 10.4 Products using gesture detection

Category 3: Unexpected Products

The products in this category were quite unexpected and completely deviated from the keyboard-video-mouse mode of interaction. Many of these products made use of the environment or augmented the environment with electronics for enrichment. Figure 10.5 shows an example. This setup combines the Microsoft Kinect and the Philips Hue programmable LED light strips to enhance the physical facility in the special school. Children are encouraged to hold onto the overhanging rope and walk from cushion to cushion. The Kinect monitors how far they have gone, and the light strips light up as encouragement and reinforcement. A similar product, developed by another group of students, was a magic ladder with programmable LED lights and speaker, which used music and lighting effects to encourage the children to do physical exercises. Another product (Fig. 10.6) combines health monitoring with gamification. The Mi Band, which is a wearable wristband that can monitor steps and heartbeat, is used to monitor the heartbeat to ensure that the exercise session is going according to plan. Other products were a portable music player with pressure sensors to detect the posture of the body during walking, and a virtual reality (VR) application that simulated a zoo visit using a mobile phone and Google Cardboard (Figs. 10.7 and 10.8).

10.4 Quantitative Evaluation

We evaluated the efficacy of our class in several ways. For a broad overview of the class, quantitative evaluation questionnaires were designed to collect feedback from our collaborative partners and students.

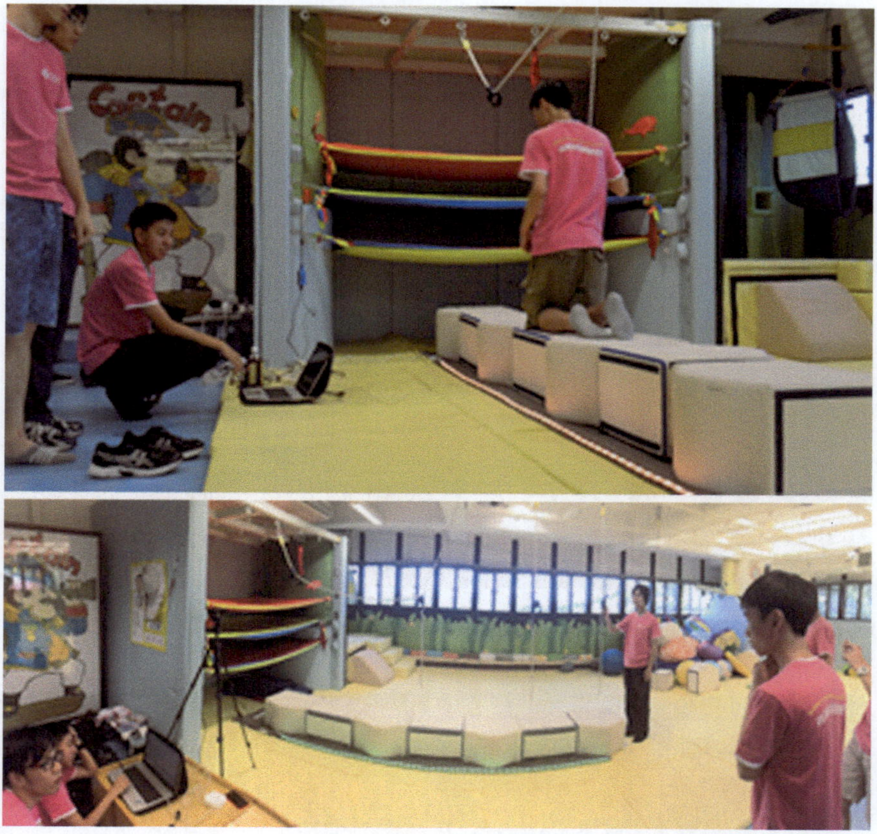

Fig. 10.5 Creative product that combines Kinect and Philips Hue

10.4.1 Feedback from Collaborative Partners

The teachers in the special schools appreciated our students' efforts. From their point of view, our students filled a much-needed service, since it was hard to find any company to create an interactive product for their children because their need was unique and the market was small. On a very encouraging note, the teachers also expressed that while they had much experience with different parties coming to do service for their children, ours was the only group that attempted to address the need for information technology and interactive training products. Figure 10.9 shows the questionnaire and the averaged feedback scores.

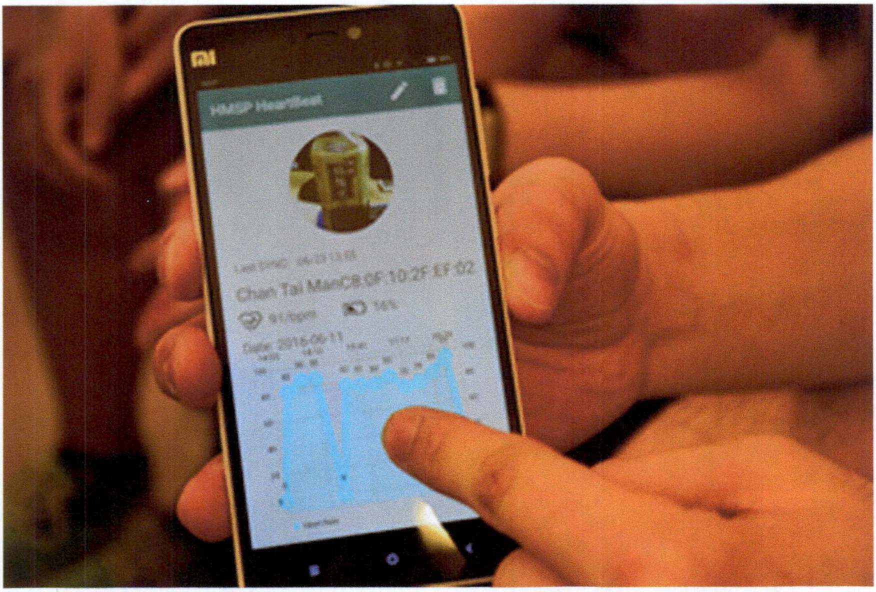

Fig. 10.6 Health monitoring application based on gamification

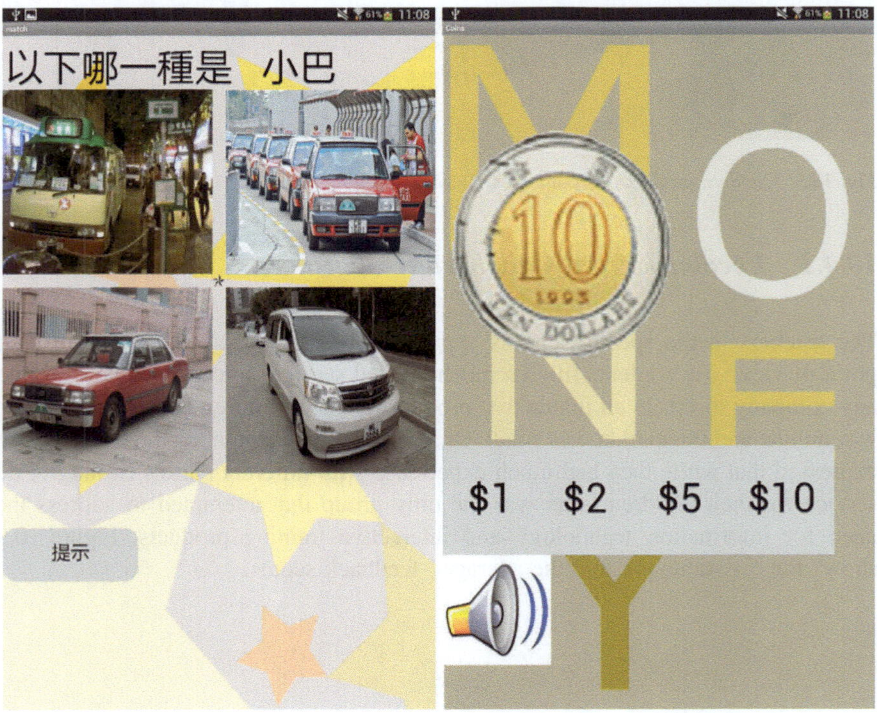

Fig. 10.7 Products in first category designed for mildly mentally disabled children

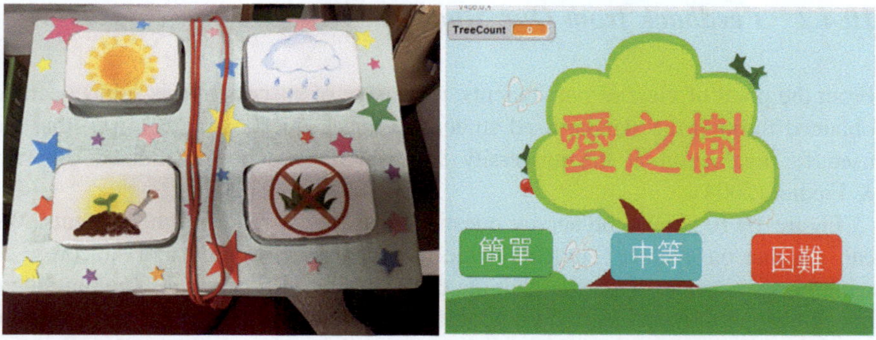

Fig. 10.8 Product of using Makey Makey in second category

	Question	Scores (2016)	Scores (2017)
Q1	Relevance of the service to the needs of your organization/clients/the community.	4	5
Q2	Interactions and communication with PolyU staff (teachers, tutors or other support staff).	5	5
Q3	Interactions and communication with PolyU students.	4	4
Q4	Responsiveness to suggestions, inputs and feedback from your organization.	4	4
Q5	Students' attitude and commitment to service.	4	4
Q6	Students' preparedness for delivering the service.	4	4
Q7	Performance of students in service delivery.	4	4
Q8	Ability of students to apply subject-related knowledge and skills to solve problems in the service setting.	3	4
Q9	Overall effectiveness of the SL Project in addressing important need(s) of your organization/clients/the community.	4	4

5=Strongly agree; 4=Agree; 3=No strong view; 2=Disagree; 1=Strongly disagree

Fig. 10.9 Collaborative partner feedback questionnaire

10.4.2 Feedback from Our Students

From the point of view of our students, a measure of success of this subject can be obtained through the standardized student feedback questionnaires (SFQ) that are used for evaluation at the university and which have been validated (Sharma & Fiedler, 2004).

Figure 10.10 shows the survey questions and the scores from the students. We can see that on average, students agree (score = 4) to strongly agree (score = 5) with the statements, suggesting that the course has been successful in helping them to achieve the intended learning outcomes. In particular, the students agree that the learning and teaching activities were helpful and that the teaching of the subject provided them with a valuable learning experience.

Figure 10.11 compares the scores across the 2 years that the subject has been offered with the department average. We note that this course tends to get higher evaluation scores than other courses in the department. We believe that part of this may well be due to the fact that students were more strongly motivated to work on this subject, as it impacted real people, which turned out to be a valuable experience for our students and assisted to create a strong connection in the relationship between student and teacher. The latter can be evidenced in the high scores of Question 6 (The staff member was helpful.) and Question 10. (The teaching of the staff member has provided me with a valuable learning experience.)

10.5 Discussion

From the quantitative evaluation results, it appears that the course objectives have been fulfilled. This section will provide a more in-depth discussion with illustrative anecdotes.

10.5.1 Building Empathy

One of the most impactful factors in this course was the internality environment. Our students were shocked during the first visit to the special schools. An example anecdote can best describe this situation. One group of students was assigned to observe and provide basic assistance for a physical education lesson for the PMLD children. The objective of the lesson was to involve the PMLD children in back-strengthening exercises to maintain the shape of their spines.

The room was colorful, relaxing music was playing, and the physical therapist and helpers were singing a song while pushing the body of the children to keep the muscles and spine elastic. This situation was supposed to be a happy moment. However, the children were screaming and crying, as they felt pain when they were

Question		2016 Mean	2017 Mean
About Subject			
Q1	I have a clear understanding of what I am expected to learn from this subject.	3.9	4.4
Q2	The teaching and learning activities (e.g., lectures, discussions, case studies, projects, etc.) have helped me to achieve the subject learning outcomes.	4	4.4
Q3	The assessments require me to demonstrate my knowledge, skills, and understanding of the subject.	4	4.4
Q4	I understand the criteria according to which I will be graded.	4	4.1
About the Staff			
Q5	The staff member's teaching was well organized with clear presentations.	4.3	4.5
Q6	The staff member was helpful.	4.4	4.6
Q7	The staff member gave useful and timely feedback on my work.	4.2	4.5
Q8	The staff member encouraged students to ask questions and discuss ideas in class.	4.2	4.5
Q9	The staff member encouraged students to find information on their own and learn independently.	4.2	4.5
Q10	The teaching of the staff member has provided me with a valuable learning experience.	4.2	4.6
Q11	Overall, I think that the staff member is an effective teacher.	4.2	4.5
Q12	Grand mean of items on Overall View	4.2	4.6
Feedback on Achievement of Learning Objects/ Outcomes			
Q13	I can link the service learning activities and experiences with the academic content of the subject.	3.9	4.3
Q14	I have learned to apply the knowledge and skills I acquired at the university to deal with complex issues in the service setting.	4.0	4.5
Q15	This subject has enabled me to reflect on my role and responsibilities both as a professional and as a responsible citizen.	3.9	4.4
Q16	I have felt more empathy towards people in need as a result of studying this subject.	3.9	4.4
Q17	I have developed a stronger sense of civic responsibility.	3.7	4.6

Fig. 10.10 Questions of the Student Feedback Questionnaire (SFQ)

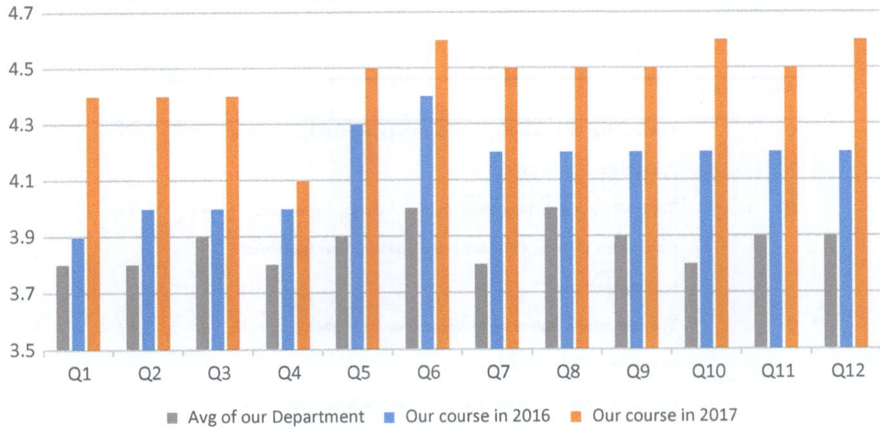

Fig. 10.11 Compared with department average—subject-based scores

forced to do the exercises. Our students were stunned and speechless when faced with this dissonant situation. Reflecting back on how even they are often reluctant to exercise, which is not always enjoyable for them, even with their healthy bodies, motivated them to think of methods that would better motivate the children to do the exercises. This example shows how this uncomfortable, dissonant environment helped our students to developed empathy for children who are very dissimilar from themselves.

In their reflective journal, most of our students wrote that they were encouraged and motivated after the first test deployment, when their prototypes were tested by the mentally impaired children. The children were happy when they were playing with our students' prototypes, which helped our students to see the impact and meaning underlying the course. This motivated them to further improve their product for the second test deployment and to polish up their prototypes into finished final products.

Another anecdote can be used to describe this situation. The product shown in Fig. 10.2 is a very simple action game. An egg is shown on the screen. The child clicked the button; then, the egg became a bird. Click the button again and the bird flies away. The group of students who developed this game had a very low level of technical expertise and, at the very beginning of the course, were completely lacking in confidence, even saying that all they wanted was just to scrape through and get a pass! However, at the first test prototype deployment, their game was a hit with the children, who were all laughing and clapping their hands after playing the game. One of the parents, who happened to be on-site helping that day, was extremely happy and spent more than 15 min talking with our students. She shared that her child had not expressed any signs of happiness for a long time, but this game had apparently got through to her. She told our students that she was so glad that she found that Hong Kong students were full of empathy and caring. Our students were a little ashamed, as they had not put the best effort into the game and had simply wanted to create something that would pass muster, but at the same time, motivated and encouraged. Their response was to put in extra effort to improve their game, adding in more meaningful content and better graphics.

10.5.2 Active Learning

To our delight, completion of the projects (and the course) did not put a full stop to students' learning. Most of our students continued to improve their prototypes for real use. One of our first-year students, Zelca, created the health monitoring application in Fig. 10.6. After the course was over, he kept improving his application, introducing a database system for persistent storage, and an enhanced version was delivered after 6 months. Zelca is a good example of how this course has nurtured students to become active learners. Some of our students have returned to the special schools and to help with their Open Day activities (Fig. 10.12).

10.6 Reflections on the Impact of the Subject

10.6.1 Learning and Teaching in Computer Science

Learning is never an effortless process. Ideally, learning should involve active reflection where students take ownership of their own learning. The high-pressure, exam-driven environment of Hong Kong, however, has produced lots of students who only study lecture slides, are passive in class, and who seek only to fulfill the basic learning objectives for a grade. Many students are neither motivated nor engaged in a lecture setting, and teaching and learning are not connected. It is extremely rare to have students combining knowledge in different subjects or demonstrate reflective thinking for transdisciplinary learning.

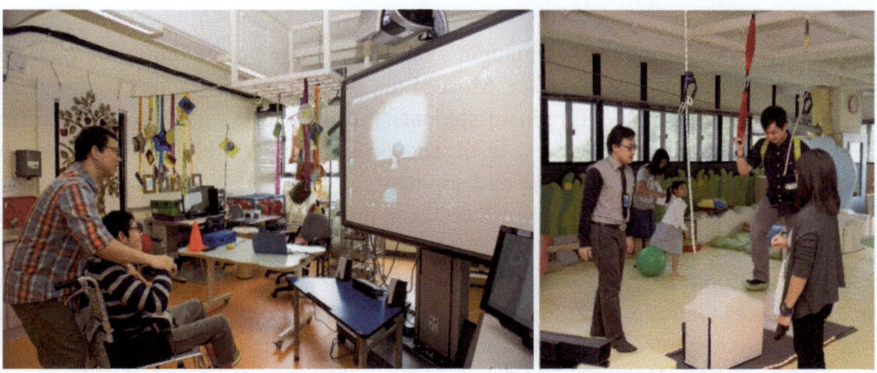

Fig. 10.12 Our students helping out at open day

Constructivist teaching is perhaps a potential solution. Constructivist teaching explains the process of how people construct knowledge through interactions with their environment. One of the core ideas is that knowledge construction is different for each person (Astin, 1996; Biggs & Tang, 2007; Hallinger & Lu, 2012). They believe that teaching is not the only channel by which knowledge is delivered. Rather, knowledge is constructed by investigation, hands-on experience, and self-reflection. Learners are the makers of meaning and knowledge. The students were put forward in real situations to observe, think, and learn.

This is relevant to us as many students think that our teaching materials and theory do not reveal knowledge to them (Perkins, 1991). This is especially true for us. Our students find it difficult to transfer and apply the theory to real-world contexts. Technology Beyond Borders provided an opportunity to facilitate our students to apply computational thinking to real-world problems, thus providing a meaningful learning cycle and a good environment. Therefore, the motivation of our students is increased. It has been shown that successful active construction of knowledge builds upon the motivation of learners (Paris & Paris, 2001). Our experience in this subject demonstrates that when students acquire information that is meaningful and important to them, they will be better motivated to connect the new information with their prior knowledge to develop better, larger, and more linked conceptual understanding (Krajcik & Blumenfeld, 2006; Pintrich, 2000). The situated learning in our subject provided students with a learning environment embedded in an authentic, real-world context. It allowed students to see the value and meaning of the project and to find interest and excitement on their own. Moreover, the knowledge acquired in a real-world situation also generalized better to a wider range of situations (Zimmerman, 2008). Solving real-world problems required transdisciplinary knowledge, and this reinforces the need for students to work interdependently with others. Through sharing, using, and debating ideas with the others, students constructed their experience and knowledge.

10.6.2 Learning and Teaching in Game Programming

The lecturers in this course have taught a course in game programming in the same department for more than 10 years. Most of the students in this game programming class were final year undergraduate students. In these 10 years, we used the traditional lecture setting. Lectures, tests, and programming exercises were used to teach the game design and game development.

From our experience, there are three common problems when teaching game programming.

First, the topic of game programming is too broad for a single subject in computer science. Game programming should be a transdisciplinary subject. It is not only about computer science. It also included design, mathematics, psychology. The techniques for developing an action game and a tile-based game are different. It is hard to cover all of the topics on one subject.

Second, the concept of game design and human-centric computing cannot be delivered to our students easily. Game programming is commonly seen as a computer science subject and attracts computer science students. It is hard to study player characteristics, reinforcement model, and cognitive system in the classroom without any real examples. It is difficult to observe real players and learn the psychology of reward, luck, and stimulus. Game development is also a huge project. Even in a simple mobile game, its gameplay and design are too complicated for a single person to learn and develop. As a result, most of the students create "copycat-like" projects, based on their own favorite games. There is little or no analysis of a target audience and its characteristics.

Third, most of our students are not motivated or engaged. Although game programming is an interesting topic, one single subject is too short. Most of their products were traditional games, such as simple action games or adventure games to fulfill the need of subject assessment and their interests. Their passion and creativity cannot be unlocked in this setting.

One way to keep students engaged is to involve them in hands-on projects, rather than working only on the problem posed in the lecture setting. However, working on an industrial project in the class is not feasible, especially for undergraduate students. It is impossible to start studio-based learning as the game development would be too complicated.

In Technology Beyond Borders, we collaborated with a real community organization serving real people. These types of community service programs are more inspiring to students and provide them with a concrete example of the relevance and importance of programming and game development. In fact, the quality of the student's projects far exceeded our expectation. They applied techniques from human–computer interaction, gesture detection, and gamification to create different game-based learning application, health monitoring application, motor, and cognitive training application. For example, the motor training game for mentally impaired people shown in Fig. 10.3 combines game development, motion detection, tangible interaction, and the physical equipment in the special school. This subject therefore demonstrates that game programming is not only for entertainment. Our students were motivated and educated about how technology can be helpful, even for severely mentally impaired individuals. Our students were also facilitated in reflecting on their roles in society, especially in the context of being an information technology professional in an increasingly digital and information society.

This course has one additional benefit. Gaming is often perceived by the general public as being a waste of time and unimportant. Gamers, and game developers, are often labeled as being antisocial outcasts who do not contribute meaningful value to society. Through this course, however, we have the opportunity to improve the public's awareness of the importance of programming and the contribution of computer games.

References

Anderson-Patton, V., & Bass, L. (2000). How well did we structure and model a self-study stance? Two self-studies of imposing self-studies using teaching portfolios. In J. Loughran & T. Russell (Eds.), *Exploring myths and legends of teacher education: Proceedings of the third international conference on self-study of teacher education practices* (pp. 10–14). Kingston Canada: Queen's University.

Astin, A. (1996). Involvement in learning revisited: Lessons we have learned. *Journal of College Student Development, 37*(2), 123–134.

Bergmann, J., & Sams, A. (2012). *Flip your classroom: Reach every student in every class every day*. Washington, DC: International Society for Technology in Education; Association for Supervision and Curriculum Development.

Biggs, J., & Tang, C. (2007). *Teaching for quality learning at university* (3rd ed.). Buckingham: Open University Press/ Society for Research in Higher Education.

Hallinger, P., & Lu, J. F. (2012). Overcoming the Walmart syndrome: Adapting problem-based management education in East Asia. *Interdisciplinary Journal of problem-Based Learning, 6*(1), 16–42.

Krajcik, J. S., & Blumenfeld, P. (2006). Project-based learning. In *The Cambridge handbook of the learning sciences.* New York: Cambridge.

Paris, S. G., & Paris, A. H. (2001). Classroom applications of research on self-regulated learning. *Educational Psychologist, 36*(2), 89–101. https://doi.org/10.1207/S15326985EP3602_4.

Perkins, D. N. (1991). What constructivism demands of the learner. *Educational Technology, 31*(9), 18–23.

Pintrich, P. R. (2000). The role of goal orientation in self-regulated learning. *Handbook of self-regulation* (pp. 451–502). San Diego, CA: Academic Press.

Sharma, P., & Fiedler, S. (2004). Introducing technologies and practices for supporting self-organzied learning in a hybrid environment. In K. Tochtermann & H. Maurer (Eds.), *Proceedings of i-Know* (pp. 543–550).

Zimmerman, B. J. (2008). Investigating self-regulation and motivation: Historical background, methodological developments, and future prospects. *American Educational Research Journal, 45*(1), 166–183. https://doi.org/10.3102/0002831207312909.

Chapter 11
Promoting Quality of Life Through Fashion for Function and Design

Charlotte S. Y. Lai, Patrick C. L. Hui and Frency S. F. Ng

Abstract This study investigates the impacts on promoting quality of life to university students and program teacher whom participated in a fashion-related service learning after they have been experienced in a series of planned activities. Qualitative research approach is adopted in this research through the reflection reports submitted by each student and an interview with the program teacher. The results reflected that there is promotion of quality of life for students in three major areas: social well-being, emotional well-being, and development and activity while there is no impact on material well-being and physical well-being. The findings indicate the service-learning program provides a platform for students' development on relationship with others, self-emotional training and the ability development which match with the objective of the service-learning program. Fashion element is also a key focus of this study as a communication medium between participated students and service recipients in various tasks and activities.

Keywords Service-learning · Quality of life · Qualitative analysis
Student development · Fashion program

11.1 Introduction

In recent years, experiential teaching methods have been widely used in all levels of education in order to provide more opportunities for students of different ages to engage hands-on with various situations. The most common types of experiential

C. S. Y. Lai (✉) · P. C. L. Hui · F. S. F. Ng
Institute of Textiles and Clothing, The Hong Kong Polytechnic University,
Hunghom, Hong Kong
e-mail: charlotte-sy.lai@connect.polyu.hk

P. C. L. Hui
e-mail: tchuip@polyu.edu.hk

F. S. F. Ng
e-mail: tcngsf@connect.polyu.hk

D. T. L. Shek et al. (eds.), *Service-Learning for Youth Leadership*,
Quality of Life in Asia 12, https://doi.org/10.1007/978-981-13-0448-4_11

learning methods are project-based activities, work-integrated education, internships, and service learning (SL) (Jackson & Wilton, 2016; Ngai, Moon, & Poon, 2012; Smith, 2012). Research into experiential learning has been done on students' benefits from adding this type of program to traditional classroom learning. According to some previous studies (Deeley, 2010; Sandaran, 2012), SL is described as a kind of education, a philosophy, and a phenomenon.

Among of all other experiential learning programs, SL programs are the most effective experiential-based pedagogy, with the major difference being the inclusion of a social/civic service element in the well-designed activities/exercises (Deeley, 2010; Hebert & Hauf, 2015). The learning process of students participating in an SL program takes place not only from the instruction given by the teaching staff or by any teaching materials, but also from students' own direct experiences through undertaking the various well-planned activities. These experiences are able to provide students immediate feelings and strengthen their learning memory; this is the major difference between traditional classroom teaching and experiential teaching.

Apart from the differences from the traditional teaching methods, an SL program also, unlike other forms of experiential-based teaching, includes social/civic services in the activities designed together with educational training objectives (Bringle & Hatcher, 1999). A SL program providing institute has to partner with organization(s) in society in planning in order to design suitable activities for the participating students to meet and work with people in need and, at the same time, let students apply hands-on their professional knowledge in real-life cases (Bruce-Davis & Chancey, 2012; Mahasneh, Tawalbeh, Al-Smadi, Ghaith, & Dajani, 2012). Because there are two main elements in an SL program, social/civic service and educational goals, detailed and well-planned activities are essential, so that students can simultaneously obtain subject knowledge and skills and provide social services to a community. Such direct experiences inevitably benefit the students' professional and personal development, in turn, to promote and enhance their quality of life in the future.

11.2 Learning Experience and Reflection

The critical part of an experiential-based learning program is the direct experience given to the students in their hands-on tasks and in facing the different challenges they may encounter in the learning process (Deeley, 2010). Through the direct involvement in the well-planned activities/exercises, students in an SL program are able to develop their ability in delivering social services, in acquiring knowledge and skill, and in being aware their roles and responsibilities to the society or community they live in; and thus, the targeted educational goals can be achieved (Watson, 2002).

Reflection is a kind of expression to show the result of the learning objective of a well-planned program (Bringle & Hatcher, 1999). Students' learning through experiences in an SL program is considered as a transformation process from the direct feeling of their experience during the process of undertaking the planned activities to achieve the stipulated learning objectives. Self-evaluation or reflection can be used to examine the effectiveness of the learning experience given to the students. According to Dewey (1916), experience could be defined as educative in four specific conditions: "(a) it must generate interest in the learner; (b) it must be intrinsically worthwhile to the learner; (c) it must present problems that awaken new curiosity and create a demand for information; and (d) it must cover a considerable time span and foster development over time" (Bringle & Hatcher, 1999, p. 114). Therefore, reflection for a well-planned program should not only refer to the knowledge given to the participating students, but also refer to the experiences related to the enhancement of their quality of life in the future. Indeed, it is the foundation to assess the effectiveness of achieving the targeted learning objectives by the program providers.

11.3 Quality of Life

Different people have their own explanations of the meaning of "quality of life." According to Felce and Perry (1995), five main domains were used to define this meaning. The first domain is social well-being, which further refers to two main sub-domains: interpersonal relationships and community involvement. Interpersonal relationships include one's relationship with the people around them, including family, friends, and acquaintances; while community involvement identifies the level of acceptance and support of one's society and community as well as the involvement in the activities/events that are accomplished with it. The second domain is emotional well-being, which can be divided into six factors: satisfaction, fulfillment, status and respect, faith and belief, positive affect, and self-esteem. The third dimension is development and activity, which refers to productivity and contributions from competence and independence, job, homelife and housework, leisure and hobbies, and education. The fourth domain is material well-being, which is considered to be the stability and security from financial assets, housing quality and neighborhood, personal privacy, transportation, possessions, and quality of food. The last domain is physical well-being, which refers to one's health, fitness, mobility, and personal safety. Based on these five domains, this study investigates how students' and service recipients' quality of life can be promoted after participating in a fashion-related SL program.

11.4 Methodology

The objective of this study is to investigate whether participating in a fashion-related service-learning program can enhance the students' and service recipients' quality of life in the future. To achieve this research aim, a qualitative research approach was adopted to analyze the gains of the SL program from the perspectives of the students who participant in a fashion-related service-learning program. In addition, the subject lecturers would be reflected the impact of the quality of life on service recipients upon they joined this SL program.

11.5 The Fashion-Related Service-Learning Program

The program under study is titled "Engaging Fashion as a Communication Media for the Needy" and held at the Hong Kong Polytechnic University. Its main feature is to give an opportunity for the student participants to co-work with the service recipients (i.e., people with different disabilities) to develop the recipients' fashion and design talents. In this program, students will work closely with these needy people in outfit design, fashion illustration, material selection and preparation, and garment making; and finally in showcasing the final products. The whole program will be held for two academic semesters with four phases. Different well-designed activities are planned for each of these phases. Students will be guided to make use of their learned subject-related knowledge and technical skills to implement those required tasks. Throughout the four phases, intensive communications and close interpersonal relationships will be necessary for students to develop with various stakeholders in the program and, beyond doubt, with the service recipients.

In Phase 1, the program organizing department will work with the nongovernmental organizations (NGO) to access to the potential service recipients, referring to the people in need, who are interested in participating in this program. In Phase 2, the program organizer will arrange workshops either on the university campus or on site of the NGO's venues in order to provide students opportunities to meet the service recipients in person. Students and the service recipients will work on the designs and illustrations for the outfits they are going to create, so communication is crucial during the time they are given to work on the task. After collecting all the designs from this phase, a committee is setup by the program organizer to select twenty designs by considering the concept of the designs and the appearance of the outfits, as well as the background story of the designers (service recipients).

In Phase 3, the best 20 designs will proceed to the garment-making process. In this phase, students will be formed into groups to complete the entire garment-making process from fabric selection, pattern development, and cutting and sewing to the final fitting procedures. The designers (i.e., service recipients) will take less part in this phase, as they might not able to participate due to their disability, but they would keep working with the students to ensure the design keeps in line with their original ideas. Professional training is required in this phase, which will provide students with subject-related knowledge and technical skills to handle a complete garment-making process. In Phase 4, a show performance will be conducted, allowing the outfit designers and students to showcase their final products onstage. This specially arranged fashion show gives a chance for members of both sides of the groups to communicate and cooperate to work out the performance.

The activities designed across all four phases are targeted to give special training to students to combine the knowledge and skills they have acquired in the classroom with real-life challenges, and with additional skill sets they could further developed.

11.6 Data Collections

In this study, a qualitative research approach is adopted in which the reflection reports from the participating students were collected after they have completed the program. The use of reflective reports is common in evaluating experiential learning programs, including SL programs (Bringle & Hatcher, 1999); hence, students can express their personal feelings and thoughts about program activities as well as their direct experiences in detail. All the information in the reports is relatively in-depth and thus provides the program organizer with more details to understand what the students experienced during the program. Insights from the findings not only benefit the program design and activity planning but also the understanding of the various benefits the students can obtain, particularly those related to the enhancement of their quality of life in the future.

In the current study, each of all students who participated in the SL program, "Engaging Fashion as a Communication Media for the Needy," in the academic year of 2016–2017 was required to submit a reflection report to record their activities undertaken in the entire learning process as well as to express their feelings about the learning experiences during and after participating in the well-designed activities of the SL program. A total of 92 reports (representing 92 students' reflection of mentioned program) were received and reviewed for data analysis.

Prior to undertake the content review, a set of common codes was developed in line with the five major domains of quality of life as suggested by Felce and Perry (1995), that is, social well-being, emotional well-being, development and activity, material well-being, and physical well-being. Based on the words, concepts, and ideas the students had written in the reflective reports, their feelings on these areas were identified. A set of induced keywords were generated for each domain/sub-domain of the above-mentioned quality of life (see Table 11.1). The provided information in the reports was then analyzed to explore the values of the SL program students perceived, particularly in promotion of their quality of life.

Through an intensive review, the pre-set codes were assigned to the relevant content of each report, so as to identify and classify the feelings of the participating students toward the gains from the SL program.

11.7 Data Analysis and Results

The content of the reflective reports were analyzed based on Felce and Perry's (1995) five major domains of quality of life. Various sub-domains under each of the five domains are further elaborated upon the meaning of each area. In the coding process, the contents in each report were scrutinized. Corresponding codes were assigned to the relevant words, concepts, and ideas the students had written in their reflection reports. For individual reports, once a code was assigned to reflect a domain/sub-domain, irrespective of number of times, it would be counted as one and only one.

The coding results are summarized in Table 11.1, with a total of 383 reflection results included. In which, 193 reflection results from the reports were coded for the major domain of "social well-being." Of which, 78 reflections were recorded a positive feedback on the first sub-domain of interpersonal relationships—including eight (8.7% of all students) on the gains of interpersonal relationships with family and household life and 70 (76.1%) on the gains with friends and social life; while 115 positive reflections were recorded for the other sub-domain of community involvement—including 57 students (62%) agreed that they have benefits from the community involvement through the relevant activities and events, and 58 students (63%) reported the acceptance and support of community involvement increased.

For the second major domain of "emotional well-being," there are six sub-domains (i.e., positive affect, status/respect, satisfaction, fulfillment, faith/belief, and self-esteem). Result shows that there are a total of 102 reflections representing these six sub-domains. In which, 21 students (22.8%) revealed that they benefited from the positive affect during the SL program, seven reports (7.6%) indicated that students benefited from status and respect, 31 students (33.7%) showed their gains from satisfaction during the program, 12 reports (13%) mentioned the increase of quality of life from the program fulfillment; while 15 (16.3%) from faith/belief and 16 (17.4%) from self-esteem.

Third, a total of 88 reports indicated improvements on the quality of life in regard to the "development and activity" domain; including 56 (60.9%) on the improvement of competence and independence, one (1.1%) on the house-life and housework, and another one (1.1%) on the leisure/hobbies; while 10 (10.9%) reported the gains on education-related issues and 20 (21.7%) on the productivity/contribution.

For the other two domains of quality of life—material well-being and physical well-being—unexpectedly, no report was reported, implying the gains for the enhancement of the quality of life in these two areas was not existed.

Table 11.1 Impact on quality of life in SL program based on the students' perceptives

Domain	Sub-domain	Element	Code	Induced keywords	No. of students $N = 92$
Social well-being	Interpersonal relationships	Family/ household life	A11	Family, better relationships with family members	8 (8.7%)
		Relatives	A12	–	0 (0%)
		Friends and social life	A13	Teamwork, communication, cooperate, discussion	70 (76.1%)
	Community involvement	Activities and events	A21	Social service, visit people in need, meaning activities, volunteer work	57 (62%)
		Acceptance and support	A22	"feel the love," understand, patient, effort	58 (63%)
Emotional well-being	Positive affect		B1	Feel positive, "can do," happiness, meaningful, grateful, thankful	21 (22.8%)
	Status/respect		B2	Citizen	7 (7.6%)
	Satisfaction		B3	Satisfy, satisfaction, achievement, valuable experience	31 (33.7%)
	Fulfillment		B4	Fulfill, fulfillment, complete the tasks, responsible, experience	12 (13%)
	Faith/belief		B5	Support, positive	15 (16.3%)
	Self-esteem		B6	Gained, stronger, improve	16 (17.4%)
Development and activity	Competence/ Independence		C1	Complete independently, finish by myself, responsibility, task	56 (60.9%)
	Job		C2	–	0 (0%)
	Homelife/ housework		C3	Living environment	1 (1.1%)
	Leisure/ hobbies		C4	Interest	1 (1.1%)
	Education		C5	Learn, knowledge, professional	10 (10.9%)
		Productivity/ contribution	C6	Contribute, complete, solve problem	20 (21.7%)

(continued)

Table 11.1 (continued)

Domain	Sub-domain	Element	Code	Induced keywords	No. of students $N = 92$
Material well-being	Finance/ income		D1	–	0 (0%)
	Housing quality		D2	–	0 (0%)
	Neighborhood		D3	–	0 (0%)
	Privacy		D4	–	0 (0%)
	Transport		D5	–	0 (0%)
	Possessions		D6	–	0 (0%)
	Meals/food		D7	–	0 (0%)
Physical well-being	Health		E1	–	0 (0%)
	Fitness		E2	–	0 (0%)
	Mobility		E3	–	0 (0%)
	Personal safety		E4	–	0 (0%)

11.8 Discussions and Implications

According to the data analysis results, a number of implications were generated toward the understanding of how participation in a SL program may benefit a student's professional and personal development, particularly in the enhancement of quality of life in his/her future.

11.9 Implications of Social Well-Being

The perceived gains in view of social well-being of the life quality attracted the highest attention. From the result in the reflective reports, the students who participated in the SL program under study showed that they have mostly gained on the domain of social well-being specifically in the enhancement of interpersonal relationships and the community involvement.

11.10 Interpersonal Relationships

Through the planned activities and events of the SL program, students were required to become involved in the interpersonal communications with different parties, that is, service recipients, teammates, program leader, teaching helpers, and the staff working in the corresponding organizations. In the two semesters, students have first to meet with the service recipients to confirm the design; then, to select suitable materials and work out the garment with the teammates as well as the program helpers; and, finally, to prepare the final runway show with the designers. During this process, students have to build strong relationships and to conduct close communication with all stakeholders in order to complete the tasks.

Most of the reflection reports (i.e., 70 reports) showed that students most benefited from the communication with their teammates as well as with the service recipients. Students described their experiences from the first time meeting with the service recipients to the end of the program of conducting the performance show. Through the experiences along the entire learning process, they were required to communicate and cooperate with their teammates to achieve the assigned tasks. Since the teams were formed with students from different countries (i.e., nonlocal students) and different study disciplines (i.e., students who have no fashion and textiles background), the participating students have a chance to work with teammates of different backgrounds. The intention of mixing students in a team is to prepare them for their future working environment in meeting clients and colleagues from different cultures and backgrounds. Through the feedback from the 70 reports, the learning objective is confirmed successful, as students have experienced in problem-solving together with peers who were having different abilities and opinions. The high score in this aspect implies that students obtained positive experience in this domain of quality of life.

The interpersonal relationships in friends and social life refers not only to the peer groups but also to the social circle involved in the program, including the various participating parties in the program, especially those needy service recipients. Most of all students admitted that they did not have experience of getting along with this kind of needy people before. This program provided them a valuable experience to know and spend time with these people. In this perspective, students' communication skills to work with people who required special attention and communication methods can be enhanced. Also, students expressed that such experience might help them to develop communication skills toward clients with special requirements for their future career.

In addition, some students also mentioned that during the process of making the outfit their communications with the program leader as well as with program helpers were also enhanced. In the garment-making process, the program leader and helpers provided many comments and experience-sharing with the students, which built a positive communication channel and environment for students to absorb their valuable experiences. Students not only appreciated their immediate help but also developed a way of working with experienced people in their future working environments.

11.11 Community Involvement

There are two sub-domains under community involvement: activities and events and acceptance and support. A total of 115 positive feedbacks were found, demonstrating the quality of life in these two areas can be promoted. For the first sub-domain of activities and events, students reported that they have zero or rare chances of connecting with people in need prior to joining the program. This is their first experience of working closely with this group of people; their feeling was positive. The students also mentioned that they used to know the information from major media but not directly from these groups of people being neglected. In this program, they gained experience with more understanding of the society they are living in and the needs of the minorities. Moreover, this experience is not only a one-off chance getting along with the people in need but enhanced the chance of students to participate in relevant social services and civic activities.

For the second sub-domain of "acceptance and support," students mentioned that the assigned activities in the SL program provided considerable time for them and the service recipients to get to know each other. After the work, 58 students revealed that they had changed their perceptions of the service recipients in certain ways, for example, their talent in design, their optimism toward their own disabilities, and their love with their families/caretakers as well as with other disadvantages people. In cosmopolitan places, like Hong Kong, the relationship between the majority and the people with special needs is distant; thus, this is a valuable experience for university students to know more about a group of people that is often ignored.

11.12 Implications of Emotional Well-Being

There are six sub-domains under emotional well-being, which all represent students' emotional gains in different areas to promote their quality of life after they completed the SL program. The first sub-domain is positive affect; for which, 21 students (22.8%) mentioned in their reflective reports that they have a positive attitude toward this sub-domain. Further, two types of positive affect were mentioned by the students. For the first type, students were having a positive attitude toward different kinds of difficulties, as they were impressed by the people in need after they spent time with them; while for the second type, students have discovered their problem-solving abilities, as they have to handle different tasks with people not familiar to them. The quality of life was promoted as students having a positive attitude toward the handling of future problems; thus, they would remain positive to deal with those issues.

The second sub-domain under emotional well-being refers to status and respect. Seven students (7.6%) reported that they have positive results of respecting the others' status and abilities. Indeed, the SL program provided students opportunities to appreciate and respect others' abilities (including disadvantage people) and the help offered during different stages of the program. For the third sub-domain of satisfaction, 31 (33.7%) students reported that they have gained satisfied feeling after participating the activities and events in the program in the following two major areas. One satisfaction feeling comes from students who feel they were able to offer help to the people in need; this means that they have positive feelings in helping people as well as in knowing the people they helped were happy. Another satisfaction feeling came from the completion of the tasks in the planned program activities and events; for example, students confirmed their ability to handle different problems in real-life cases.

In relation to the fourth sub-domain of "fulfillment," 12 students reported that they felt good after fulfilled the tasks and activities, as the achievement on the tasks completion give them positive encouragement. The fifth sub-domain is "faith and belief." In the students' reflection reports, 15 students showed there were changes on their faiths and believes toward different issues, like the situations of the society, the positive encouragements by and the abilities of people in need, and the students' own abilities. The last sub-domain of emotion well-being is "self-esteem." The SL program had brought the students positive changes on how they perceive their self-esteem after the participation of the activities and working with different corresponding parties. Sixteen students reported their confidence, and self-esteem was enhanced through the completion of the outfit, the help for the people in need, and even the awards they won.

11.13 Implications of Development and Activity

Five sub-domains fall under the "development and activity" domain in the promotion of quality of life; they are: competence/independence, job, homelife/housework, leisure/hobbies, and education. There is another construct that representing the result and/or outcome generated by the above-mentioned five sub-domains which is productivity/contribution.

The first sub-domain, competence/independence, was reflecting the students' self-feeling on the promotion of quality of life by their confidence on completing the tasks successfully especially on their own ability. Fifty-six students have the positive reflection on this sub-domain. However, there is no student showing their gains on the second sub-domain of "job"; this is probably because they do not consider the activities in the program as a formal job but service. Only one student mentioned his/her perception in the area of the third sub-domain—homelife/housework, and one other student on the fourth sub-domain of leisure/hobbies. This result represents that only a limit of students has benefits from these two areas. Nonetheless, ten students showed their attitude toward the gains in education-related issues, considered as the fifth sub-domain, from participating in the activities and events of the program. Most of the gains of this sub-domain were from the practical skillsets of garment-making process, while some others are related to the problem-solving skills. The sixth elements—productivity/contribution—is referring to the result of the five sub-domains, and 20 students have positive feeling on the promotion of quality of life on their productivity and contribution on the tasks given in the SL program.

11.14 Implications of Material Well-Being and Physical Well-Being

Unexpectedly, no student mentions any gains in view of the last two domains—material well-being and physical well-being. It is probably because the captured SL program is planned to provide students training on promoting quality of life in the other three areas—that is, social well-being, emotional well-being, and development and activities—through the provision of social services to people in need. In the design of the SL program, there is no connection to the finance, food, housing, and transportation issues which fall under the material well-being; nor the health, fitness, mobility, and personal safety issues that fall into the physical well-being category.

11.15 Teachers' Reflection

From our observation, we believe that the SL experience has broadened students' horizon to encompass societal concerns. The students have become more mature at the end of the course, and their views about the needy have become more positive too. We also observed that the tangible benefits to the service recipients in the SL program are that through working with our students they can acquire some basic ideas and skills for the creation of a fashion design, and improves communication with their relatives and caretakers. They become aware that they have their own abilities, and their dream can be realized with assistance. We believe that the process is important to the service recipients. The fashion design process has served as a means for them to demonstrate their creativity and therefore helps them rebuild their self-confidence and self-esteem. Through interacting with students, the service recipients also improve their communication capability and hence are able to better collaborate with others and better integrate into the community. Many of the service recipients told us that this fashion-related SL subject was an important and happy event for them in their life. We believe that we have fulfilled our goal of using fashion as a medium for communicating with and caring for the needy.

11.16 Conclusion

This study is focusing on a fashion-related SL program, which means fashion is a very critical element in this program in generating special learning experiences to the students. Fashion and clothing are very important and special products in people's daily lives. It can refer either to essential items or to luxury elements to enhance one's image (Goldsmith, Flynn, & Moore, 1996; O'Cass, 2004; Woodward, 2007). People have different explanations of "fashion" in terms of the function, use of fabrication, design, price, brand, and the representing style. These differences of meanings in fashion create rooms for people to exchange their ideas about various areas of garment development. As fashion is considered essential to people's daily lives, it can be used as a common communication bridge to link people with different backgrounds; therefore, fashion is an ideal topic for organizing an SL program.

Through the activities of the fashion-related SL program, the topics around fashion can be used to bridge any communication gaps between the participated students, service recipients, and teaching staff. In the meanwhile, the making process of an outfit is accessible with some basic background of knowledge and skills, unlike some other programs that required heavy duty machinery or highly professional skillset that is not easy acquire for other program setup. The unique fashion and textile-making process is also considered as an ideal medium for program design; students and service recipient can enjoy and participate in different stages from outfit design and illustration, pattern making and material selection, cutting and sewing, and garment fitting to the running of the final fashion show. This advantage of the uniqueness of the garment making could help the students, service recipients, program leader and helpers, as well as the staff from NGOs to development strong interpersonal relationships; this is verified by the students as 76.1% of students agreed with that through the reflection report.

From the results of data analysis by reviewing students' and teachers' reflections, the promotion of quality of life through the SL program is reached, especially in the three areas—social well-being, emotional well-being, and development and activities. These three domains are the major objectives in planning of an SL program, which are aimed to provide students opportunities to reach out trainings not only from academics requirements but also more from on mental developments. The developments in interpersonal and social skills, community involvement, emotional developments are consider as very important in this era, as students are easier to get the acquired information and professional training from various sources especially through the Internet. In addition, the service recipients improve their communication with their relatives and caretakers through fashion. It is good for improving the quality of life on the elderly and the disabled.

References

Bringle, R., & Hatcher, J.A. (1999). Reflection in service learning: Making meaning of experience. *Educational Horizons*, 179–185.

Bruce-Davis, M. N., & Chancey, J. M. (2012). Connecting students to the real world: Developing gifted behaviours through service learning. *Psychology in the Schools, 49*(7), 716–723.

Deeley, S. J. (2010). Service-learning: Thinking outside the box. *Active Learning in Higher Education, 11,* 43–53.

Dewey, J. (1916). *Democracy and Education*. New York: Macmillan Inc.

Felce, D., & Perry, J. (1995). Quality of life: Its definition and measurement. *Research in Development Disabilities, 16*(1), 51–74.

Goldsmith, R. E., Flynn, L. R., & Moore, M. (1996). The self-concept of fashion leaders. *Clothing and Textiles Research Journal, 4*(4), 242–248.

Hebert, A., & Hauf, P. (2015). Student learning through service learning: Effects on academic development, civic responsibilty, interpersonal skills and practical skills. *Active Learning in Higher Education, 16*(1), 37–49.

Jackson, D., & Wilton, N. (2016). Developing career management competencies among undergraduates and the role of work-integrated learning. *Teaching in Higher Education, 21*(3), 266–286.

Mahasneh, P., Tawalbeh, A., Al-Smadi, R., Ghaith, S., & Dajani, R. (2012). Integrating service learning in Jordanian higher education. *Innovations in Education and Teaching International, 49*(4), 415–425.

Ngai, E. W., Moon, K. K., & Poon, J. K. (2012). Design and implementation of a supply chain learning platform. *Journal of Educational Computing Research, 47*(3), 293–327.

O'Cass, A. (2004). Fashion clothing consumption: Antecedents and consequences of fashion clothing involvement. *European Journal of Marketing, 38*(7), 869–882.

Sandaran, S. C. (2012). Service learning: Transforming students, communities and universities. *Procedia-Social and Behavioral Science*, *66*, 380–390.

Smith, C. (2012). Evaluating the quality of work-integrated learning curricula: A comprehensive framework. *Higher Education Research & Developement, 31*(2), 247–262.

Watson, P. (2002). The role and integration of learning outcomes into the educational process. *Active Learning in Higher Education, 3*(3), 205–219.

Woodward, S. (2007). *Why women wear what they wear*. Oxford: Berg.

Chapter 12
Expressive Textile Arts as a Caring Medium for the Vulnerable Groups

Jin C. H. Lam and Joe S. C. Au

Abstract "Participation in the arts and accessed to a range of arts opportunities can dramatically improve health outcomes and increase well-being" (Betsi Cadwaladr University Health Board in Arts in health and well-being: Annual report 2010–11, p. 3, 2012). By integrating the expressive textile arts processes and allowing one to flow into another, the service users including ex-mentally ill patients and ex-offenders in this service-learning project gained access to their inner resources for healing, self-awareness and creativity. This study provides an overview of the service-learning subject "Community engagement through expressive textile arts and fashion" including the concepts and practice of expressive textiles arts. The project implementation of the interactive textile arts and fashion creativity workshops delivered by the subject lecturers is further elaborated. The quantitative research method is adopted to evaluate the impact of the expressive textile arts on service recipients and students, and the reflections from the students are also discussed.

Keywords Arts and health · Expressive textile arts · Fashion creativity
Vulnerable people · Service-learning

12.1 Introduction

In recent years, a growing body of evidence has been compiled exploring the potential of the arts to impact on health and well-being in a variety of social contexts, to counter inequalities and increase engagement. "Participation in the arts and access to a range of arts opportunities can dramatically improve health

J. C. H. Lam (✉) · J. S. C. Au
Institute of Textiles and Clothing, The Hong Kong Polytechnic University, Hunghom, Hong Kong
e-mail: jin.lam@polyu.edu.hk

J. S. C. Au
e-mail: joe.au@polyu.edu.hk

D. T. L. Shek et al. (eds.), *Service-Learning for Youth Leadership*,
Quality of Life in Asia 12, https://doi.org/10.1007/978-981-13-0448-4_12

outcomes and increase well-being" (Betsi Cadwaladr University Health Board, 2012, p. 3). This study aimed to investigate the impact of expressive textile arts on people with special needs, namely former mental patients and ex-offenders after taking a series of interactive textile arts and fashion creativity workshops from a service-learning subject, "Engaging Fashion as a Communication Media for the Needy" offered by the Hong Kong Polytechnic University in 2016 and 2017. In this service-learning subject, subject lecturers and students co-designed with the service recipients to enhance their self-confidence and rebuild a satisfactory identity through practising expressive textile arts. A total of 20 textile arts prototypes were created in each cohort of 2016 and 2017 and were presented in a mini-fashion show and a static exhibition both at the Hong Kong Polytechnic University in July 2016 and July 2017, respectively. A quantitative research method was adopted, and a questionnaire survey was conducted to evaluate the impact of expressive textile arts on service recipients and students taking the service-learning subject and students' reflections on the service-learning project. The service project of this service-learning subject was found to be able to improve the health of people who experience mental health problems. Besides, the static exhibition and fashion show effectively disseminated the expressive textile artworks jointly created by the service recipients; students and subject lecturers were able to draw the social issue of the people with special needs to the attention of the public.

12.2 What Are Expressive Arts, Textile Arts and Expressive Textile Arts

"Expressive arts is the practice of using imagery, storytelling, dance, music, drama, poetry, writing, movement, dream work and visual arts in an integrated way to foster human growth, development and healing" (Atkins, 2002, p. 3). This suggests that each human being is inherently creative and infused with the gift of imagination.

The textile arts making process is a multi-dimensional experience and can be used as a healing process for people suffering from mental and/or physical discomforts (Meadow & Beyerle-Rutherford, 1999). Reynolds first demonstrated findings based on a study of 35 women involved in illness management by using textile arts (Reynolds, 1997). They were asked to process needlework to distract their attention away from worries or pain, and the results showed that participants agreed the textile arts making process helped them to block out the symptoms by focusing the attention on the textile working process. Textile arts can calm people themselves and feel centred when they become immersed in the sheer pleasure of the creative process.

In this service-learning project, the service recipients practised textile arts as a form of expressive arts for self-expression and reflection. Textile arts can give people a sense of place and enhance the sense of self with a collective identity

(Collier, 2011). It can also link people to previous traditions and rituals and let them feel release from previous lives and relationships (Reynolds, 1997). Through this creative capacity, everyone can express and shape their experience into creative expression. The service recipients can rebuild their identity and restore the quality of life by stimulating personal development through the process of creating expressive textile arts. Besides, it can enable service recipients to find new interests and skills. This kind of experience is able to carry out positive change in their lives (Reynold & Prior, 2003). "Many forms of textile art-making are highly time-consuming, fostering a future orientation, and the creative process is often socially visible within the home, with positive consequences for self-image" (Reynolds, 2004, p. 58).

12.3 About the Service-Learning Subject

The service site mainly focused on the districts including Yaumatei, Tsimshatsui and Mongkok. The agencies were "The Society of Rehabilitation and Crime Prevention" and "The New Life Psychiatric Rehabilitation Association" in 2016 and 2017, respectively. The service recipients were mainly ex-offenders and ex-mental ill patients. In each cohort, there were 20 service recipients and 76 and 74 students joining this service-learning project in 2016 and 2017, respectively.

The objectives of the service-learning subject are to:

(a) Introduce the concept, theories and practice of expressive arts, textiles arts and expressive textile arts;
(b) Develop students' practical skills of developing expressive textile artworks, and its application for contemporary fashion;
(c) Enable students to use expressive textile arts making process as a healing medium to help needy people in a wider community;
(d) Enhance students' skills of problem-solving, communication and teamwork in the context of art and design;
(e) Introduce the concept and practice of service-learning for needy people locally and overseas; and
(f) Nurture students' sense of social awareness, responsibility and engagement.

Upon completion of the subject, students will be able to:

(a) Recognise the concept and theories of expressive arts, textiles arts, and expressive textile arts in different contexts;
(b) Develop and implement the skills and techniques of practising expressive textile arts as a healing medium and its application in contemporary fashion;
(c) Effectively link the service-learning activities with the academic content of the subject;
(d) Reflect on their role and responsibilities both as a professional in their chosen discipline and as a responsible citizen; and

(e) Demonstrate empathy for needy people and develop a sense of social awareness, responsibility and engagement.

The academic focus of this subject will cover the following areas:
Concept and practice of service-learning

(a) Definition and principles of service-learning
(b) Benefits of service-learning
(c) Responsibilities, attitudes and ethics in service-learning
(d) Planning and delivering the service-learning project
(e) Reflecting on the service-learning experience

Concepts, theories and practice of expressive textile arts

(a) Theory and principles of expressive arts, textile arts and expressive textile arts
(b) Skills and techniques of practising expressive textile arts as a healing medium and as a multi-dimensional experience for people suffering from mental and/or physical discomforts
(c) Using colour, textures and patterns in expressive textile artworks to interpret recipients' memories and personal narratives for self-discovery and healing
(d) Appreciations of expressive textile arts on contemporary fashion
(e) Basic expressive textile arts techniques, such as stamping, fabric collaging, hand embroidery and painting

Project-specific concepts and practice

(a) Understanding the background of service recipients
(b) Health, safety and other issues relevant to the service project
(c) Moral and ethical concerns specific to the project and beneficiaries

12.4 Implementation of the Service-Learning Project

The service-learning subject was taught using a combination of lectures and interactive workshops and aimed at developing students' practical skills of creating expressive textile arts together with the service recipients. The students gained basic skills and techniques of creating expressive textile arts and its applications for contemporary fashion. The students co-designed and co-developed expressive textile artworks with the service recipients and subject lecturers.

The local community partner was invited to deliver a seminar about its background and the skills required in communicating and working with the service recipients before the commencement of the service rendering sessions. During the service rendering sessions, a mutual learning experience between students and recipients was promoted. Students were team up with service recipients to discuss and co-design expressive textile artworks under subject instructors' supervisions. Emphasis was placed on using colours, textures and patterns for creating expressive textile artworks so as to interpret recipients' memories and personal narratives to self-discovery and healing.

The final expressive textile artworks were showcased in a styling presentation, a static exhibition and a mini-fashion show within the university. A professional hair and makeup sponsor was sourced, and a professional show production house was appointed for the fashion show. During the styling presentation and mini-fashion show, the service recipients presented their expressive textile artworks by modelling their creations themselves and their personal expressions and inner confidences were further encouraged. The fashion show served as a social platform where the results of the service-learning project were disseminated to a wide public audience effectively. In addition, the expressive textile artworks were also presented in static exhibition in the Hong Kong Polytechnic University in 2016 and 2017 in order to further raise the academic and public awareness about the expressive textile arts created by the people with special needs in Hong Kong.

12.5 Methods of Evaluating Impact of the Project

A quantitative research method was adopted in this study. A questionnaire survey was conducted before and during the expressive textile arts making workshops for the service recipients. The design of the questionnaire was based on the 'Art-based Intervention (ABI) Questionnaire' (Snir & Regey, 2013). Variables regarding "feelings and thoughts before attending the workshops", "feelings and thoughts during the workshops", "attitude towards the textile arts materials" and "attitude towards the expressive textile artworks" were obtained through a self-administered questionnaire survey, subjects being 20 service recipients from a community partner in each cohort. There were 10 ex-mentally ill people and 10 ex-offenders from "The Society of Rehabilitation" and 20 ex-mentally ill people from "The New Life Psychiatric Rehabilitation Association" joining this service-learning project in 2016 and 2017, respectively.

For students taking the service-learning subject, a questionnaire survey was conducted before and after taking the subject. The major three parts were: (i) students ratings on attainment of learning outcomes as a result of attending an service-learning subject, (ii) student ratings on learning experience of their service-learning subject and project and (iii) student ratings on intention for continual engagement in community service after taking the service-learning subject. There were 76 students and 74 students joining this service-learning project in 2016 and 2017, respectively.

A 7-point Likert scaling was adopted for various items of the surveys for service recipients and students. The ranking scales were: the scale of 1 for "entirely disagree", 4 for "neither agree nor disagree" and 7 for "entirely agree". Respondents took an average of 45 min to complete a questionnaire. The software package SPSS 22.0 was employed to facilitate the quantitative data analysis.

12.6 Impact on the Service Recipients

In cohort 2017 and 2016, the research findings suggest that positive impacts were found on the service recipients' perceptions of "feelings and thoughts before attending the workshops", "feelings and thoughts during the workshops", "attitude towards the textile arts materials" and "attitude towards the expressive textile artworks". In response to service recipients' perceptions of "feelings and thoughts before the workshops", 95% of the service recipients claimed that they felt "much excited" to participate in the textile art creative workshops in both cohorts. 70 and 75% of the respondents were "much confident" in their ability to perform well in the expressive textile arts workshops in 2017 and 2016, respectively. Only 10% of the respondents were "much reluctant" to get involved in the workshops, and all respondents felt "much peaceful and pleased" to participate the workshops in 2017 and 2016. Regarding respondents' perceptions of "feelings and thoughts during the workshops", positive results were obtained from both cohorts of service recipients. Over 85% of respondents felt "much pleased" and "much relaxed and concentrated" to create the textile artwork during the creating process. 95% of the respondents "enjoyed" working on the expressive textile artworks, and less than 10% of them claimed that they could not "overcome the failure" of their creative process. Positive "attitude towards the expressive textile artworks and the textile arts materials" is presented from both cohorts of service recipients. Over 95% of the respondents felt "much satisfied" with their created textile artworks, and 90% of respondents were "much interested" in creating textile arts materials.

12.7 Impact on the Students

In cohort 2017 and 2016, the research findings suggest that positive impacts were found on the students' ratings on: (i) attainment of learning outcomes as a result of attending an service-learning subject, (ii) learning experience of their service-learning subject and project and (iii) intention for continual engagement in community service after taking the service-learning subject.

12.7.1 Attainment of Learning Outcomes

(a) More than 82% of the students claimed that there was a "deeper understanding of the linkage between service-learning and the academic content of the subject". Student A (2016), "The most treasurable experience was developing the outfit with my team and the service user. He was an extremely quiet person. When getting along with him, as a talkative person, I still defeated by his tough mouth. This was challenging because we needed to not only serve him, but also cooperate with him to complete an outfit. Fortunately, I had three excellent teammates. We encouraged and supported each other in relay melting the user's iceberg gradually".

(b) More than 85% of the students claimed that they were able to "applying and integrating knowledge to deal with complex issues". Student B (2017), "The first time be in touch with fashion was in my secondary school time. I remember I was making a stylish clothing by plastic bags with my classmates. Unlikely in this course, we are not only designing the garments, but also serving the participant attentively". Student C (2017), "In this service-learning subject, I attended different workshops and lectures which prepared me to acquire fresh knowledge and skills. I have learned useful fashion and textile knowledge through the lectures. For example, different clothing and design are suitable for various people who have different body shapes. This kind of knowledge definitely helped me in designing the clothing for our user in the later stage".

(c) It was found that at less 90% of them could "work effectively in teams" and "communicate effectively with peers, collaborators and service recipients". Student D (2016), "To me, sharing with and learning from the user in these days is one of the most meaningful and unforgettable experiences this year. No matter the fact that communicating with him was a big challenge, thanks to my patient group mates, he smiled and talked more. In this course, we, as a team, helped each other and built complementarity". Student E (2017), "Talent wins games, but teamwork and intelligence win championships. It is the best quote from Michael Jordan for me to sum up what I experienced in this service-learning subject. Throughout the one and a half months, we have been facing so many ticklish situations. Although I used to believe in my artistic ability on creating fine works, the strength of each member is actually from the whole team". Student F (2017), "Meeting with our user was the most thankful part in the whole activity. She is a warm-hearted person who always take care about us. In the very first beginning, I was a bit shy and nervous to talk with her and I tried my best to get closer with her. Unexpectedly, our user was very friendly to chat with us and was willing to share her own experience to us. Through the workshops and the show rehearsals, I could know more and more about her. Almost every time when we met together, she brought some snacks to share with us. She undoubtedly was a warm-hearted person and I was so touching".

(d) There are more than 90% of the students suggested that they had a "better understanding of the problems facing underprivileged members of the community" and "become a more responsible member of your community". Student G (2017), "I have participated lots of voluntary works to serve the community, such as visiting the elderly residents who are living alone and playing golf with mental health users. However, those voluntary works did not last a long period, most of them were organised once off only. Therefore, it was difficult for me to have a deeper understanding of the users. This service-learning project was different from my previous experiences and provided a chance for me to understand the needy in my community". Student H (2016), "If we have the power to make other happy, we should do it, as the world needs it. Undoubtedly, I have learned so much this service-learning subject".

(e) More than 84% of them had a "better understanding of their own strengths and weaknesses". 90% of the students suggested that the "overall learning outcome was gained". Student I (2016), "I mainly acted as a communicator with the user in team. I felt difficult to find a topic to chat with him in the beginning. However, I got a special method to communicate with him and he can remember my name now. I may be not that good in painting on the garment because I am not good at drawing and design. Thus, I would contribute some stamping ideas to my group mates and practiced with the user". Student J (2016), "This service learning programme not only provides the chance for ex-offenders and ex-mental health users to rebuild their confidence and re-develop the positive value toward the community, but it also let us adopt what we have learnt at PolyU to fulfill our social responsibility. Last but not least, we would like to quote a word from the user to sum up this event – Good"!

12.7.2 Learning Experience of Their Service-Learning Subject and Project

(a) More than 75% of the students claimed that "they took this subject because they were very interested in the service-learning project of the subject". Student K (2017), "Taking this service-learning subject absolutely is a very special and meaningful experience to me. As a business management student, honestly I was a little bit worried about my own ability in this area. However, I regard this as a precious chance for me to try some new thing that I have not been get in touch with my academic study. I have not tried designing garments for others before. I felt very excited to acquire this new kind of knowledge. Though the help from tutors and my group mates, I found it very interesting".

(b) 85% of them "believed that the service they performed in the service-learning project had benefited the people they served" and "felt that their services were appreciated by the collaborating agency and service recipients". Student L (2017), "At the end of the course, I recognised the most invaluable thing was that we built up a close relationship with the user. We believed that we were not only helping him to produce a satisfactory outfit, but we also improve his quality of life to some extent. Looking back to our first meeting, my team still hardly believed that we could cooperate with the user so well. Even though our outfit was not the best among the others, I considered our team had obtained the greatest achievement in this course". In 2017, after completing the service-learning project with the community partner, "New Life Psychiatric

Rehabilitation Association", its representative indicated that their organisation would "like to continue collaborating with PolyU in organising service-learning projects and added that: "The outcome of the project is significant on the change in our persons-in-residents. The project benefited them in enhancing their self-esteem and reducing their self-stigma too. The persons-in-residents stated that the project gave them a memorable and valuable experience. The students showed their caring and understanding about the person suffered from mental illness, and they learn to work with different people".

(c) Over 82% of them found that the "instructors and teaching assistants prepared them appropriately for performing the service" and "could feel the enthusiasm and passion of their instructors and teaching assistants in delivering the subject and the service". Student M (2017), "Unlike last year, we are required to engage in the Catwalk Show with the element of Laughing Yoga with the user. I am not confident with the show and know little about fashion design. Being an engineering student, I am worried about the effort that I can spare during the design workshops in the beginning of executing the service-learning project. However, the adverse situations have been ameliorated gradually through the collaboration with teammates and the guidance from the tutors". Student N, "As a fashion design student, it is a precious time to achieve the service-learning goal by fashion based knowledge, such as basic design principles, textile arts, skills of body measurement and fashion styling. Under tutors' supervisions, our group got applicable recommendations in particularly improvement of the visual effects of the designed outfit. It also helped us to gain new branches of knowledge and practical experiences in fashion styling and design".

(d) 81% of them claimed that "their team mates in the service-learning project were generally motivated and supportive". Student O (2017), "When it comes to the interaction between the user and us. I think this is the most precious and memorable part. We have meetings for more than two weeks. These are quite different from those volunteer works that usually only has one meeting with the target group for each function. Thus, I can interact with the user more so as to have a more thorough acquaintance with her".

(e) 90% of them claimed that "there were a lot of opportunities for them to meet and interact with the people they served". Student P (2017), "As I am not that talkative, it is quite hard to find some topics to chat with her at first. However, the user is willing to share lots of her past experience and things she daily loves to do. Different kinds of topics were developed through her sharing. This impressed me most as we chat like friends. Not only do I interact with her in our group, but I also make friends with users in other groups. When she and other users share their design with each other, I join in the discussion and chat together. They always tell many jokes and we laugh together. These are undoubtedly unforgettable memories".

(f) More than 85% of them found that "the service-learning project provided challenging and meaningful tasks for them to accomplish" and the "project challenged them to try things that they had never done before". Student Q

(2017), "Taking this service-learning subject definitely is an empathy challenge for me. As an interactive media design student working with in a group with students in other disciplines, I learned that every design has its weaknesses and strengths. I learned to discover what the user preference and what type of body shape she is. We challenged each other's preconceptions about what would and would not work. For example, the way to draw the pattern on the garment. At the first, we tried to use the painting brushes to draw the graphic pattern, however, it was too hard for the user to control. Then, we suggested using the clothing maker and paper molding technique to create the graphic design works. I realised that we have numerous ways to execute the design progress with appropriate outcome. In experiencing design, empathy and understanding of the user are very important. It is a huge practical advantage for me to learn about it. We can also see the reality of the way changing a design actually affects its performance".

(g) 90% of the students indicated that they "found the experience of studying this service-learning subject highly useful and rewarding". Student R (2016), "I think my service-learning course ended successfully and happily. In this course, my group mates and I designed a satisfactory outfit and communicated well with the user. Although the user is a little bit reticent, I still believe and feel that he love to stay with us. And I felt very happy that our relationship was developed day by day". Student S (2016), "I have experienced many new things. From the lectures and workshops, I acquired the knowledge of textile arts and its application on fashion as well as the design skills of mix-and-match frequently used in fashion, which indeed, it helped me a lot to build up a fashion sense. As an engineering student, such sense may not bring benefit to my academic study directly, but it can definitely assist me to how to solve a design problem in the context of fashion and can also enhance my interpersonal skills potentially". Student T (2017), "It is really a memorable and precious experience to work with the users and make contribution to society. We all do enjoy the workshop and the show".

12.7.3 Intention for Continual Engagement in Community Service

More than 72 and 11% of the students claimed that they were "quite likely" and "definitely" to "plan to participate in other community service or civic engagement activities after completing this service-learning subject" and 11% of them were "definitely", respectively.

12.8 Conclusion

After running this service-learning subject with the emphasis of expressive textile arts for two cohorts, as subject lecturers, we witnessed the impact of the subject and project on the development of the students in the domains of "social well-being" and "emotional well-being" (Felce & Perry, 1995, p. 60).

(a) Community involvement: We noticed that our students have developed sound personal relationship with the users as well as the students from other academic disciplines. The students have also demonstrated their acceptance and support to the vulnerable groups, such as ex-mentally ill people and ex-offenders in every stage of the service project starting from the preliminary work, design prototyping, and to the fashion show. "After taking this subject, I have a better understanding of those people in needs. I do not think they are any difference between us. This service-learning subject is very meaningful, and I will remember this excellent learning experience" (Student U, 2016).

Some of the users were quite shy and reserved in the beginning. Students' passionate support and heartfelt acceptance allowed them to be more willing to express their feelings and thoughts. Through those sincere communications between the users and students, the students understood more about their innermost world. "I even started to treat the user as a normal person. In my eyes, he is a gentleman. Each time when he spotted the door, he always showed his courtesy to open and hold the door for us and let us go first. After this experience, I believe that ex-mentally ill people can go back to the community if we can give them a chance" (Student V, 2017).

The students understood the fact that one should never judge a person before really knowing him or her and they should think critically. People with mental illness learn to and strive to manage their symptoms and live their own life. They are normal, just like everyone else. They believed that the users can recover from mental illness in one day. "What the users want the most are not our excellent design skills, or outstanding outfits made, but our sincerity, caring and developing friendship with them" (Student W, 2017).

(b) Interpersonal relationship: Throughout the service-learning project, the students had plenty of chances to understand and communicate with the users of different backgrounds. The close interactions could enhance students' interpersonal experiences and give them positive vibes. In this circumstance, the students had developed positive social relationships with them and demonstrated themselves as having a valued place in a social network. "When I knew more about the user's own story, I should cherish what I have. From the user's experiences, it was even not easy for him to go out to street normally in daily life. At the end, I hope he felt joyful to be with us and more importantly, he can get well soon. I really have a great time with him" (Stduent X, 2016).

(c) Satisfaction, Fulfilment, Belief, Self-esteem: After completing the service project, the students presented positive emotions about their achievements made in the service-learning project and they were able to pursue valued goals and opportunities for learning and personal development. "In the beginning of this service-learning subject, I did not have high expectation since I only wanted to fulfil the service-learning requirement honestly. However, I found that I gained a lot in such a precious process by having a more in-depth understanding of the ex-mentally ill people. I should contribute more to our society, as well as to put aside the stereotypes and prejudice towards different parties. I am very delighted as I can involve in this meaningful activity" (Student Y, 2017).

Finally, as the subject lecturers of this service-learning subject, we realised that the people who have recovered from mental illness or the ex-offender is not that unreachable. They need huge amount of care but, in the meanwhile, they desire to be treated equally as a normal person. The key element will never be changed and it is empathy!

References

Atkins, S. S. (2002). *Expressive arts therapy: Creative process in art and life*. Blowing Rock, NC: Parkway Publishers.

Betsi Cadwaladr University Health Board. (2012). *Arts in health and well-being: Annual report 2010–11*. Retrieved 10, 2017, from http://www.wales.nhs.uk/sitesplus/documents/861/CF12.013%20AiHWB%20Annual%20report%202010%5F11.pdf.

Collier, A. F. (2011). The well-being of women who create with textiles: Implications for art therapy. *Art Therapy, 28*(3), 104–112.

Felce, D., & Perry, J. (1995). Quality of Life: Its definition and measurement. *Research in Developmental Disabilities, 16*(1), 51–74.

Meadow, M., & Beyerle-Rutherford, E. (1999). Becoming whole: A pastoral story. *Health Care for Women International, 20*(4), 427–432.

Reynold, F., & Prior, S. (2003). "A lifestyle coat-hanger": A phenomenological study of the meanings of artwork for women coping with chronic illness and disability. *Disability and Rehabilitation, 25*(14), 785–794.

Reynolds, F. (1997). Coping with chronic illness and disability through creative needlecraft. *The British Journal of Occupational Therapy, 60*(8), 352–356.

Reynolds, F. (2004). Textile art promoting well-being in long-term illness: Some general and specific influences. *Journal of Occupational Science, 11*(2), 58–67.

Snir, S., & Regey, D. (2013). ABI—Art-based intervention questionnaire. *The Arts in Psychotherapy, 40,* 338–346.

Chapter 13
The Journey of Service-Learning: Promoting Health and Quality of Life for Slum Residents in Cambodia

Phyllis C. P. Pang and Cynthia S. T. Wu

Abstract The World Health Organization (WHO) updates and enriches the accessible resources and measures, such as tools for well-being, the global index of happiness, and global quality of life. Seeing that health is a basic human right as well as a key indicator of quality of life, the School of Nursing in the Hong Kong Polytechnic University (PolyU) has developed the Service-Learning (SL) programme namely "Healthy lifestyle challenges in developing communities". Cambodia is the first service site, where access and resources on health care are limited and expensive. The teaching team believes that some of the risk factors leading to the top ten causes of death can be reduced through health promotion activities. Experiential learning and outcome assessments are the methods of teaching and learning in SL, putting emphasis on how students can learn to serve and serve to learn. The challenges of the SL programme are the sustainability of service and empowerment of local stakeholders for committing to developing their own SL programme in meeting the needs of Cambodians. Meanwhile, our vision is one of developing PolyU students in global citizenship and leadership through provision of scholarships with the necessary resources and support in real-world practice.

Keyword Service-Learning · Global quality of life · Healthy lifestyle
Health promotion · Cambodia

P. C. P. Pang (✉)
School of Nursing, The Polytechnic University of Hong Kong,
Hunghom, Hong Kong
e-mail: phyllis.pang@polyu.edu.hk

C. S. T. Wu
Senior Teaching Fellow School of Nursing, The Polytechnic University
of Hong Kong, Hunghom, Hong Kong
e-mail: cynthia.wu@polyu.edu.hk

D. T. L. Shek et al. (eds.), *Service-Learning for Youth Leadership*,
Quality of Life in Asia 12, https://doi.org/10.1007/978-981-13-0448-4_13

13.1 Background

With a population of 15.33 million, the people of Cambodia have a life expectancy of age 68.66 (2015). Hospital bed density is 0.1 bed per 1000 people, and the poverty index is at 0.251 (World Health Rankings, 2017b). Even 42 years after the Khmer Rouge 1975–1979 civil war, Cambodia is still seriously traumatized as a result and remains a developing country. Of the top 10 causes of death in Cambodia, coronary heart disease is ranked as top, tuberculosis as 2, stroke as 3, influenza and pneumonia as 4, HIV as 5, diabetes mellitus as 9, and hypertension as 10 (World Health Rankings, 2017a). Among these figures, many of the risk factors, such as those leading to coronary heart diseases, stroke, diabetes, and hypertension, can be reduced by health education and living in a more healthy lifestyle. With a flight time of less than 3 h from Hong Kong, Cambodia was chosen as a suitable location, a "service site" for the training of Hong Kong student nurses undertaking the Service-Learning (SL) course "*Health Lifestyle Challenges in developing communities*"

The "service site" initially chosen was in the Sen Sok slum of Phnom Penh, with an estimated 500 households in 2015. In 2017, an extension of service was made to the Angtumlorb Village of Kampong Speu of Cambodia with an estimated 200 households. Service-recipients are families/households (mainly adult) living in the slum or rural areas where health facilities are remote and limited. Collaborating NGOs agencies are the Youth Men's Christian Association (YMCA), Human Resource Development Institute (HRDI), New Life Fellowship (NLF), Young People Do (YPD), and the Royal University of Phnom Penh (RUPP). These NGOs provide a good network and support locally for the SL project. Students involved in SL provision are undergraduate students from a variety of faculties of the Hong Kong Polytechnic University (the PolyU), who apply for the SL subject as the designated Service-Learning subject.

13.2 Health as the Key Indicator of Quality of Life

With the advancement in Internet technology, both members of the public and professionals alike are increasingly able to access the free and reliable health resources and medical knowledge for improving health. Health knowledge is no more the privileged access of professionals. With the improvement of the economy and education levels of a society, the level of collaboration and partnership between public and professionals may become the success indicator of the quality of health of a society. World Health Organization (WHO) and many other global health authorities have been updating and enriching the accessible resources and measures such as tools for well-being, the global index of happiness, global quality of life (QoL). People and professionals across countries work together in developing further comprehensive and essential materials for the local and national health needs (WHO, 2015, 2016). This work-together strategy has been considered as one of the cost-effective approaches for achieving the global health.

Health is a basic human right as well as a key indicator of quality of life (QoL). The Cambodia SL subject hosted by the School of Nursing of the Hong Kong Polytechnic University has been included as one of the General University Requirement (GUR) subjects under the theme of Service-Learning. The course has been providing opportunities for faculty students from healthcare and non-healthcare departments, to work together for the health of less resourceful communities in developing countries. Students, after acquiring the basic health concepts, health promotion techniques and assessment skills of taking blood pressure, vital signs of TPR as temperature (T), pulse (P), and respiration (R), work as a service team of 4–6 to develop deliverable action plans to modify health risk behaviours for a target community.

The subjectivity of health dimensions on quality of life to an individual can be influenced by the resources available to people and their access. This perception may also affect one's sense of control over one's own health, and act as a self-motivator. Throughout the service in Cambodia, faculty students and teachers from both sides are working together for the development of a sustainable service model for the health of the slum residents. Strategies of engaging the related parties and stakeholders for supporting the mission of care and following the service impact will be developed.

13.3 The Course Description

The Service-Learning (SL) course "*Health Lifestyle Challenges in Developing Communities*" has set the objectives as: "…. *developing and educating students in provision of service on health promotion regarding lifestyle modification based on the need assessment of the validated health survey*". Students would be equipped with knowledge and skills in assessing health status, examining lifestyle pattern and living environment of families in the slums. Based on the health assessment, students would develop a health profile of the families and explore factors leading to health issues. They would write a health promotion plan, thus motivating the families towards modifying their behaviours leading to a healthier lifestyle. This avoids advocating drastic lifestyle changes, making it difficult to sustain.

Upon completion of the subject, students would be expected to understand the challenges and needs in maintaining a healthy lifestyle in developing communities. At the same time, they would learn the techniques to interview people on their health status, conduct basic health assessments, and develop a personalized health promotion plan. They would learn to behave sensitively, and appreciate cultural and religious diversity. This fits the concept of "serve to learn, learn to serve" by facilitating students to realize that health behaviour can be modified through goal-oriented health promotion plans and compassionate care in service areas/villages where the healthcare resources are limited. Meanwhile, this SL subject aims at facilitating students' personal growth through on-site coaching, debriefing, and reflective learning, by applying and considering ethical dilemmas, professional competences, global citizenship, and social responsibility.

13.4 The Methodology of Teaching and Learning

The process of the experiential learning and outcome assessment helps develop students' capacity of caring for the health of the people. Students design their health promotion plans using the ABC framework of outcome measures for their clients in home visits. In this framework, A stands for the Affection—the emotional and psychological outcomes of the lifestyle modification; B represents the Behavioural outcomes which focus on the change of the habitual behaviour; and C denotes the cognitive learning outcomes which emphasize the changes more on knowledge or concepts. The faculty students, also the service-providers, acquire knowledge and skills for the basic health screening such as taking body temperature and blood pressure using the digital devices. Eventually, they need to get along with new classmates who come from different faculties and work as a team to design the appropriate health promotion plans for the target residents.

This SL course started when the first author, Phyllis, joined the fact-finding trip with Office of Service-Learning (OSL) to Cambodia in 2013. Her inspiration of launching this SL course was to empower people who live in the resource-scarce regions, with their associated problems of poor hygiene condition, scarce water supply, no proper sewage system, and poor concept of garbage disposal. All these conditions had impacts on health outcomes. There are cultural differences and beliefs with respect to lifestyle and health behaviour. The SL course also aims to prepare and empower faculty students, who live in a better-off place like Hong Kong in terms of resources and healthcare system, to care about their international neighbourhood. The teacher and student ratio (1:6) assures the quality mentoring process takes place. This experiential learning can further enhance the students' early adulthood development in aspect of relationships, work ethic and career choice (Harcourt, 2017) and being equipped with empathy skills and readiness to work in the harsh conditions, with scarce resources, cultural differences, hot weather, etc. Moreover, students can choose to continue to serve the needy people in the context of their own professional development in the future.

Most of the PolyU students, who have grown up in the developed city of Hong Kong, were psychologically shocked when they first saw people living in rural and slum areas in Cambodia. Performing home visits in the slums in extremely hot weather without air conditioning, staying with homestay in a village with limited access to Internet tested their endurance and demanded the need to adjust. Students were encouraged to communicate by both verbal and non-verbal means, where they needed to learn to be tolerant and put aside their personal views during service.

The classroom activities also equipped students with the simple basic health assessment techniques and health education skills for promoting a healthy lifestyle and bridging cultural differences. Students, on arrival to Cambodia, are continuously exposed to stimulations and challenges of cultural diversity: with communities still in shock of the historical genocide during the Khmer Rouge period; with demands for being responsive in relation to problems arising during the SL trip; and the need to seek alternative solutions when facing barriers during their period of service.

Since the launching of the SL project in Cambodia, there has been a total of 20 student leaders recruited, engaged, and developed in joining the teaching team and providing support as peer mentors for students of the SL project. In 2016–2017, Phyllis acted as an advisor for 11 student leaders, who had joined the SL trip in the previous year, in submitting a proposal as a Self-Initiated Project (SIP) named "Empowerment on fundamental health concepts in developing countries". Eventually, the SIP project was funded under the PolyU Community Service Fund Student Service-Learning Grants 2016/17. The students took their own initiative in drafting, submitting, presenting, planning, implementing, and evaluating the entire project on their own. It was a great success of the students of SIP in terms of service-provision, leadership development and their professional exposure in humanitarian application on promoting fundamental health concepts to people living in deprived communities, such as the slums and HIV orphanage. The Cambodia teaching team and the local students were inspired and emotionally touched in working with the service team which included students, graduates, and teachers to support the delivery of the service for the slum residents. Phyllis and her team share the vision of developing future leaders who have the heart to care for people and the needy population. Students continue to be encouraged and empowered in search of their personal development through leadership and service-provision to the health vulnerable groups.

13.5 Evaluation of the Service-Learning

Various measures are used to evaluate the impacts on students' learning. The pre- and post-comparison of a PolyU-wide Service-Learning Survey (SLS) is based on a 19-item scale to elaborate interpersonal effectiveness, teamwork, problem-solving, and social responsibility. The SLS has been validated in a pilot Service-Learning programme in 2012 on 25 PolyU students (Office of Service-Learning, 2013). The internal consistency of the SLS was tested with alpha values for the four dimensions (i.e. interpersonal effectiveness, teamwork, problem-solving, and social responsibility) as 0.67, 0.77, 0.83, and 0.85, respectively. The programme also showed that the students had significant improvement in all the four dimensions after programme completion (Office of Service-Learning, 2013) (see Appendix for Student Educational Assessment Details).

At the time of writing, in total, there were 81 students joining the SL project serving a total of 455 service-recipients in Cambodia during the course of SL trips since 2015. According to the students' reflective journals, nearly all our students perceived the SL experience as a meaningful community caring service, as it started new initiatives for service-recipients in slum areas to care about their own health. Students experienced happiness, friendship, and interpersonal development/ enhancement through overcoming challenges, problems, or barriers in implementing the SL project in Cambodia. Their problem-solving abilities were enhanced, and sense of civic responsibility was cultivated by deeper understanding of the service-recipients and the problems. A relatively high proportion of them indicated willingness/interests in continuing their commitment in such services.

13.5.1 Impacts on Student Learning

Outcomes of students' learning were measured by a 19-item Service-Learning Survey (SLS); a 30-item Global Citizenship Scale (GCS); and an evaluation of students' pre- and post-reflective journals. Overall, the results were very encouraging:

- Students (96.6%) perceived the SL experience as a rewarding and useful experience in starting new initiatives for service-recipients in slum areas and caring about their own health.
- Students (89.7%) valued and benefitted from the experienced through overcoming challenges, problems, or barriers in implementing the SL project in Cambodia.
- Students (89.7%) developed themselves through dealing with unexpected situations, challenges, by being given autonomy and chances for reflection.
- Sense of civic responsibility among students (91.3%) was cultivated by their deeper understanding of the service-recipients and the problems they encountered.
- Students (91.3%) indicated willingness/interests in a continual commitment in service.

Two external reviewers, from the School of Nursing (PolyU) and Office of Service-Learning of PolyU, were invited to help collect feedback from PolyU students about the SL subject in 2015. Their findings were that students expressed that it was a rewarding and meaningful service, a happy experience, and showing their intention to continuous service engagement. Meanwhile, students reflected on the major challenges of dealing with unexpected situations and feasibility of the teaching plan (Pang & Wu, 2016a). The service-recipients were happy with the health assessments. Some older people (recipients) found it difficult to finish all their exercises, which indicated that the health promotion plan really needed further elaboration to fit it with the residents' ability (Pang & Wu, 2016a, b).

An external reporter, Ms Blanca Garcia, stayed together with the team and interviewed the students and the teaching team in 2016. She expressed that the experience and exposure to the slums of Cambodia clearly have impacts on the students. One student noted, "*I am very lucky to be a Hong Kong student. In Hong Kong, I can seek medical health very easily and I can find clean water very easily*". Another student wrote: "*We should feel really fortunate. We should have more goals in life and do more things which have a purpose and to help more people because we are more privileged, so I want to apply what I have and what I can do to help more people*," (Garcia, 2016). She interviewed a local volunteer, with nursing background, she added, "*I like to learn more about health education*" (Garcia, 2016). The Teaching Assistant, Sylvia, shared, "*…most of them (students), … the first time to Cambodia, might have some culture shock or adaptation problems*". Sylvia further elaborated, "*They are really touched by how warm the people (in the slums) are, despite with lack of resources, however, they are still really generous. The students can take this away and when back in Hong Kong, they can incorporate this into nursing, as a serving profession, when they can serve the needs of others*" (Garcia, 2016).

13.5.2 Challenges and Learning Opportunities

The major challenge of the Cambodia team would be the language barrier and cultural differences. As the team was required to conduct the health survey in the slum area where most of the service-recipients did not understand any English, we heavily relied on the local volunteers/students who were doing the translation for us. Misunderstandings happened affecting the progress and quality of the SL project. In the future, we plan to finalize the teaching material in advance and send to the local collaborators for translation and acknowledgement. Both local volunteers and students will have better understanding and preparation of the SL project so that we can have a better service impact to the service-recipients. Regretfully, there were, on and off, incidents that students got sick due to food or personal health concerns, requiring extra effort and time in taking care of them. The teaching team and student leaders needed to work closely on contingency plans in buffering the incidents.

In addition, the involvement of NGOs, especially local Cambodian students acting as translators for the team, kept changing every year. Stable collaborators of the local NGOs may enable the programme to be more effective and sustainable. With the newly established collaboration with RUPP in 2017, we would like to explore the possibility of empowering local stakeholders and the participation of local students. Moreover, the Cambodia team would like to collaborate and involve volunteers from RUPP. The approach adopted the concept of a community empowerment model, which refers to a process to re-negotiate power in order to gain more control. As defined by WHO (2016), "Community empowerment" is more than simply the involvement, participation, or engagement of communities. Instead, it is a process along a continuum, offering insights in enabling people through the SL programme, maximizing their potential and progressing actions into collective social and political changes (Laverack & Wallerstein, 2001).

It recognizes the empowerment of people sharing their existing power and giving up some of it (WHO, 2016). Community empowerment addresses the social, cultural, political, and economic determinants that underpin health. Thus, building up partnerships with local stakeholders in finding solutions necessarily is crucial in sustaining the project and programmes (WHO, 2016). The Cambodia team understands it takes time and effort in empowering local stakeholders and communities. We will work closely together continuously until they are empowered and ready to develop their own SL projects relating to healthy lifestyle and promoting them to the needy people on their own.

13.5.3 The Framework of Guiding the Service and Practice

The framework guides the process of health learning, health teaching, and evaluating its feasibility and efficacy of achieving the ABC learning outcomes. The framework encourages students as well as teachers to set a common goal and focus on the process of health enhancement. There is a commitment to motivating the ABC changes, which require collaborative team efforts of seeking practical and innovative solutions, to communicate effectively on the health problems in visual and sensible images. This becomes a high challenge.

The slum areas to the service team are new. Establishing the trust and empathy relationship with the people is a challenge to both students and teachers. The pre-service orientation of the field visits and historical culture programme help the service team to integrate the socio-demographic and cultural background of the target residents into the service plan. For the evaluation, a set of observable, measurable indicators for the health outcomes were developed from the WHO guidelines. Throughout the process of analysing the feasibility of the ABC intervention plan, students become more able to argue with the teachers as the students were more familiar with their plans. Teachers were also more willing to "let-go" as the residents are community dwellings who are able to participate and advocate their own health. The diversity and possibilities of motivating changes in health behaviours can be very creative and innovative. Through this brainstorming and discussion session, the authors are becoming more open-minded and creative in designing health promotion events. For students, they become more aware of the benefits of integrating their knowledge with the literature and evidences from research and scientific papers in supporting the accuracy of their observations and proposition. Students highlight their value for, and appreciation of, having the opportunities of applying knowledge in actions for the health benefits of people. They are aware of transferring the problem-solving skills and formulating healthcare solutions to real situations that are so much different from the classroom settings. Students learnt very much of the importance of building trust and empathy with their serving residents for their willingness to receive them as the home visitors. One student felt so frustrated after being rejected by two homes. After seeking the underlying reasons, students learnt how they should accommodate their lifestyle and pattern of working, and finding a suitable time for the home visits and health teaching. We emphasize that we should work with the residents and not "on" them for the sustainability of the health outcomes. Students experienced the differences in the quality of care while integrating the principle of health care in real life. Reflections from students highlighting their appreciation and value of the opportunities of integrating knowledge in action throughout the service may further explain the intrinsic means of SL. The 10-day SL trip also offered students the chance of living and working together with the shared missions and goals of health care.

13.5.4 The Intrinsic Motivation of Learning

Students become independent learners and self-motivated for learning with a self-initiated purpose. From this SL project, when students become more familiar with the community needs and with the clear mission and service goals, they are much more driven by the goal of achievement instead of relating the performance with merely the scores and grades they could gain.

The cross-disciplinary learning settings provide a social network for faculty students to establish friendship and connections in future. Students regard this offshore service as one of their valuable authentic challenges as people they were helping are having different cultures and living in poor hygiene environments with limited social resources.

For the service planning, students received information on global health issues and selected the focus of intervention. Students when contributing to the plans and actions of modifying health risk behaviours for the service target, their passions, talents and abilities were being observed by the teachers and supervisors. For example, the quit-smoking home visit event may involve the design of the card games, the instructor and the evaluator. Students with an interest in technology might want to consult their disciplinary supervisor for further technical input. A student who wants to explore the level of the safety and bacterial growth of the tap water in the slum areas, volunteers to make extra efforts of conducting scientific investigation in the faculty laboratory. The non-government volunteer association in the serving Cambodian region also starts to attract more local youth from universities and high schools to participate in developing healthier living habits in slum areas. The local university students from the non-health disciplines in engineering acted as the translators during the home interview found this service programme meaningful. It is also the first time for them to visit the slum areas and broaden their understanding of the living conditions there. The involvement enhanced their understanding of this vulnerable community, and they may consider building up their service and following the interventions if they could be supported and equipped with resources, knowledge, and skills.

Students seem to have more confidence and initiations to strive for excellence, not really for simply their academic grade, but ultimately for improving the health of the target population. When students serve as a pair-up team, they are totally immersed in observing whether their teaching could be well received and accepted by their residents in reducing their health risk behaviours such as the intake of salt and cigarettes. Students and teachers shared observations from the fieldwork daily, and the difficulties and successful skills were evaluated and exchanged among each other. One group of students shared the joy of the success of a home visit after being rejected for three times. The team reflected that they should not give up; meanwhile, they should try again to arrange the home visit at a more appropriate time; for example, they should seek a time when the residents are not playing card games or other leisure activities, not doing housework nor sleeping. They were not aware of motivating the interest of learning from the residents' perspectives until they were frustrated by repeatedly being declined by the residents. They reflected that the residents could be touched by their patience, their repeated trials of visiting as well as they being willing to listen to their concerns of health needs and select the appropriate contents for their learning and practice.

During the post-service reflection, each team exchanged their experiences of reinforcing the health-promoting behaviour and adjustments, for example the habits of cooking and smoking. Students felt excited when the house owners promised to allow the second visit, which implied they were satisfied with their last home teaching. Students reflected on the efficacy of their work and shared in their success and failures of the home teaching in terms of activity design and materials. One service team found the residents lacked interest in doing the towel exercise on their own at home. They proposed to invite people in their neighbourhood and discussed a suitable time so that they can remind each other in future for the regular practice. This intuitive response came through their personal experience of doing regular exercise that should involve more fun and less effort through being with others. The reasons of health barriers could be common. When students could be empathetic, they may foresee many possibilities of overcoming the reasons of non-participation and be well prepared for the techniques of enhancing health.

From a health education perspective, when learners are able to translate knowledge to an action of a health-promoting behaviour, the impact of health learning exists. It is through the practice in the real world, in addressing barriers in life and living, that we see the challenges of health education and health promotion. While transfer of learning will not happen in one moment of teaching and learning, it exists when the application and integration of the knowledge and practice in new situations can be rigorous and continuous within the transfer tasks. The framework of SL and its underlying pedagogic principles of designing and implementing the transfer tasks of practice learning provide the curriculum space in higher education for developing innovative and critical thinkers in promoting quality of health and life in the real world.

13.5.5 From Service to Empathy and Achieving

Experience itself does not lead to deep learning and critical thinking. Through the reflection on the service challenges, students are engaged in evaluating the action plans and analysing the appropriateness of the actions for the health problems. During the reflection on the service experience, students relate their observations to the meaning of their prior learning. Students further elaborate their thoughts and feelings of addressing the challenging incidents in their reflective writings. A student found the challenge of teaching health for the people with visual and hearing problems. She found herself being not equipped with the communication skills they have learnt in class and become more aware of the importance of learning non-verbal communication skills for improving the service quality for this special group of people. She observed their specific learning needs and advocated the need of adopting alternative media and non-verbal communication approaches for this vulnerable group. The act of writing provides opportunities for students to transfer the learning from service to empathetic thinking. Teachers are impressed by students achieving the goals of learning for the health of others.

A student mentioned the importance of understanding the culture of the people they serve in order to conduct the health promotion successfully. In her journal, she wrote "… the *people (in Cambodia) would not consider the intake of 24 cans of beer in party time be a problem of excessive drinking as it happens occasionally. We need to be cultural(ly) and social(ly)* (sic) *sensitive to facilitate better outcomes*".

A nursing student also said, "*as a future nurse, being sensitive to social, cultural and economic situations in the planning process can better enhance the outcomes of health promotion. Thus, putting ourselves into their shoes (situations) may generate significant outcomes*".

A student expressed her gratitude and appreciation for the support provided by the local trainers. In the journal, she wrote "*… from their (teachers of Learning Village) facial expressions, body languages and the teaching materials that they have prepared for us, I know from the bottom of my heart that they did prepare the best for us. I could actually see the passion in them when they teach* (sic) *us. This made me feel so impressed …*".

13.5.6 Developing the Sensitivity of Life

For analysing the clinical incidents in quality of care, quite often, teachers may place an emphasis on whether there exists any professional negligence and seeking solutions of prevention. The role of a caregiver in listening to psychological needs and providing the psychological support for people suffering from the incidents may be less focused. As teachers, we were impressed by one of the student's sharing which focused more on the psychological comfort from the physical harm.

He appreciated the positive attitudes of forgiving rather than blaming in life when he recalled the life values shared by his resident. He stated, "... *if we can focus more on what we own, but not being stubborn highlighting what we had lost, we would be happier and satisfied, so we can enjoy and make the most from our life ... I also learnt forgiveness from him. His deafness was thought to be caused by the doctors, but he did not blame anyone. Our living attitude determines what we deserve. Forgiving others means setting myself free from misery and constraints. We put ourselves in jail if we keep reminding ourselves of the past*".

We, as humans, share uniqueness in our own body, mind, and soul, while the quality of life can be facilitated by every single effort. Our emotional responses to health and illness experience could be common as well as very much different. While the resident shared their healthcare experiences and emotions with our students, they are interpreting their views towards life with them. Students by listening to their residents' stories and how they cope with their negative life experiences further developed the sensitivity towards health and life.

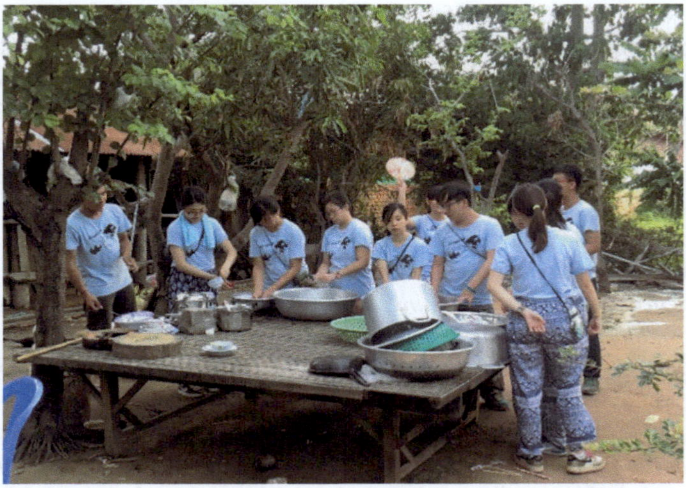

Students of PolyU, who have grown up in an urban city like Hong Kong, enjoyed washing dishes together and sharing of team-work

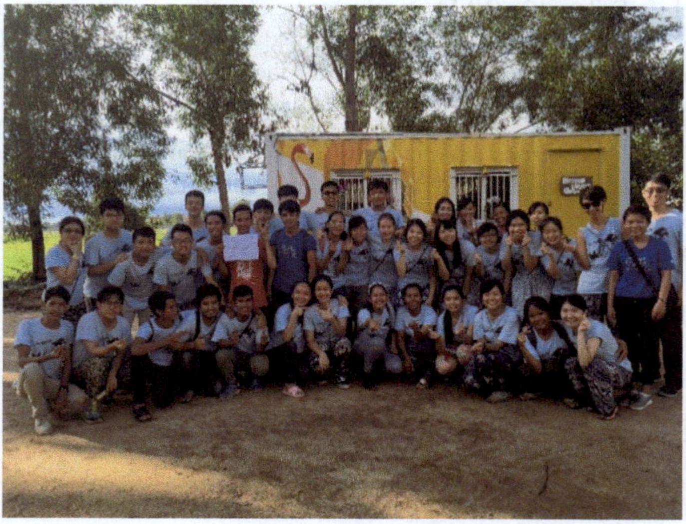

Group photos of students in the homestay, Cambodia on 2016–2017

13.6 Feedback from the Stakeholders

The role of Office of Service-Learning is crucial in connecting the local stakeholders in Cambodia. It would not be so successful without these NGOs' participation and facilitation. The stakeholders highly regard the values and the significant impacts on the target communities as listed.

(1) The Human Resource Development Institute (HRDI) reported they were shocked to witness people living in such a poor conditions in the slums in 2015. The volunteers indicated their willingness to help the underprivileged community and learn more about their poverty continuously.
(2) The Young Men's Christian Association (YMCA) indicated students from PolyU were good partners, understood each other well, and had the same vision and mission in serving the needy people in Cambodian for a better healthy lifestyle.
(3) Young People Do (YPD) reported and agreed that the SL project has provided new activities or services addressing the service gap in the community, and the service was relevant to the needs of the service-recipients. They found the service-providers are developing personal health for the slum residents as well as enhancing the personality development of the volunteers. They greatly appreciate the service team to bring in the wonderful programmes to help the poor communities in Cambodia.

(4) New Life Fellowship (NLF) greatly appreciates the commitment and attitudes of the faculty students. The service could bring in medical resources and materials that were scarce but needed for the health promotion.

In summary, the impacts and feedback from the collaborating NGOs are encouraging. This Service-Learning provides opportunities for the Hong Kong faculty students and teachers to work with the Cambodian students in providing home teaching service for health. The future plan will involve more local students and teachers of the servicing regions and with the NGOs to develop their own SL projects, connecting more of the stakeholders in contributing to this service programme for the slum residents.

13.7 Sustainability and Future Opportunities

The sustainability of the service and the connections of the stakeholders for the long-term impacts on the target community will be challenging. This service trip can be viewed as a seeding project for the students, our next generations to grow, inspire, and motivate each other in realizing the practice of "serving to learn and learning to serve". In the near future, the School of Nursing will provide scholarships for student development in global citizenship and leadership through providing the necessary resources and support for the real-world practice. Throughout the process, the students' caring attributes could be developed and nurtured. With this financial support, more students will have the opportunities of contributing to the quality of life for people who live in areas which have less access to the health resources.

Appendix—Assessment Details of PolyU Students

(1) The Global Citizenship Scale (GCS) is a 30-item scale measures global citizenship from three dimensions: social responsibility, global competence, and global civic engagement. The reliability measure was conducted in the US and HK studies. The alpha value obtained for the subscales ranges from 0.74 to 0.86 in the Hong Kong study and with less than 0.1 differences among 2 samples, which are generally accepted as good (Lo, Kwan, Ngai, & Chan 2014).
(2) Pre- and post-comparison of the reflective journal on service and experience from PolyU students. Reflective journal assessment criteria were adopted from Office of Service-Learning, PolyU with rubrics in assessing the level of reflection and learning. Guidelines for reflective journal writing are being provided to students matching with the intended learning outcomes.
(3) Feedback from teaching staff/external observer(s).
(4) Feedback from collaborators (NGOs).

References

Garcia, B. (2016). *Healthy lifestyle challenges for developing communities, international service-learning at PolyU 2016 selected case studies* (pp. 97–111).
Harcourt. (2017). *Development in early & middle adulthood,* https://www.cliffsnotes.com/studyguides/psychology/psychology/developmental-psychology-age-13-to-65/development-in-early–middle-adulthood on 15 July 2017.
Laverack, G., & Wallerstein, N. (2001). Measuring community empowerment: A fresh look at organization domains. *Health Promotion International, 16*(2), 179–185.
Lo, K. W. K., Kwan, K. P., Ngai, G., & Chan, S. C. F. (2014). An initial exploration of the cross-cultural validity of the global citizenship scale in the Hong Kong setting. In *Proceedings of the 1st International Conference on Service-Learning*, Nov 20–21, 2014, Hong Kong.
Office of Service-Learning. (2013). *Student Learning Statistics*. The Hong Kong Polytechnic University, Hong Kong.
Pang, P. C. P., & Wu, S. T. C. (2016a), Shaping future nurse leaders: Service-learning experience of promoting healthy lifestyle in developing community, Hong Kong College of Gerontology Nursing, Scientific Meeting Cum AGM 2016, on 28 May 2016.
Pang, P. C. P., & Wu, S. T. C. (2016b), Learning through reflection: Students' service-learning experiences in Cambodia, 2nd International Service-Learning at PolyU 2016, Office of Service-Learning, The Hong Kong Polytechnic University, 1–2 Dec 2016.
WHO. (2015). *What is health promotion*. Retrieved February 17, 2015, from http://www.who.int/topics/health_promotion/en/.
WHO. (2016). *Community empowerment* http://www.who.int/healthpromotion/conferences/7gchp/track1/en/http://www.who.int/healthpromotion/conferences/7gchp/track1/en/.
World Health Rankings. (2017a). *Top 50 causes of death in Cambodia*. Retrieved September 27, 2017, from http://www.worldlifeexpectancy.com/country-health-profile/cambodia.
World Health Rankings. (2017b). *Cambodia: life Expectancy*. Retrieved July 15, 2017, from http://www.worldlifeexpectancy.com/cambodia-life-expectancy.

Chapter 14
Designing a Better Environment Through Analysing the Built Environment

Barbara W. Y. Siu

Abstract According to its oldest definitions, civil engineering is a very broad discipline that deals with the design, construction and maintenance of the physical and naturally built environment. It has been widely accepted that built environment is one of the major supports to public health and quality of life. This chapter is dedicated to a service learning subject lead by the Department of Civil and Environmental Engineering at the Hong Kong Polytechnic University that engages students in studies of the built environment. Students work alongside with the service clients to gain first-hand understanding of the problems faced by the end-users, which helps them to reflect on the conventional top-down design approach. The quantitative and qualitative data obtained by students not only helped them in devising improvement suggestions to service clients and public authorities, these data also forms part of district database and can be used in setting performance targets and monitoring progress. Apart from the benefits to community, there has been observations in students' academic, professional, and personal developments, as well as positive impacts in service clients' quality of life attributes.

Keywords Service learning · Age-friendly city · Built environment Engineering education · University students

14.1 Background—Human and Built Environment

The word "built environment" has been defined in different ways. Most generally, it is the part of the physical environment that is constructed by human activity. By one definition, the built environment consists of the following elements: (1) land use patterns, the distribution across space of activities and the buildings that house

B. W. Y. Siu (✉)
Department of Civil and Environmental Engineering, The Hong Kong Polytechnic University, Hunghom, Hong Kong
e-mail: barbara.siu@polyu.edu.hk

D. T. L. Shek et al. (eds.), *Service-Learning for Youth Leadership*,
Quality of Life in Asia 12, https://doi.org/10.1007/978-981-13-0448-4_14

them; (2) the transportation system, the physical infrastructure of roads, sidewalk, bike paths, etc., as well as the services this system provides; and (3) urban design, the arrangement and appearance of the physical elements in a community (Cunningham & Michael, 2004; Roof & Oleru, 2008; Saelens & Handy, 2008). The built environment has a strong correlation with public health (Cunningham & Michael, 2004; Koohsari, Badland, & Giles-Corti, 2013; Roof & Oleru, 2008; Saelens & Handy, 2008) and quality of life (Engel et al., 2016).

According to one of its oldest definitions dated back in 1828, a civil engineering's work is "*the art of directing the great sources of power in nature for the use and convenience of man*" (The Institution of Civil Engineers, 2017). Civil engineering is a very broad professional engineering discipline that applies the knowledge of mathematics and physical sciences to deal with the design, construction and maintenance of the physical and naturally built environment. The Department of Civil and Environmental Engineering is thus the best candidate at the university to take the lead in introducing a service learning subject that focus on the linkage between human and built environment.

Students from the science and engineering disciplines are expected to apply their knowledge in science and technology in improving the built environment for the well-being of the community. The service learning subject described in this chapter serves as a platform for students from these disciplines to work in a multidisciplinary team to identify and investigate built-environment-related problems faced by the underprivileged group with quantitative and qualitative techniques, and devise solutions from a *human-centred approach*.

14.2 Subject and Service Design

The service learning subject, "CSE3S01—Built Environment Enhancement for Underprivileged Communities", was first introduced in summer, 2013/14, with initial intake of 50 students. This subject has been offered once or twice per academic year since then, and 285 students have taken this subject up to date (end of 2017). The objectives and intended learning outcomes for students are highlighted in Box 1 and Box 2 below.

Box 1. Objectives of CSE3S01
The objectives of this subject are:

1. To introduce to students the concept and practice of service learning.
2. To raise students' awareness of the problem with the build environment in Hong Kong and educate them on the challenges and needs of the underprivileged communities.
3. To provide students' an opportunity to apply their classroom knowledge in solving real-life problems in local communities.

4. To raise students' awareness of their role as a professional in society.
5. To enhance students' generic competence of innovative problem solving, communication and teamwork.

Box 2. Intended Learning Outcomes of CSE3S01
Upon completion of the subject, students will be able to:

a. Demonstrate an understanding of how built environment enhancement improves the welfare of the community.
b. Propose and evaluate alternative solutions to address the needs of the underprivileged.
c. Reflect on their role and responsibilities as a professional.
d. Work effectively in a multidisciplinary team to solve problems and communicate effectively with clients and stakeholders.
e. Demonstrate empathy for the underprivileged and a strong sense of civic responsibility.

14.2.1 Nature of Service Activities

The educational benefits and community benefits are realized through service activities which requires students to:

- Identify built-environment-related problems that underprivileged people (or communities) are facing with quantitative and qualitative techniques.
- Develop feasible solution(s) to address the problems identified together with the beneficiaries.
- Communicate their proposals to community partners and/or beneficiaries through reports/exhibition/talks.

14.2.1.1 Service Deliverables

Apart from improvement proposals/plans, alternative kinds of deliverables may be produced to suit the objectives of the community partner and the needs of the service clients, for example a thematic report after a more extensive research-type study, which will form as an important source of information for the community partner or even the policy-maker to identify service improvement opportunities, and the results of this kind of thematic study can be disseminated to the general public as a social awareness exercise. In principle, the outcome of the service project should either directly serve the needs of the beneficiaries, aid the community partner to improve their service provided to the beneficiaries, or advise the policy-makers on better decision-making process to improve the welfare of the beneficiaries in a long run.

14.2.2 Flexible Types of Service Projects

The overall subject and service project framework has been set in a generic way so as to accommodate a wide range of built-environment-related community projects. For example, potential projects/topics may include:

- Age-friendly community.
- Indoor air quality monitoring and improvement strategies which is helping elderly with chronic respiratory diseases.
- Roadside pollutant exposure and health studies to make recommendations on changing walking path choice for school children who mainly go to school on foot.
- Investigation on the locations of addition of footbridges or at-grade road crossing facilities to improve the mobility of the elderly and disabled persons in the community.
- Walkability survey (availability and quality of pedestrian infrastructures) and walking behaviour study (origin, destination, duration, path, conditions of walking environment) of the elderly or low-income group that will lead to suggestions in improving town planning and pedestrian facilities design and services standards (such as width of walkways, shelter/trees, pavement condition, green time of pedestrian crossings).
- Public transport affordability and travel pattern of the low-income groups to make suggestions to alleviate the situation of transport poverty and social exclusion.

14.2.3 Educational Benefits

Through interaction with the service clients during the service projects, the students would be more aware of their professional role, i.e. to build a better world for people to live in, in which *human element* is an indispensable part. Students would gain personal experience in the mismatch between the outcomes of the top-down approach in the design and operation of the built environment and actual needs of the end-users. During the project, students would develop empathy on the underprivileged and contribute their professional knowledge to improve the design and management of the built environment to suit the needs of their service clients. The benefits of service projects extend beyond the semester. As students graduate and take on a career in the planning and management of the built environment, their experience of applying professional skills to address human needs would be converted to a positive attitude, and this is going to benefit the community in a fundamental way.

14.3 Ageing and Age-Friendly City

As introduced in Sect. 14.2.2, the subject framework has been made rather flexible in addressing various kinds of built-environment-related community issues; the subject's major focus has been set on *age-friendly city* since its first offering in summer, 2013/14, because the subject team sees "How Hong Kong is going to embrace the rapidly ageing population?" as our major challenge in the coming decades.

Ageing population and urbanization are two important forces shaping in the twenty-first century. The percentage of world's population over 60 will double from 11% in 2006 to 22% in 2050; also, by 2030, about 3 out of every 5 in the world will live in cities (World Health Organization, 2007). As of 2016, out of the 7.33million total population of Hong Kong, 15.9% are aged 65 and above. 32.3% (or 811,645) of households in Hong Kong are with elderly persons, and around one-third of these households are elderly only households (Census and Statistic Department, Hong Kong Special Administrative Region Government, 2016). The percentage of elderly population (aged 65 and above) is expected to increase from 15% in 2014 to 28% in 2034 and 33% in 2064 (Census and Statistics Department, Hong Kong Special Administrative Region Government, 2015). How to adequately serve the needs and enhance the quality of life of elderlies in the urban setting is thus an urgent challenge.

To cope with the increasing elderly population in cities, WHO introduced the active ageing policy framework in 2002 and adopted the definition of active ageing as: "*Active ageing is the process of optimizing opportunities for health, participation and security in order to enhance quality of life as people age*" (World Health Organization, 2002). Subsequently, the age-friendly city framework was introduced in 2007 that spelt out more explicitly the eight important elements to active ageing: "1. Housing", "2. Transportation", "3. Outdoor space and building", "4. Social participation", "5. Respect and social inclusion", "6. Civic participation and employment", "7. Communication and information" and "8. Community support and health services". The first three elements are related to the *physical environment* and overlaps with the academic focus of the Faculty of Construction and Environment. These common areas make "age-friendly city" an ideal platform to design a service learning subject that bring benefits to the community while realizing the intended educational outcomes.

14.3.1 Service Site—Yau Tsim Mong District

The age-friendly city project is implemented in an old urban district—Yau Tsim Mong district through close collaboration with the major elderly service centre in the area (Salvation Army Yaumatei Multi-service Centre for Senior Citizens).

Yau Tsim Mong district is situated in the Kowloon Peninsula. In its compact area of 6.99 km^2 (Survey and Mapping Office, Lands Department, Hong Kong Special Administrative Region Government, 2016), it houses 342,970 people, that is a population density of 49,065 person per km^2, the second highest in Hong Kong. Despite of its high residential density, Yau Tsim Mong district is also a major business and tourism centre. Yau Tsim Mong district is a mix of the old with the new, while some older areas are undergoing urban renewal, there are new developments as well, and it offers excellent opportunities to bring in and to enhance age-friendly elements in this district.

14.3.2 Service Projects

As described in Sect. 14.3 and Fig. 14.1, there are eight focus areas in the concept of age-friendly city, and this subject is directly related to the three elements related to built environment summarized in Box 3 below (Fig. 14.2).

Box 3—The three AFC focus area in CSE3S01 (adapted from World Health Organization, 2007)

AFC Focus Area #1—Outdoor Spaces and Buildings

- Characteristics of urban landscape and built environment
- It has major impact on *mobility, independence and quality of life*
- Directly related to the ability to "age in place"
- *AFC Focus Area #2—Transportation*
- Accessible and affordable public transport is a key factor influencing active ageing
- Being able to move about the city is essential to *social and civic participation*, as well as access to *community and health services*
- *AFC Focus Area #3—Housing*
- Essential to safety and well-being
- Housing structure, location and choice
- Appropriate housing and access to community and social services
- *Independence and quality of life* of older people

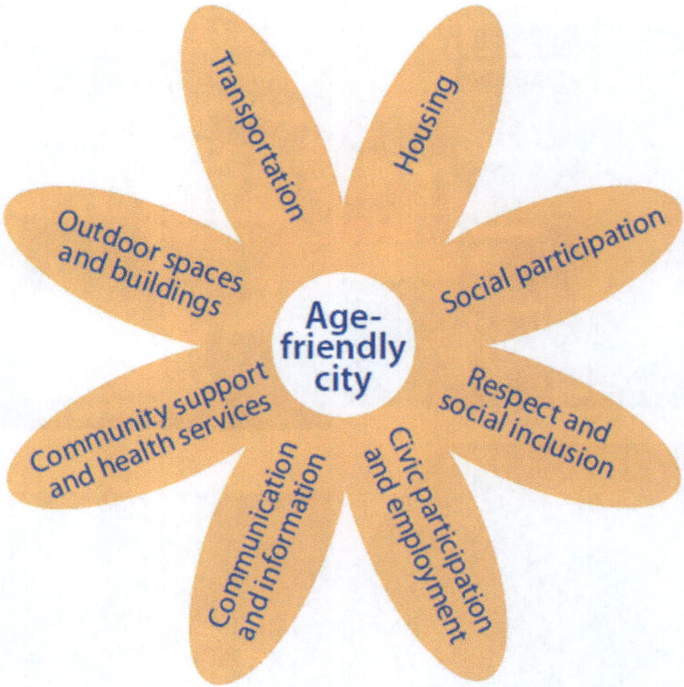

Fig. 14.1 Age-friendly city topic areas (World Health Organization, 2007)

The actual service activities have been carefully planned to achieve the educational objectives of this subject and to address society needs. Table 14.1 highlights the various service activities and deliverables to address the three AFC areas in Box 3 above.

All the service activities have been designed for students to

- Understand the habits and activity patterns of the elderly and their constraints.
- Understand the difficulties in ageing in place.
- Assess the age-friendliness of Yau Tsim Mong district/Hong Kong.
- Help students the enhance communication skills, cultivate empathy and sense of respect for the elderly.

When the subject was first offered in summer, 2013/14, the 50 students had home visits as well as focus study with elderlies in order to develop a holistic understanding on age-friendly issues from both individual and community perspectives. Later on, with preliminary understanding gained from service projects, the subject spun off into two lecture groups of 60 students each in 2016/17.

In one of the lecture groups, students do home visits to elderlies who are more physically infirm and/or live alone (or as couple), and take their client on tours which they plan together. Students in this lecture group are looking at the age-friendly city issues at a more individual or personal level, since they have very

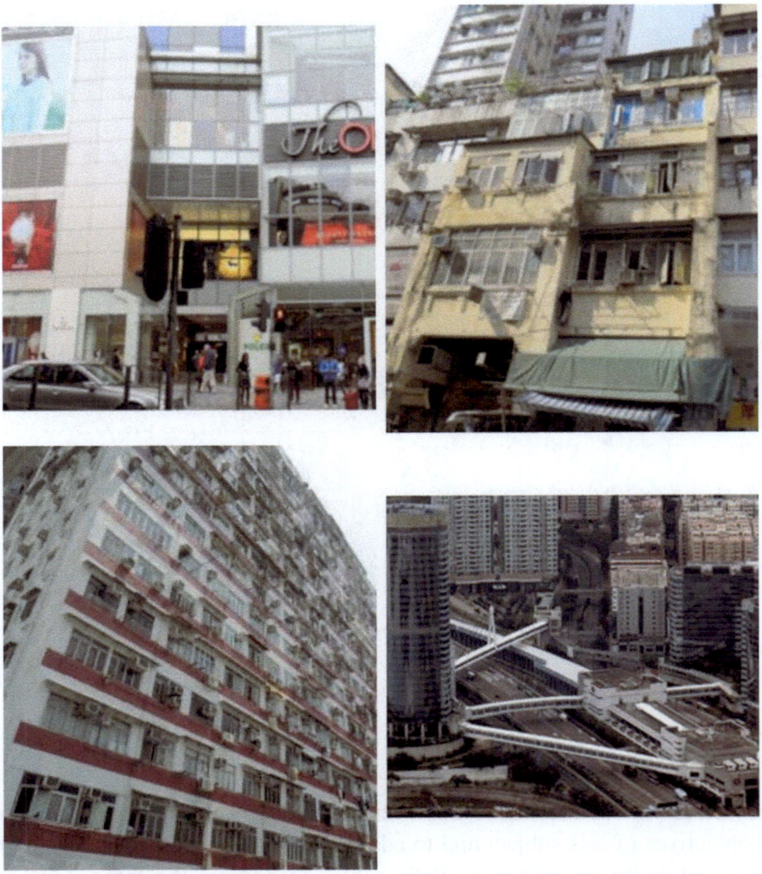

Fig. 14.2 Yau Tsim Mong District—A Mix of Business, Residential, Tourism, Old, and New

close interaction with their clients; yet, their scope of understanding may be rather limited.

The other lecture group team up with more active elderlies from community centres to perform focus study, i.e. to look at more problematic spots in their local community. Students in this lecture group would also perform objective and systematic assessment of age-friendliness using indicators adapted from WHO guidelines (World Health Organizations, 2015). Students in this lecture group would be able to look at age-friendly issues from a wider, community perspective, but they have limited opportunities to hear the voices directly from the neediest group of old people who are not so visible in the community setting. Therefore, at the end of the subject, students of both groups come together in the debriefing session to share what they have done and how they perceived the difficulties faced by elderlies differently.

Table 14.1 Teaching and service activities

Class		Lectures/seminars: – Subject introduction, age-friendly city concepts – Elderly simulation – Elderly in Hong Kong, per-service training – Design standards, data collection methods Project meetings: – Discuss study plan – Project progress and findings – Debriefing/reflection on academic learning and personal development Debriefing: – End-of-subject – Reflection and sharing of experience
Service components	Home visits	Activities: – Identify areas of improvements (Age-friendly Housing) – Discuss improvement suggestions with clients – Implementation Deliverables: – Improvements in living environment, or improvement plans passed to social worker for follow-up in case of more complex improvement suggestion – Case report
	Tours	Activities: – Plan a half-day outing/tour with home visit client – Examine age-friendliness of transportation and outdoor spaces and buildings during tour Deliverables: – Tour recommendations for elderly – Photographs/memoir for elderly
	Age-friendly city Focus study	Activities: – PolyU students team up with elderlies – Identification of study theme/problematic spot – Field visits to collect data for problem identification and analysis – Devise improvement suggestions with elderlies – Engagement workshop/presentations at community centres Deliverables: – Presentation at community centre—raise awareness of age-friendly concepts – Report—include study findings, recommendations for improvement and monitoring, e.g. submission to district council
	Age-friendly city community assessment	Activities: – Use defined indicators to perform baselines assessment baseline assessment of age-friendliness using core indicators adapted from WHO guidelines – Objective data collected – For evaluation, progress monitoring, setting goals and targets Deliverables: – Data sheets and assessment report

14.4 Impacts on Elderlies

The built environment is one determining element that contributes to active ageing or older people's quality of life. To put the professional knowledge and skills of the Department of Civil and Environmental Engineering into service, the service activities are focusing on improvements in the built environment. Some of the improvements are immediate (typically the small-scale improvements in living environment), but those in the public realm (outdoor space and building, transportation) takes a long deliberation process before the improvement plans are being realized. By now, it should be apparent on how the service activities are oriented towards the elements of "Housing", "Outdoor spaces and buildings" and "Transportation" among the eight age-friendly city topic areas highlighted in Fig. 14.1.

Yet, from the feedbacks collected directly from elderlies, community partner and observations made during the service projects throughout years, the subject brings about other benefits.

In the age-friendly city focus study, elderlies work with students as a team to identify problems in their community, devise solution and prepare presentations at community centres (as engagement activity). Through this collaboration with students, the following outcomes have been observed:

- Increase in competence: Elderlies gained knowledge in age-friendly city and are more capable of digesting and interpreting quantitative and qualitative information due to the joint field study with students.
- Empowerment: With the gain in competence and the platform being set up to follow-up the improvement suggestions at district council, elderlies are functioning as change agent; they felt empowered, and they are able to make some changes to the community.
- Social participation: Through the engagement talks at community centres, a lot of elderlies who felt passive and pessimistic became eager to express their views towards age-friendly city issues.
- Social acceptance and respect: Apart from elderlies who participated directly in the focus study found acceptance and respect from students and officers at the district council, elderly participants at the engagement talks realized that their voices are being listened to and accepted.
- Empathy: The close collaboration with students for one semester provided opportunities for elderlies to expand their social network to a group of young people whom are usually not part of their social circle. During the process, they understood the perspectives and values of one another, instead of being very critical about young people, elderlies began to understand and empathize the challenges faced by young people nowadays.

The service projects and the way that the projects are delivered contributed the quality of life of elderlies, the project deliverables (home improvements, proposals on improving age-friendliness of community) are contributing to the "material well-being", while the process which the service project is delivered brings about increase in competence, empowerment, etc., as mentioned above contributes to "social well-being", "development" and "emotional well-being" of elderlies (Flece & Perry, 1995), these aspects are highlighted in yellow in Fig. 14.3.

14.5 Impact on Students

While the overall gains of service learning in PolyU students' learning are contended in Chap. 19, this section discusses more qualitatively the observations in reading students' reflective journals, observations in students' field service. Since students' consent has not been obtained when they submitted their reflective journals, students' works are not directly quoted here. Discussions are going to be made in both positive and negative aspects.

14.5.1 Independent Learning

After several introductory lectures on the basic concepts, students looked up other references online, such as design standards in Hong Kong and overseas, or examples of good practices in other countries (such as intersection layout as in Fig. 14.4, or new technology in tacking uneven pavement surface). In problem identification, they researched what are the appropriate approaches in data collection (e.g. how to evaluate the effects of illegal parking (Fig. 14.5), which kinds of devices are needed in measuring indoor air quality (Fig. 14.6)). There are some negative examples, such as students did not plan carefully about the field investigation, did not bring any equipment (not even a tape rule) when they are supposed to measure the widths of walkways in a specific task.

14.5.2 Problem-Solving

There are a lot of ad hoc problems in project works, in which not every situation can be covered in lectures or they can be warned ahead. Some students were able to identify a good solution while some could not.

- For example, students are supposed to plan a half-day tour with their service clients, but some clients later on refused the proposal. Some students tried to look for the reason and convince the client to change their mind, or come up with some alternative activities that are meaningful and less physically demanding, while some just gave up and ask the subject lecturers on how to fulfil the service hours otherwise.

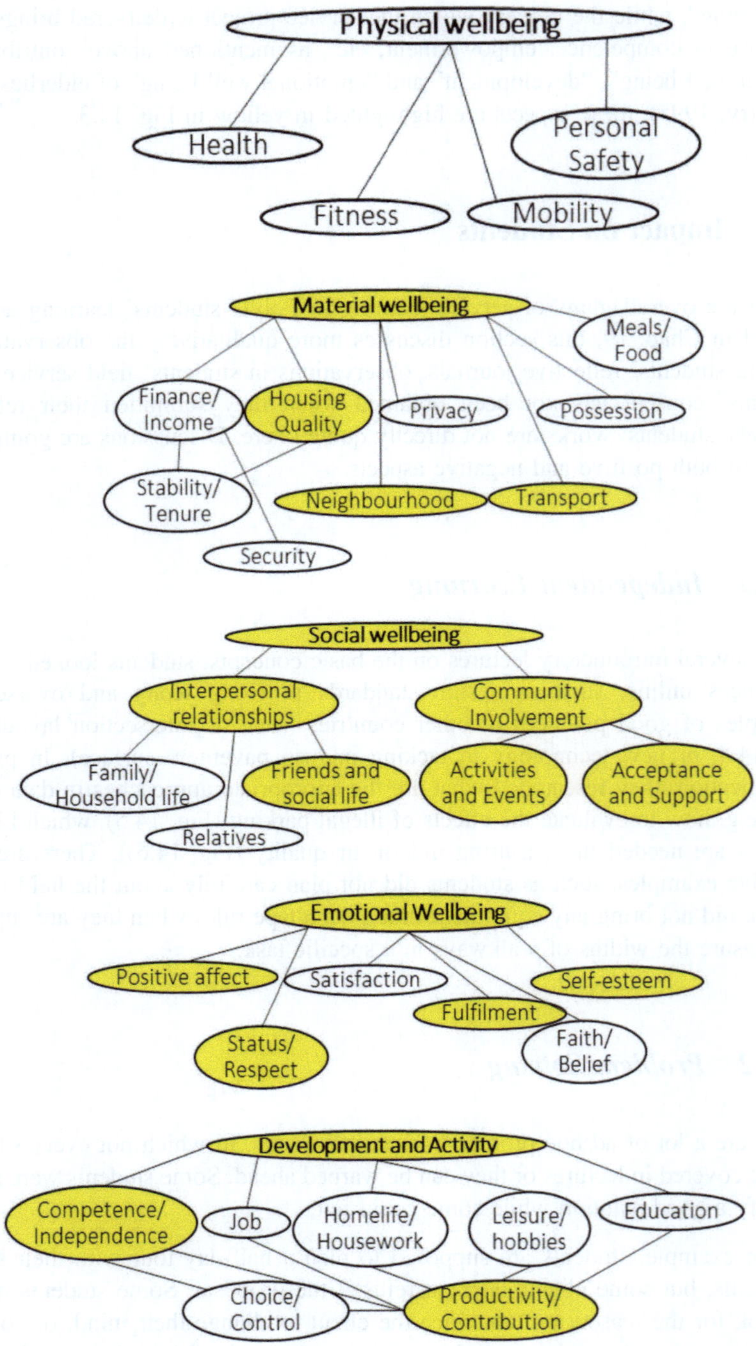

Fig. 14.3 Service Project intervention in quality of life aspects of elderlies. Adapted from (Flece & Perry, 1995)

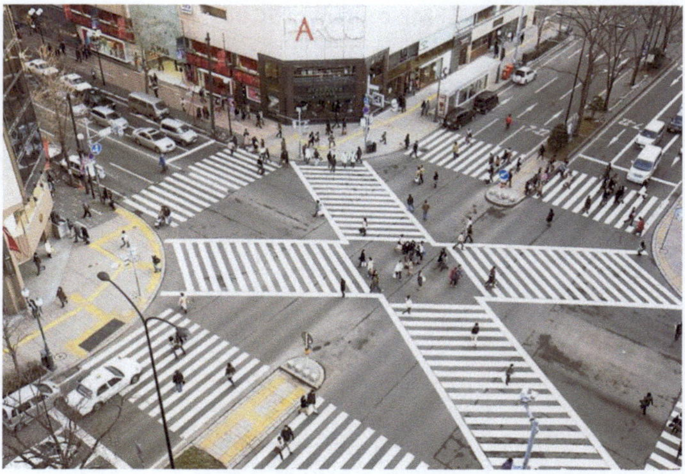

Fig. 14.4 Suggestion to shorten the distance of pedestrian crossing, example taken from Tokyo, Japan

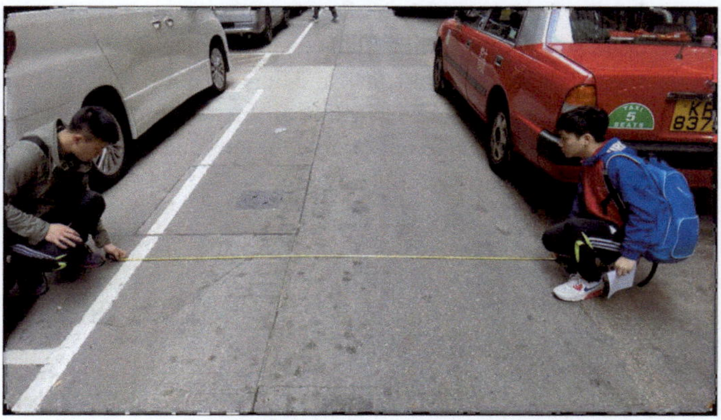

Fig. 14.5 Students checking whether remaining width of carriageway is wide enough for emergency vehicles

– Another example would be students are supposed to remind their clients of the upcoming home visit on phones. Some student did not do it, did it too long before, or just half hour before showing up at the doorsteps, these are instances of poor planning. Sometimes, they called several times and could not reach their clients and then just gave up. While discussing this kind of situation in the project meeting, some students admitted that they were not aware of the possibility of this client being alone at home and needed help. However, they felt that they could not enter the building anyway because there is a gate. Students could have waited at the gate for someone to come out or explained the situation and asked the guard to

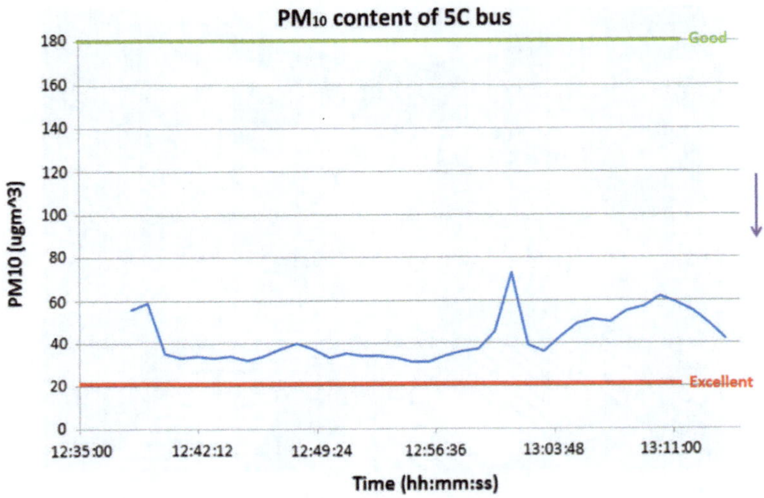

Fig. 14.6 Air quality inside public transport measured by students against air quality objective

accompany them to the home of their client, even policemen or the social worker would have done something similar. This example may be an indication of students seeing the service activity as a task and they do not care about the client that much, despite it is more likely to be a lack of problem-solving skills and the entire group was not aware of the range of possible reasons and how the problem can be tackled better rather than simply going away.

14.5.3 Empathy

In the service projects, no matter through the close interaction with elderlies in home visits and tours, or in the age-friendly city focus studies, students learnt a lot more about the lives of old people. Some students felt very sorry for elderlies who worked hard for decades, but being exploited by their employers and thus has not much saving, living in very unfavourable conditions (Fig. 14.7), students started to think about social injustice. When students visited the elderly community centres, they saw discrimination; the staffs there knew the names of the more affluent elderlies who regularly enrol in various classes that require course fees, but did not really welcome other members who just come to pass time, read newspapers and socialize. A group of students from the first cohort, after they finished the subject and went to Shanghai for study tour, they made a long-distance call to remind one of their clients of her upcoming medical appointment. Seeing students moving from focusing on their own grades in this course to showing care for others is also a rewarding experience for teachers. Empathy is not something that would develop very naturally in some students, and they needed some reminder in project meetings with subject lecturers.

14.5.4 Deep Learning

The service learning subject has brought students some eye-opening experience, despite most of them are not so pleasant ones, that is what stimulated reflection and deep learning.

- While students were conducting questionnaire survey, they were shocked at many old people are illiterate. It caused some hurdles because students thought they can simply print out the questionnaire and let elderlies finish themselves. Moreover, students found the respondents are quite gloomy, they saw themselves as useless (low self-esteem), being ignored, and thought that the questionnaire might be scam. These are all something student have never thought of and really moved them while conducting field service.
- In students' field studies, they had a very strong impression that private developers/facilities operators (especially the high-end ones) purposely do not want elderly to hang around in their premises by removing seats, closing down the escalator, etc. These no-too-pleasant encounters often triggered students to think deeper about what could be done. For example, students reflected the conflict between personal interest and social responsibility, or on the housing problems in Hong Kong, seeing how impractical it is for Hong Kong people to live with their old parents and what can be done as a professional who are going to build houses.

14.5.5 Mutual Respect and Understanding

Before this project, elderlies and young people do not have much chance to interact. They had some impressions derived from mass media or Internet. Through service, students changed their views about elderlies, instead of being stubborn and conservative they can be very well-educated, open-minded. Elderlies often think young people as arrogant and selfish, but they found our students are in fact very caring and respecting old people. It is rather interesting to observe students' interaction with elderlies in the subject. In Chinese culture, we were taught to respect the elders, and it is often translated to being submissive. Some students just followed what the elderlies suggested, while some were willing to challenge their views with reasons. As expected, most of the elderlies were grateful to and appreciated what the students have done in the home visits, tours, field visits or preparing presentation at community centres; sometimes they had high expectations on students and were rather critical about students' level of enthusiasm and performance.

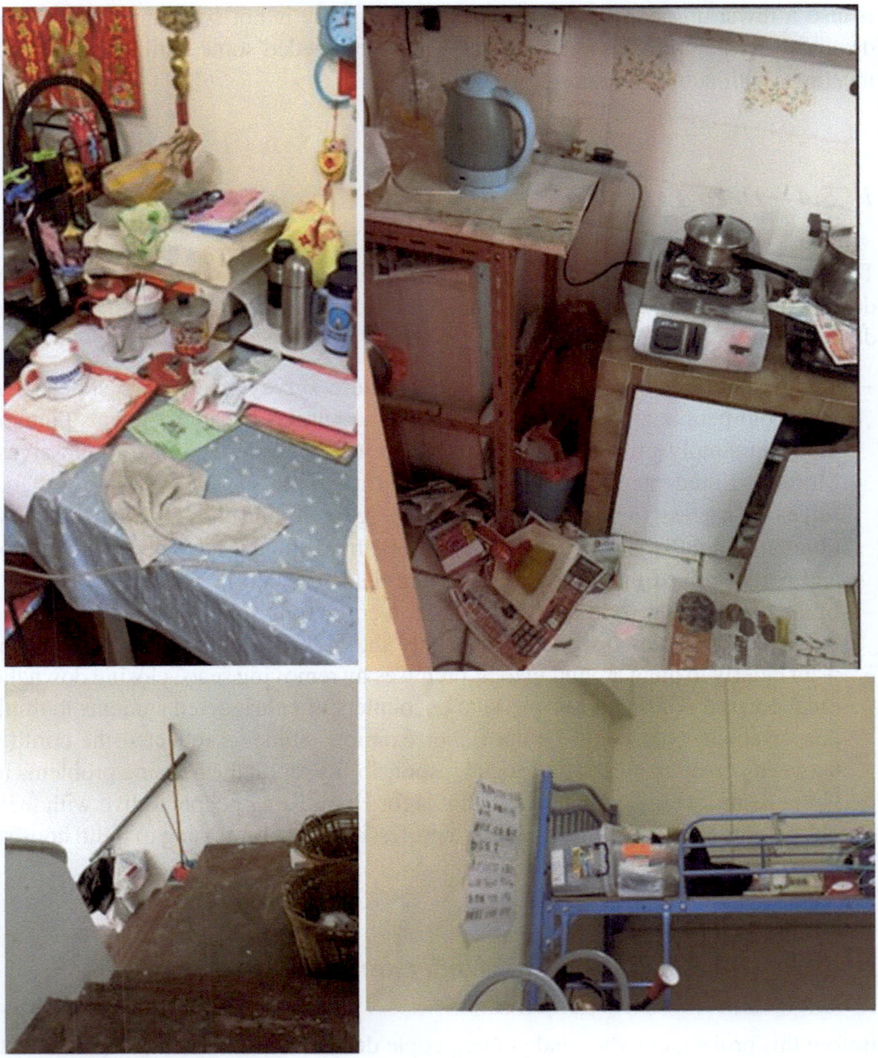

Fig. 14.7 Pictures of living environment of typical elderly only households

14.6 Reflection as Subject Leader

The above sections qualitatively discussed the subject/service's impacts on elderlies and students, and these sections are some reflections as a subject lecturer.

14.6.1 Adaptation to Experiential Learning

Service learning is an experiential learning approach in which students' learning comes from their action and reflection. This is very unfamiliar to students and teachers. Students in Hong Kong came from a very examination-oriented system, and they are very accustomed to highly structured, lecture-based learning. Students felt confused and were not comfortable at the beginning of the subject when they were planning what they would do in order to achieve the desired service and learning outcomes, and they felt a lack of guidance when given too much freedom to chart their own learning. Despite there is a widespread trend of active learning approaches in higher-education, teaching and learning in science and engineering disciplines remain rather traditional, at least at PolyU. Experiential learning not only caused a cultural shock in students, but subject lecturers as well. Engineering teachers' adaptation to a new teaching and learning style that have not been experienced before in our own education or career is also painstaking. With limited training and support, teachers are also going through an experiential learning process in how to teach a service learning subject: to provide guidance instead of instructions, to facilitate reflections rather than demonstration of technical knowledge and to assess students' level of achievement in various qualitative criteria rather than awarding marks to right or wrong answer.

14.6.2 Students' Acceptance in Service Learning

At PolyU, service learning is a graduation requirement, and students only have a choice of which service learning subject to take but not forgoing service learning entirely. In students' reflective journals and debriefing meetings, most students admitted that they do service learning because they do not have a choice, they are not too interested in spending the time and effort in community service, and most students started off with a negative feeling about service learning. In time, some students found satisfaction in service and discovered some learning and changes in perspectives, and these students normally demonstrate higher level of engagement and are more proactive in service. Some students, on the other hand, could not shake off the feeling that they are forced to do this, they displayed continuous resistance and felt that the subject and service activities are poorly organized, and there is too much work and would like to fulfil the requirements using minimum effort. This group of students lacked engagement throughout and could sometimes jeopardize the teamwork, which required extra mentoring by the subject lecturers.

14.6.3 Awareness of Social Needs

Aside of the work, service learning provided an opportunity for faculty members to reflect the relationship between research and community, to help us to keep our feet on the ground. Expert knowledge in a subject area and research skills can be directly applied in service through student. One example would be, students and elderlies involved in the project (or the community in general) are looking for improvements in walking environment, they can all subjectively tell what is good and what is not so good, but they need help from faculty members in identifying what are the defining elements of walking environment to facilitate objective data collection and analysis. Another example would be, in community meetings or focus group interviews, elderlies might have expressed a lot of views, but with proper data transcription and qualitative analysis technique, further insights could be generated.

Through engaging in service activities with students, faculty members can see the deficiencies in existing standards, guidelines, and policy; just to list two examples: (1) in the current town planning standard (Planning Department, Hong Kong Special Administrative Region Government, 2016), the population-based provision of recreational facilities encompasses active sports like badminton, squash, swimming, football, but there is no explicit standard provision of exercise facilities for elderlies; (2) in transport planning guidelines (Transport Department, Hong Kong Special Administrative Region Government, 2013), it assumed pedestrian walking speed as 1.2 m/s in traffic signal calculation and stated that engineers might consider using a walking speed of 0.9 m/s in case of high portion of elderly users; there is no additional consideration or guidelines on traffic signal design in view of ageing population. The service experienced allowed faculty members to voice out observation when they are being consulted as experts in government committees.

14.6.4 Challenges

Teaching service learning subject can be a rewarding experience when we see the students showing high level of engagement and self-initiative, reflecting on own room of improvements, and observing their change in attitude or perceptions. Moreover, the project setting allowed students to demonstrate their creativity and talents that often surprised the teachers. Yet, there are other challenges associated with the delivery of service learning courses.

14.6.4.1 From Passionate to Burnout

The first thing would be the workload. Service learning subjects are usually delivered in form of small group projects, regular field supervision and debriefing/

meetings with students and are essential to ensure quality of service as well as students' learning. Each service session is typically 3–4 h and off-campus. This leads to timetabling problems with students and tremendous amount of coordination work compared with a typical lecture-based subject. As a result, service activities are often scheduled in evenings and weekends. The extra work in coordination and also work outside normal hours often cannot be completely recognized in the university's framework. Service learning teachers are passionate about what they are doing and find satisfaction and sense of fulfilment in seeing students' growth and doing good to the community. However, when consistently high workload and pressure over semesters eventually go beyond the tipping point, there begin feelings of burn out, low morale and resistance. This introduces extra difficulties in subject coordination.

14.6.4.2 Coordination Among Subject Team

Due to the small group project nature of the subject, a much higher student–staff ratio is needed, and it means the subject is often delivered in a subject team. When the subject team is getting large, coordination among lecturers would be necessary to ensure consistency. Most faculty members used to work independently with high level of autonomy and are now required to communicate a shared vision or work according to something he/she might not totally agree to, and it leads to pressure or even conflicts among colleagues. Coordination among colleague is often much taxing than the workload itself, and it is even more so when some team members felt overloaded with the service learning subject.

14.7 Conclusion

This service learning subject has been an experiential process for both students and teachers. The subject has been designed for students to gain subject knowledge, develop professional skills, awareness of social problems, empathy to people in need and personal development. These learning outcomes are realized through service projects that target certain community needs. The subject framework has been defined in a flexible way to accommodate different community needs. In view of the trend of ageing population in Hong Kong and the relationship between built environment and quality of life of older people, this subject has been focusing on the theme of age-friendly city since its first offering in 2013/14. Throughout years, there has been organic growth in the subject with increased class size, more diverse and in-depth service activities. Looking back, the subject has made positive contribution to the service clients (elderlies) through improvement in the physical environment, and enhancement in other aspects that contributes to their quality of life, such as respect, acceptance, social participation, empowerment, and fulfilment. To students, this service learning experience effectively fostered independent learning and problem-solving. Students are being introduced to a social group whom they are not familiar with and developed semester-long relationship with the same group of service recipients; from this, students truly understand and appreciate the complexity of the problems (not limited to age-friendly issues) faced by elderlies and developed empathy based on these relationships. Not only forming bonds with new people, often students encountered things that are out of their expectation in service, and these new experiences provoked deep reflection. Service learning teachers are passionate in teaching and found great satisfaction and sense of fulfilment in witnessing students' growth, change in attitude and doing good to the community. The experiential learning approach has been a new thing to both students and teachers which required adjustments; thus, there are development in teachers while engaging in the subject. Teachers are overwhelmed by the workload due to group-based field work, and subject coordination among the teaching team is challenging as faculty members used to enjoy high autonomy in teaching and research. The engagement in service activities with students provided faculty members with opportunities to reflect on the relationship between research and community. This service learning subject acted as a conduit for us to apply our expert knowledge and research skills in service and to advice government on setting of policies, guidelines and standards.

References

Census and Statistic Department, Hong Kong Special Administrative Region Government. (2016). *2016 Population by-census main results*. Hong Kong: Census and Statistic Department, Hong Kong Special Administrative Region Government.

Census and Statistics Department, Hong Kong Special Administrative Region Government. (2015). *Hong Kong population projections 2015–2064*. Hong Kong: Census and Statistics Department, Hong Kong Special Administrative Region Government.

Cunningham, G. O., & Michael, Y. L. (2004). Concepts guiding the study of the impact of the built environment on physical activity for older adults: A review of the literature. *American Journal of Health Promotion, 18*(6), 435–443.

Engel, L., Chudyk, A. M., Ashe, M. C., McKay, H. A., Whitehurst, D. G., & Bryan, S. (2016). Older adults' quality of life—Exploring the role of the built environment and social cohesion in community-dwelling seniors on low income. *Social Science and Medicine, 164*(Supplement C), 1–11. https://doi.org/10.1016/j.socscimed.2016.07.008.

Flece, D., & Perry, J. (1995). Quality of life: Its definition and measurement. *Research in Developmental Disabilities, 16*(1), 51–74.

Koohsari, M. J., Badland, H., & Giles-Corti, B. (2013). (Re)Designing the built environment to support physical activity: Bringing public health back into urban design and planning. *Cities, 35*(Supplement C), 294–298. https://doi.org/10.1016/j.cities.2013.07.001.

Planning Department, Hong Kong Special Administrative Region Government. (2016). *Hong Kong planning standards and guidelines*. Hong Kong: Planning Department, Hong Kong Special Administrative Region Government.

Roof, K. M., & Oleru, N. P. (2008). Public health: Seattle and king county's push for the built environment. *Journal of Environmental Health, 71*(1), 24–27.

Saelens, B. E., & Handy, S. L. (2008). Built environment correlates of walking: A review. *Medicine and Science in Sports and Exercise, 40*(Supplement 7), S550. https://doi.org/10.1249/MSS.0b013e31817c67a4.

Survey and Mapping Office, Lands Department, Hong Kong Special Administrative Region Government. (2016). *Area by district council (Based on 2016 district council)*. Retrieved from https://www.landsd.gov.hk/mapping/en/publications/district.htm.

The Institution of Civil Engineers. (2017). *Royal charter, by laws, regulations and rules*. London: The Institution of Civil Engineers.

Transport Department, Hong Kong Special Administrative Region Government. (2013). *Transport planning and design manual*. Hong Kong: Transport Department, Hong Kong Special Administrative Region Government.

World Health Organization. (2002). *Active ageing: A policy framework*. Retrieved from https://apps.who.int/iris/bitstream/10665/67215/1/WHO_NMH/NPH_02.8.pdf.

World Health Organization. (2007). *Global age-friendly cities: A guide*. France: World Health Organization.

World Health Organizations. (2015). *Measuring the age-friendliness of cities: A guide to using core indicators*. Kobe, Japan: World Health Organizations.

Chapter 15 Merging the Professional with the Layperson: Optometric Services for the Community

Chi-wai Do, Henry H. L. Chan, Lily Y. L. Chan, Geoffrey Chu, Horace H. Y. Wong, Natalie Y. Y. Chan, Vivian W. Y. Lo, Savio Lee, Ann Chan and Ada H. T. Ma

Abstract In this subject, we aim to integrate community services with students' learning opportunities. Students work in groups and organize and implement a vision screening project by themselves under supervision. Through this subject, students are given opportunities to act upon their roles as community service providers, care, work, and communicate with various disciplines to bridge together knowledge they have acquired during their university studies and then share and apply their special interests with others. The project not only benefits service users,

C. Do (✉) · H. H. L. Chan · L. Y. L. Chan · G. Chu · H. H. Y. Wong
N. Y. Y. Chan · V. W. Y. Lo · S. Lee · A. Chan · A. H. T. Ma
School of Optometry, The Hong Kong Polytechnic University,
Hunghom, Hong Kong
e-mail: chi_wai.do@polyu.edu.hk

H. H. L. Chan
e-mail: henryhl.chan@polyu.edu.hk

L. Y. L. Chan
e-mail: lily.yl.chan@polyu.edu.hk

G. Chu
e-mail: geoffrey.chu@polyu.edu.hk

H. H. Y. Wong
e-mail: horace.wong@polyu.edu.hk

N. Y. Y. Chan
e-mail: natalie.yy.chan@polyu.edu.hk

V. W. Y. Lo
e-mail: vivian.wy.lo@polyu.edu.hk

S. Lee
e-mail: savio.lee@polyu.edu.hk

A. Chan
e-mail: ann.chan@polyu.edu.hk

A. H. T. Ma
e-mail: ada.ht.ma@polyu.edu.hk

D. T. L. Shek et al. (eds.), *Service-Learning for Youth Leadership*,
Quality of Life in Asia 12, https://doi.org/10.1007/978-981-13-0448-4_15

but also provides a very structured learning environment for students to gain experience working with a number of people in different levels of the community and to better understand societal needs, especially in this major public health concern of blindness prevention.

Keywords Optometry · Service-learning · Eye · Special needs
Geriatrics · Pediatrics · Uncorrected refractive errors

15.1 Introduction

15.2 What Is Optometric Services?

Optometrists are primary healthcare providers who are the primary contact source for the public experiencing eye problems. According to the World Council of Optometry, "*Optometry is a healthcare profession that is autonomous, educated and regulated (licensed/registered), and optometrists are the primary healthcare practitioners of the eye and visual system who provide comprehensive eye and vision care, which includes refraction and dispensing, detection/diagnosis and management of disease in the eye, and the rehabilitation of conditions of the visual system* (World Council of Optometry, 2015)." Since many conditions and diseases of the human eye and visual system are the hallmark of underlying systemic health conditions, optometry is a healthcare field which involves extensive teamwork, elaborate communication, and collaboration to connect and coordinate their patients to particular healthcare specialties needed for their health conditions.

When a healthcare team is composed of talents from multidisciplinary fields, there is a synergy created that merges knowledge base and skills of the team as a whole in practicing more efficiently and effectively to provide the medical workup, diagnosis, management, and follow-up on their patient's health problems. Optometry is not only limited to eye healthcare diagnosis and management. Optometrists work with a spectrum of age groups. The populations they served range from young children to older adults, people with special needs from various facilities, families from different walks of life and requirements. Because of this broad range of people skills connection and services provided to the public, this gives the profession a "head start" on social responsibility and to practice community service early on in their careers as part of their normal every day-to-day work.

15.3 What's the Goal of Merging This Profession with the Layperson?

Eye diseases and visual disorders span across all age groups and are major public health problems evident within our community. Hong Kong is one of the most densely populated cities in the world. Our published literature has reported a concern regarding constricted living space as a possible environmental threat for myopia development in schoolchildren (Choi et al., 2017). Additionally, the prevalence and degree of myopia are high among Hong Kong Chinese schoolchildren. By the time a child is 12 years old, it is expected that more than 60% of their classmates are myopic (Lam, Lam, Cheng, & Chan, 2012). On the other extreme, the United Nations have reported that Hong Kong ranked top on the longest average life expectancy scale of 83.7 years old. As the chances of getting eye diseases such as glaucoma, diabetic retinopathy increase as we age, this poses a major public health issue for our health system (Woo, Chan, Lam, & Yeo, 2010). According to the World Health Organization, the estimated number of blind people will double by 2020 (World Health Organization, 2006). In our profession, we work with the community to increase awareness, and try to develop adequate human resources to lessen the strain on this major public health concern. The School of Optometry at HKPolyU is the only local university in Hong Kong to provide accredited training for optometrists (http://www.polyu.edu.hk/so). As part of our teaching and internship training endeavor, there had always been an engagement of optometrists and students organizing and participating in vision screening and eye care promotion missions for the disadvantaged, whether locally and/or internationally. It was a particularly significant and valued component in the education of optometry students in order to train them to gain an awareness of underserved communities and encourage them to provide for these neglected populations as they practice optometry in the future. Our manpower had, however, been bound to only optometry students participating in vision screenings, limiting our resources to serve the needy. On average, among 100 optometry students who were involved with vision screening activities annually, we attended to only a handful of NGO groups, serving a few hundreds of beneficiaries. As it was clear that this gap cannot be served by optometry students alone, when HKPolyU introduced a compulsory 3-credit service-learning component in their graduation requirements, it was a logical step for optometrists to extend this work for non-optometry students, given our history in community care projects. With the participation from layperson, our missions to service this need for eye care in the community helped narrow this gap in the limited number of optometry students we can only train. By the time, we merged different disciplines into vision screening activities, and we were able to cater our services to a lot more people in need. Without doubt, it was a distinctive decision to expose more students to this effort, furthering collaborative and cross-disciplinary applications to service-learning work on what optometry had done long before. We do believe that this will bring potential educational benefits to the faculty and students as it can be regarded as a broadening of teaching and learning as well as a strategic approach to collect big data for improving community healthcare settings. This was in line with World Health Organization's Prevention of Blindness Vision 2020 initiative: (1) increase awareness, (2) partner with organizations, and (3) develop adequate human resources (World Health Organization, 2006). The intended purpose, in fact, was to design a subject to educate students about the importance of vision during their learning process, while fostering leadership, community services, and cultural acceptance. As a whole for the students and the profession, it had significant potential public health benefits. For optometry students, it provides the clinical experience needed for community care to the underserved and nurture their competencies to continue this practice after their graduation.

From our previous experience in overseas vision screening projects (Chin et al., 2015), we realized our students have the potential to engage in international projects with impact on the local ethnic groups. We were further encouraged through pilot projects (made possible by the PolyU Community Service Fund and the Global Youth Leadership Institute) to test trial this concept to serve on international missions. Here, we brought students outside our discipline to participate in vision screenings in Mainland China and in overseas missions to developing countries such as Cambodia, Vietnam, and Kyrgyzstan. Our servicing initiative had the intent to serve more people and expose students to appreciate cultural diversity was well received with positive feedback from participating students and supervisors. As a student described in his reflective journal, "*It was meaningful to help people in need by utilizing the clinical and practical skills he learned at school. Apart from providing eye care services and optical aids to them, he had culture exchange with the local people as well as the interpreters. They cooperated with the local university students, shared, talked with each other with plenty of time for them to get to know each other and learn more their country and the people after their screening trip.*" It was an eye-opening experience for the students to learn about different living styles, their historical roots, standards of living, and their languages. At first, they thought they were only a service provider but actually they realized they were also the service beneficiaries. These students demonstrated a greater satisfaction in their own living conditions yet at the same time learned to value the close social and family dynamics observed in other cultures while on these overseas vision screening projects. Students who joined these overseas experiences expressed that they regarded their service trip as, "*one of their most unforgettable experiences in their university life,*" and reported a high likelihood of wanting to join similar services in the future. There were students who applied for student scholarships to initiate their own projects after serving in these projects. For example, a selected group of students who went on an overseas vision screening in Kyrgyzstan demonstrated reciprocation in proactive action. They invited their project supervisor back to assist them in providing further constructive work in their self-initiated service mission. Their project involved improving the quality of life for a certain family they had encountered. They also collaborated with the local university students on these activities in order to provide a peer influence and support on their active citizenship platform. New ties were established with the local orphanage to explore new initiatives to help their future development. We are also exploring the possibility to help the local blind schools by offering low vision services for their schoolchildren in the future. Our students became advocates to improve the quality of lives of others. This gave us an optimistic strategy to further our initiative in not limiting their service-learning potential to local projects but extending it more broadly to serve the underserved worldwide because of the strong impact these projects potentially serve to cultivate students' self-initiatives.

In 2014, we started this concept and expanded our teaching philosophy for a different undergraduate student base. More than a hundred undergraduate students started this milestone, "*to learn about eyes.*" This subject (Do et al., 2016) had thus continued to welcome new students every semester, which included future professionals-to-be from various faculties including those from the other faculties and schools. The class was also not limited to local students. There were students from Mainland China, Korea, Japan, Taiwan, and Malaysia to name a few.

15.3.1 How Has the Educational Context of This Subject Cultivated an Appreciation on Quality of Life?

More than 314 million people suffer from poor vision worldwide because they do not have access to proper eye care service. With the advance of health technologies, people are surviving longer than before. Yet, extending one's life expectancy (survival) does not necessarily equate to a good quality of life (Woo & Chan, 2015). For general undergraduate students without having seen nursing homes or experienced the constraints of wheelchair users, quality of life measures are not easy views to conceptualize. Thus, in order to ensure a good foundation of basic knowledge and application, our teaching timeframe involves a two-semester balance of education and application in vision and eye care-focused topics. This will give students enough time for a deeper reflection on their position in society and visualize how they may undertake community engagement through their specialty areas in the future. The curriculum has been planned according to a set of predetermined intended learning outcomes centered toward cultivating student–leadership, individual values, and social well-being. Eye care concepts are taught through lectures, laboratories, tutorials, and on-site service works. Laboratories and tutorials involve pre-designed group activities to give creative roles and tasks for students to explore and to offer opportunities for them to work with different population groups as well as different peers from various fields while learning how to conduct a vision screening.

On-site service work encompasses vision screening projects for local communities. Extensive group activities and project work are arranged for students to experience real-life teamwork cases with students from different disciplines working together. Here, students are challenged in their subgroupings to learn about each other, understand their team goals, and anticipate their shortcomings.

They contacted community organizations and met service recipients from various age groups, socioeconomic, and education backgrounds. Each service recipient had individual complaints we needed to address. By giving our students these opportunities to work in different districts in Hong Kong they otherwise may never visit, they were able to evaluate the current circumstances of the more impoverished parts of Hong Kong with government-funded housing, less families with a post-secondary school education, and perhaps less public health facilities to serve them. This overall education framework is applied to increase awareness of major public health issues while providing learning opportunities for students to appreciate strategies that actively help them learn and explore about themselves. During this process, they learn about the community they live in and future challenges they may face through communication, empathy, preparation, and collaboration with their peers, the NGOs, and service recipients.

15.4 How Has This Integration Impacted the Teaching Team?

15.4.1 Interrelating Curricular Andragogy

In optometry, we educate students by relating classroom teaching to real-life clinical conditions. Our intent is to bridge and provide students with basic knowledge first and then transfer it to outside the classroom. Optometry students follow a compulsory schedule and subject selection, as they are also aware they need to use their knowledge and apply it to patient care in their future career. Thus, in the past, having a solo group of optometry students and optometrists doing community service work made logistics arrangement and on-site roles and responsibilities relatively straightforward. There is an inherent protocol and conformity to follow what has worked in the past. The presentation of our new curricula changes this environment now as the student population includes non-optometry majors. The manpower has nearly tripled in size to offer comprehensive vision screenings to more population groups, allowing optometry students to appreciate a protocol that involves cross-disciplinary ideas and assistance. To encourage students to ask questions, we have incorporated a virtual communication platform in our teaching practices to offer a convenient channel for student–teacher communications. Since the incorporation of this digital networking platform, however, we must maintain flexibility in our schedules and the ability to work outside standard hours in order to answer students' questions and share documents on an immediate basis. The supervisory role has also taken on more administrative matters requiring additional time commitment in engaged learning. Being able to impact student's development, however, is a reason why we have grown such a devotion to help our students. For example, at times, students will provide feedback regarding their realization of the strength and quality of care that can be improved in interdisciplinary care from their vision screening experience. Here, we have a student who wrote the following, "*I realize through the interrelationship among body systems, that a disease can affect more than one part of the body. So it is good for different disciplines to collaborate. Different disciplines have different roles and strengths and together we can give a more holistic picture of health conditions, compared to us working alone. I think it is good to bring this idea back to Hong Kong and I will encourage my department to organize more health screenings to engage different disciplines….I realize promoting public health is not just about improving medical knowledge but the policy of the society will also affect one's well-being. Instead of just focusing on my studies, I will actively participate more in health-related issues (e.g. Voluntary Health Insurance Scheme) by attending public consultation or conferences. I hope to make our society's policy become ones that can safeguard our health.*" It is this type of impact these interactions have, serving as their mentor and role models on reasoning and thinking and how to incorporate interdisciplinary approach to the care of patients that makes teaching this subject filled with a sense of teaching achievement. At any given time, we find ourselves balancing a range of clinical, administrative, and classroom teaching responsibilities, spending overall a significant portion of time in this role exploring an interface that can effectively balance our students' expectations to make service-learning one of their priorities. Since there are new students every semester and as an optometric educator, it is important to remind ourselves that our intent is not to train them to become optometrists. Thus, creating professional activities and exploring skills suitable for all students have been a key challenge in making this subject a rewarding experience for all. It is important that we use both evidenced-based learning and continuous assessment to guide students along the way.

15.4.2 Cultivating Student Leadership Through Team-Based Principles

Young university undergraduates share a common goal needing to fulfill all university requirements in time for graduation. When we ask senior year students why they select our subject, they sometimes reply, "I am a final year student. I have to complete a general university requirement course; otherwise, I cannot graduate in time." The motto "learn to serve, serve to learn" becomes their slogan of choice as apparent means to obtain a passing grade. After completion of the subject, it is concerning whether students will have further desire to serve the needy or maintain any social contacts with peers and NGOs they have worked with. Thus, to facilitate our responsibility to instruct without neglecting students' core attitudes, it is necessary but not easy to align all students' mindsets from one lecture and/or tutorial alone. From supervisors' experiences, majority of students lack experience in community service. What seems like a natural everyday encounter to us might be a struggle and nonproductive encounter to them as they make their first direct contact with populations in need, particularly participants with a physical or developmental disability. Much effort is required to ease these uncertainties and have them appreciate the multi-dynamic aspects of life, such as a regard for family and financial support, emotional and social well-being as well as sense of belonging (community membership) when challenged with a physical, developmental, or mental health disability. Sharing of personal experiences provides a good solution to ease students from fears. As one of the teaching team members notes, "I have to pay attention to their response during the lectures and to elaborate more in details whenever I see some puzzled faces." When students treat service-learning just as a compulsory requirement that needs a passing grade, a great deal of effort is needed to further their motivation. We try to make our contents as clear to the students as possible. When they are clear on what they have to achieve, hopefully they can visualize greater goals and future initiatives that have a greater meaning than solely earning a good grade. Indeed, we are still exploring best models of practice for this group.

There is also another subset of students enrolled in this subject because they can relate to eye health problems; either family members or themselves have had concerns about certain issues. For them, their goals are clear and they assign themselves more empathetic to questions to consider while listening to lecture contents. In order to oversee students to follow the same pace and mentality as we teach these students mixed into the same group, we need to account for the diverse learning preferences of different students.

When all these students gather in their own project groups, during the first semester, we incorporate team building activities such as "The Human Icebreaker" where team members find commonality in a series of questions related to their group. These questions are specifically assigned in order to identify peers with different key talents that will help them in project planning. Questions such as searching for group members who may know how to speak a particular Chinese dialect or who had previous experiences serving the needy, etc., can bring students to share and delegate responsibilities based on their own strengths and interests. For their teams, we purposefully excluded specific titles such as "the team leader" because these titles may often be misinterpreted and are not well received by others in the same group. When students work in a group, we want each of them to lead. That is, whenever and in whatever situation they are placed, we want to nurture their responsibility to care for their team irrespective of their assigned duty. When these characteristics do not exist within the team members, then it is hoped that team members will realize their weaknesses and eventually learn to help each other. We have adapted this strategy after a poor response seen in our initial groups where students chose hierarchy positions to lead their team members. Under that context, the group leader (*Chairman*) was most often perceived by fellow members as "bossy" and/or "a poor listener," which disrupted our intent to encourage group collaboration and cultivate harmonious social networks. Instead, we use our modified version of round tables during these preparation and planning activities where students enroll themselves into one of four subgroups with different tasks. Each subgroup caters to certain group responsibilities that have separate steps.

Subgroups include categories such as liaison contact, educational souvenir design and purchasing, data management, logistics, and video/photography design. Members of each subgroup are required to ensure they inform other team members of their progress, monitor their own team on time management, delegate, and enlist help from members in other subgroups when needed. The team as a whole will not function if they do not complete their delegated tasks in time. For example, the souvenir design team is responsible for managing items that mimic teamwork requirements when students enter the workforce in the future. They need to brainstorm with their team an initial idea on educational themes for their project. Liaison work is needed with other subgroups to gather information about their service recipients. Project expense projection and souvenir feasibility for the recipients should also be taken into consideration before finalizing their orders. It is through these preparation activities that students learn how to be more considerate of others and learn to think from the recipients' perspective in terms of their age, needs, and practicality of the items they intend to give. Other common leadership team building activities such as Salt and Pepper and Minefield have not been used as we find most students usually (though not always) show good bonding during these vision screening activities planning.

Our supervisory team includes optometrists who are practicing clinicians, vision scientists, and academics from various specialties in eye-related topics. They must take an active role in identifying strengths and various interests of students throughout the year to help enhance their educational experience for every cohort. Each student may have ideas that can be expanded into good opportunities to showcase. As their supervisors, we are their role models in service-learning, demonstrating how we have used our profession to serve others. Here, supervisors' bedside manners, generic skills are as important as their clinical experience. Our passion to serve has often been inspirations for students. In fact, students have sometimes asked our supervisors to serve as their job reference contact after their graduation because they felt a greater sense of connection with our team than their core department due to the project interaction time required in this subject.

15.5 Real-World Data Really Matter

We did not expect a one-time service experience to produce an impact strong enough to change their mentality; however, we have observed a realization of students' engagement in on-site matters relating to people interaction. Some students who shared an initial attitude of "*fulfilling the credit requirement*" have shown a change in their attitude during service rendering to the participants toward a more sympathetic approach in their actions. For example, a student from our class gave us the following feedback, "*Through performing depth perception test, I learnt that it is important to gain feedback from participants. I should be flexible to change my instructions accordingly because participants from a different culture or background may have a different understanding of instructions.*"

As an orientation to cover core issues involving a vision screening, students are first introduced to direct community care during their first semester. At these screenings, they assist as "helpers" to experience the event. In one cohort, there are approximately eight facilities providing vision screenings for various population groups in different underserved districts. The population groups were selected to reflect those in need of support. Vision screenings are conducted by the previous semester student cohort under the supervision of licensed optometrists. This provides entry students an exposure of the routine tests needed in a vision screening environment while assisting their peers, optometry students, and supervising optometrists. As a student described, "*On that day, our roles were helpers to guide the elderly while observing the whole screening take place. For example, we learnt how to set up the equipment and distribute manpower. More importantly, this was the first experience to see how a real screening was conducted. I am confident to say that it has benefited our screening a lot later.*" These students provide on-site help in vision screening activities by leading each participant from station to station. During this critical participant–helper interaction time, we have often observed a bonding and trusting engagement of the participant to their assigned helper. As a helper, our students play a "caretaker" role in order to ensure the completion of all tests for their participants as well as to provide support for them during these tests. By the time a participant–helper pair reaches the consultation station (the final testing booth) in a vision screening, it is not uncommon to see an evident synchrony in their interaction as our helpers have now successfully led and established a meaningful role for themselves in the screening project.

As a transition between lecture and actual on-site performance, we made available a multipurpose preclinical learning facility for most of the small group discussion learning, which is equipped with vision screening tools. This gives students an early orientation mindset of working and thinking in a "professional" environment. Even though students have not been taught many techniques required of optometry students nor do they have the sufficient knowledge base and ability to do a proper assessment, a student is required to achieve an optimal competency level to ensure safe and accurate delivery of vision screening tests such as visual acuity, color deficiency, eye coordination, and stereoacuity screening. Supervisors oftentimes need to remind them on the procedures and review and review again because most of them overlook or cannot remember the details.

In order to build team spirit among optometry and non-optometry students within the group, students from each cohort enroll themselves in a service group with a pre-scheduled date of service and service target/collaborative NGO/site location. As described earlier, these tutorials involve an extensive discussion of real-world challenges that are present in their project group. In this group, we have optometrists who are their supervisors and students from the School of Optometry supporting them. These tutorials can last for hours, accumulating to many weeks' worth of action–interaction. Tutorials allow supervisors to work more personally with students since the group size is small. When choosing work allocation for students, being able to connect with student's individual personality is important because we try to distribute work best suited to nurture student's strengths.

By the end, the group must deliver a proper proposal to present a screening logistics. The focus of these tutorials is to encourage leadership and team spirit. Supervisors are able to identify various student characteristics and their ability to work in groups. Individual members with strong leadership skills, those who are attentive and considerate become apparent as they work together with their peers and NGOs. Most students enjoy the group work. But having a free rider or having someone in the group who does not listen or respect others' thoughts and ideas in the group poses the most conflicts, bringing negativity in their group work experience. It is also at these times that students realize the world is not all about their own schedule. Different peers are busy at different times, and they need to respect one another's preferences and timetables. We hope that these interprofessional tutorials will transform experiences of each individual's talents and help create a group work project that improves certain aspects of the service recipients' lives. During service site visits, we want students to attend to their communication and organization styles, skills and be more people-orientated. While the School of Optometry has an established list of NGOs we have worked with in the past, it takes efforts to allow them to appreciate this new re-orientation in service provision. Our collaboration requires all NGOs to dedicate interaction time with our students for them to learn about the organization, needs in the community, and purpose of requiring their community services. Service site visits also bring upon an introduction and familiarization of the environment they will need to work in. This is the time when we encourage students to anticipate different problems and gather an overall foresight of the vision screening during preparation and coordination.

We have found that good cooperation is essential in making their project and event successful. Students who have demonstrated good adaptability are able to appreciate more opportunities for them to learn about people interaction. As optometry is a caring profession and patients usually do not fear about visiting an optometrist, the overall patient-centered experience itself is mostly curiosity or excitement rather than anxiety. The bridging of in-class concepts to on-site applications is also most evident in these scenarios. For example, during distance visual acuity screening, students often report they are surprised and later satisfied when they are able to make a difference by giving participants encouragement or connect to the service recipients through verbal or nonverbal cues. There was a sense of personal satisfaction of being able to successfully lead and change a participant's behavior based on their ability to observe and apply empathetic skills during these patient–examiner encounters. Other eye conditions such as color vision deficiency have also been a difficult concept to understand, but when they have witnessed some people indeed cannot distinguish certain colors that are evident to them, the students have reported empathy and a sense of realization on the concerns and demands of a visual impairment. It is after these service activities where students start to ask questions again. Sometimes repeating concepts they have learnt in class, but this time, it is not through rote memorization but by a natural inclination of real-life experience where they can relate to a story scenario with an actual patient encounter who can verify that it is indeed true. Non-optometry students do help a lot if they are given enough training and follow clear guidelines. Supervisors hope that the intended learning outcomes provide a positive impact on both the service population as well as the students who provide the service.

There is usually a difference in experience sharing of students serving different population groups. As a whole, we want students in each semester cohort to realize there are many groups requiring health policy changes that will give these people the social support they need. For example, students who have served senior residential homes are exposed to a higher rate of seeing eye diseases than those serving children from preschools with uncorrected refractive errors. An experience in caring for the elderly, working on how to use a wheelchair, observing subtle signs of depression may be apparent interaction for optometrists but not necessarily a routine encounter for professionals in other fields. By the end of their service activities, students often report a greater awareness of the importance for family network and realization of healthy lifestyle choices in the future.

By the end of the service, groups will create a short presentation to share their experiences through core themes such as social responsibility, empathy, cultural diversity, active citizenship, communication, and teamwork. Each group, in hopes, will combine the expertise of optometrists, students, and future professionals from many fields and be able to create an awareness, group reflect, and find ways to promote vision care. This also serves as a program evaluation to determine whether intended learning outcomes have been achieved and learn how students plan to apply leadership skills and demonstrate social responsibility in their future careers.

15.5.1 Valued Role of Reflective Journaling

During the vision screening itself, whether it be serving local or overseas mission, the work demand is high. The vision screening is busy, and the focus must be on the patient during any clinical encounters. There are participants waiting to be served, and many more waiting to be served. At this time, the supervisor to student interaction may not be ideal because students need to concentrate on their tasks and their professional time with each participant. They may often be engaged solely in the patient contact experience without having any chance to ask questions that arise. We give students an informal discussion during break time to talk about their interactions. Additionally, students are required to write journals reflecting their vision screening experiences. Reflective journals are used as an additional tool to help students develop intended learning outcome goals as they have been used in health education for professional development in critical thinking skills (Niemi, 1997). Their reports provide subjective feedback for subject improvement and allow students to express their analysis of their experience. As supervisors read their journals, they are able to evaluate whether students made any self-awareness of issues. It also provides a private media for students to ask their supervisors questions and to relate their own issues, unlike in-class lectures where students play a more passive role. When these questions arise, supervisors are given an opportunity to respond. For example, during a vision screening where local refugees were served, a student asked in their reflective journal, "*....Before this vision screening project, I just thought the purposes of taking Service Learning course are raising the awareness of university students towards the community and fulfilling the graduation criterion. I did not think doing social activities for several times can improve the lives of the needy greatly or can change their lives. However, this screening project totally changes my thoughts for having Service Learning course. In the screening, a diabetic man came. He found himself having diabetes in his hometown. After arriving Hong Kong, he did not go to hospital for regular checkup for diabetes. Last month, he was sent to intensive care unit. The SO students found the vessels in his eyes were burst which was the complication of diabetes. If this situation continues to be neglected, he may be blind. SO students and supervisors were concerned about his case and tried to think of the way to help him. On one hand, I am surprised that vision screening not only can enhance the public eye care knowledge, but can also save the future of the refugees. Without this activity, that man might not discover the diabetic retinopathy and it is already too late when he gets blind. Therefore, vision screening can serve as frontline activity to safeguard the public ocular health. On the other hand, I think SO students and supervisors are passionate about the work of vision screening. They are willing to share the knowledge and guide us to do the tests. Also, I am surprised that the glasses are free of charge for the refugees. The supervisors not only use their knowledge to contribute to the society, they also find some funding to support the needy. Their passion really inspires me and enables me to reflect myself....This activity is a wake-up call for me to do more for the needy. I am student of Medical Laboratory Science. As a part of the healthcare disciplines, I know I should be passionate and concerned about the patients. However, my passion fades out because we do not have the direct contact with the patients. After this activity, I will try to learn from the SO students and supervisors and think about what I can do more for the society by applying my knowledge. If every university student can do more, Hong Kong will be much better.*"

As the supervisor, we replied with the following comment: "*...As optometrists, although we diagnosed but it's sometimes frustrating to see patients needing to bear a chronic illness without further means to cure his underlying conditions other than raise his awareness and helping him bridge into the healthcare network. I think with your major, you will be involved in the behind the scenes work in analyzing test results. We all play different roles in caring for patients whether it be directly or behind the scenes. Hope that as you enter the work force, you will still remember this particular DM case and can explore ways to connect more economical means to monitor chronic conditions without needing patients to spend all their savings for healthcare. For yourself, I hope you gain the knowledge to better care for your diet and maintain a healthy lifestyle to avoid these nasty diseases.*"

We hope that these reflection periods will lead to an outcome that changes in the way they will think while they practice their own profession in the future, that is, to think about the consequences of their words and actions on people they work with rather than solely looking at workload output. In the case of a vision screening, do not look at just the number of service recipients served. It is about interaction with the participants and you and what you and the participants gain from the experience.

An example we share here involves one of our students who led an education booth during her service-learning work. She was inspired to start her own social media after her encounter with children who often had many misconceptions on understanding proper visual hygiene. She shared in her journal entry that although she was a biology major, she learned about optometry and educated schoolchildren about visual-related issues. She had misconceptions about eye health knowledge before but through our lectures and training she learned about core issues. During service work, she saw even more children who misunderstood many major vision and eye health concerns. In her own major, she expressed that there are also many common misunderstandings that influenced people who have no access to professional knowledge. This experience then inspired her to do some activities to make science popular and simple to understand for a layperson in the future. As her supervisor, we responded and shared with her a Harvard Commencement Speech from YouTube (Harvard University, 2016). Although they went to different universities, their reflections on childhood experiences regarding the lack of access to proper education in rural impoverished areas of China and their experiences and views about education and importance of sharing knowledge were quite similar. She became a service-learning scholar and presented some of our key project findings in a local vision science conference (The International Conference of Vision and Eye Research, 2017). Whatever path inspired her, she went on to Harvard, now completing her postgraduate studies with an aim to become an educator and research scientist in the future.

With these reflective journal submissions, it has helped supervisors realize what students have understood and their attitudes toward working with their peers and the service recipients. It keeps them in touch with our students. Even though it takes a long time to read all students' journals, the experience for supervisors in this is important because it gives them more ideas to teach when interacting with the next set of cohort and sharing similarity in experiences. This is a rewarding experience, especially for our overseas group since students spend extra time together and tend to open up about their individual feelings regarding their experiences more. The workload to read the reflective journals within the semester is a fair task and has not burdened our colleagues. It helps them learn about each student from their group, identify creative thoughts and allows them to relate more so to students' experiences than during the vision screening on-site. Attitudes about pre- and post-experiences are shared to learn about their growth.

15.5.2 Their Journey to Scholarship Opportunities

One of the initial concerns in this subject is how non-optometry students can benefit from this subject academically. This subject offers a stepping-stone to create community involvement for those interested in pursuing more service work in the future. Students are encouraged to use their own expertise to contribute to this subject as part of the achievement of intended learning outcomes. The key factor to effective implementation of scholarly engagement is to ask supervisors to note who has stood out among their peers in terms of their dedication and charisma to serve. When supervisors identify key talents in their group whereby their students have an initiative to continue their service work, we invite and encourage them to apply for service-learning scholarships offered by HKPolyU to cultivate their leadership roles in the society. Usually, in a group of 120 students, there is close to 10% of students eager to pursue further works as a scholar, with about 3% of our students successfully achieving this scholarship. As a scholar, these students serve a new role in the group to support our subject and can lead by example using their experiences and provide community service from a different viewpoint. They are also given an option to initiate and organize their own project as a service-learning scholarship recipient. We have also encouraged this selected group to think beyond to research applications and try to associate whether their "graduation thesis" (aka Final Year Projects) can incorporate any components related to service-learning. Our intent is to offer further opportunities for them to develop their research interests associated with their own disciplines with a foresight to model improvements in projects they have served.

From students' experience sharing, we often encounter these ideas. For example, a student who went on a service-learning project to serve the "left behind children" of post-earthquake survivors from the major Sichuan earthquake witnessed how poor education and living conditions were. Yet, he saw how much these children still enjoyed what remained and envisioned himself in partnership with other health disciplines to arrange body checkups for these children in the future so that they can maintain good health and be able to enjoy what they have. However, as his major is in Medical Laboratory Sciences, he understood how expensive laboratory testing can be. By modeling our platform, he realized there often needs to be a compromise between cost-effective solutions with limited resources. Whenever we encounter these types of reflections, we often try to encourage these students to further their ideas and welcomed them to initiate any collaborative projects with our department. For his interest, a joint collaboration with a local university such as the Institute for Disaster Management and Reconstruction can further his interest in pursuing these cross-collaboration health checks. We are currently helping him explore these potentials.

We have seen more case examples of creative student thinking and applications.

Case Example 1: I Can Develop an App for That!

The efficiency of electronic medical records is well established for many healthcare practices, including optometry. Technology may improve access by allowing delivery of timely information via the intranet. Here, we describe a case example of a student from this subject who took an initiative to develop an App for EMH records for vision screening. His intent was simple, but the outcome led to an overall change. Student L was enrolled in our subject due for a mission to Mainland China. We have told the group in advance based on the geographic location and service target we serve, and it is expected that there will be many participants who will need a glasses prescription. The group went on to divide tasks and responsibilities, and Student L pursued his skills from his own major to explore ways to help his group. Using his computer programming skills, Student L converted paper records into an electronic format so that data entry can be conducted directly on-site. While we provided the hardware necessary for this setup, Student L represented a software spinoff founded as a result of community engagement. To him, it was a simple act of using his professional skills in programming to lessen the after-care workload burden on his group mates who will need to do data entry input for more than 1000 participants. Student L continued his passion in service-learning and was selected as a service-learning scholar among a pool of applicants from different subjects and cohorts. He was able to use this new status to create further opportunities to serve in more projects and led more groups to incorporate EMH records. He had further created an impact on corporate social responsibility, enabling one of our partner NGOs, The Esquel-Y.L. Yang Foundation to recognize his achievements through local press coverage and invited him to give a special sharing session with their employees to explain his adaptation of e-culture while on service-learning missions. Although that may not have concluded to a job offer opportunity, for an undergraduate student, it represented a great milestone and an early leap into his future industry and social impact.

Case Example 2: A Platform to the Professional Level
On a professional level, advances in technology have led us to envision many opportunities to improve our care for patients. Many eye and vision tests can be simplified and made user-friendlier through innovative focus using computing algorithms. Today's strategy in developing and making these connections possible is through collaborative research. Upon exposing our discipline to more students outside our usual encounters, we have made research collaboration with service-learning subject leaders more accessible. For example, The Department of Computing has been a key partner in these initiatives as we have several undergraduate as well as postgraduate projects where we collaborated our ideas and their ability to transfer and transform it into a working prototype. These include the development of a refractive error screening apps using photorefraction techniques, visual acuity screening using micro-eye movements measures and hand gesture responses, a child-friendly game to conduct vision screenings, etc. Some students went on to present their works in international conferences to share with their peers, and we, no doubt, look forward to furthering their efforts into calibration and actual clinical usage.

Case Example 3: A Vision of Love- https://www.polyu.edu.hk/so/visionoflove/en
The introduction of extra manpower knowledgeable in vision screening activities has increased public awareness of the constraints poor vision and can cause and explore means to provide affordable glasses eyewear for populations from different socioeconomic levels. Through our university alumni network and philanthropist contribution made possible from the Vision of Love Fund, we were able to provide

further follow-up on all the patients who had recognized visual problems detected during our vision screening activities. In this adjunct project called, "Vision of Love," we created a mobile eye clinic where our primary eye care, optical dispensary, vision therapy, and low vision resources are custom fitted for mobility provision in schools and nursing homes. In this regard, patients no longer need to worry about access and affordability of care due to their age or background. Our target beneficiaries are people who have difficulty accessing vision and eye healthcare services, including but not limited to the older adults, school children (especially kindergarten and primary school students), new immigrants, low-income families, members of ethnic minorities, wheelchair users, people with mental illness and developmental disabilities. This enables us to invite our optometry alumni, who previously were active community service participants when they were students to join our team and further their interest in eye care missionary service provision. Further expanding our manpower, our university staff alumni and students have established a volunteer staff network (Vision Ambassadors) from our university's social responsibility initiative to work alongside these projects. Based on our curriculum offered from our service-learning subject, they underwent special advanced training sessions to ensure their quality of service while providing these optometry-related services.

15.6 Conclusion and Future Work

Optometry plays an important role in the primary healthcare system. Eye education is no longer limited to optometry and ophthalmology. Increasingly, we will see multi-level public health education by means of cross-disciplinary outreach using this platform to teach students about vision and eye health-related concerns, previously unaware of our roles in the community. This subject has gained a considerable value to students, faculties, and participants. We are providing here a chance for students from everywhere a different platform for them to serve others outside their comfort zone. It takes strong willpower to join since they know they need to work with healthcare professionals, and there will be service recipients with problems, whether physically or internally. Students are satisfied overall with their service-learning experience, with several areas needing improvement highlighted in this chapter. In optometrists serving as supervisors, they saw themselves as good role models, with a high overall satisfaction. We hope that students strengthen their social responsibility commitment as they become future assets in their communities and provide outreach services in their own careers. Community voluntarism is not limited to care by optometrist alone. Realizing public health involvement through vision screenings, education talks, and charitable contributions is various means for community contribution and helps for the disadvantaged. Future goals include implementing a multi-professional teaching team and service provision to involve the participation of secondary and tertiary eye healthcare providers in this healthcare education model.

References

Chin, M. P., Siong, K. H., Chan, K. H., Do, C. W., Chan, H. H., & Cheong, A. M. (2015). Prevalence of visual impairment and refractive errors among different ethic groups in schoolchildren in Turpan, China. *Ophthalmic Physiological Optics, 35*(3), 263–270.

Choi, K. Y., Yu, W. Y., Lam, C. H., Li, Z. C., Chin, M. P., Lakshmanan, Y., et al. (2017). Childhood exposure to constricted living space, a possible environmental threat to myopia development. *Ophthalmic Physiological Optics, 37*(5), 568–575.

Do, C. W., Chan, L. Y. L., Wong, H. H. Y., Chu, G., Yu, W. Y., Pang, P. C. K., et al. (2016). Blending community services and teaching to open vision care and eye health awareness to University students. *Higher Education Outreach and Engagement, 20*(4), 81.

Harvard University. (2016). Graduate speaker Jiang He| Harvard Commencement 2016. Retrieved from https://www.youtube.com/watch?v=BM2HMoK5aIU.

Lam, C. S., Lam, C. H., Cheng, S. C., & Chan, L. Y. (2012). Prevalence of myopia among Hong Kong Chinese schoolchildren: Changes over two decades. *Ophthalmic Physiological Optics, 32*(1), 17–24.

Niemi, P. M. (1997). Medical students' professional identity: Self-reflection during the preclinical years. *Medical Education, 31,* 408–415.

Woo, G. C., & Chan, L. Y. (2015). Chapter 11 paediatric low vision: Rehabilitation model and devices. In A. Chen & S. J. Leat (Eds.), *Paediatric vision care current practice and future challenges* (pp. 203–222). Asia: McGraw-Hill Education.

Woo, G. C., Chan, L. Y., Lam, C. S., & Yeo, K. T. (2010). Chapter 10 diabetic retinopathy screening program. In X. R. Li, J. P. Liu, X. X. Li, & Y. N. Hui (Eds.), *Diabetic Ocular Disease* (pp. 225–235). Tianjin, China: People's Medical Publishing House.

World Council of Optometry. (2015). *Why optometry? The case for delivering quality, advanced and equitable eye health and vision care for patients*. Retrieved from https://worldcouncilofoptometry.info/wp-content/uploads/2017/02/WhyOptometry-2.pdf.

World Health Organization. (2006). *Global initiative for the eliminiation of avoidable blindness: Action plan 2006–2011*. Retrieved from http://www.who.int/blindness/Vision2020_report.pdf.

Chapter 16
Turning Service-Learning Teaching into Scholarly Work

Josephine M. Csete

Abstract The main aim of this chapter is to support teachers of service-learning (SL) subjects and projects in conducting a scholarly study on some aspect of the teaching and learning process. Key principles from the Scholarship of Teaching and Learning (SoTL) are outlined with foundational references provided. Topics include: (1) the benefits of conducting SoTL studies in SL for the teacher/researcher; (2) types of scholarly studies that can be conducted on the teaching of SL; (3) basic background on SoTL including the standards applicable to all forms of scholarly work; and (4) the main stages of drafting questions, designing, conducting, analyzing, and disseminating the results of a scholarly study. The chapter contains a summary checklist of the key questions presented.

Keywords Service-learning · The Scholarship of Teaching and Learning SoTL · Designing educational research · Educational research methods Experiential learning · Career development for academics

16.1 Introduction

This entire book has been written in the belief that service-learning (SL) makes a positive difference in both the lives of the students providing the service and the clients and communities being served. What is being learned at the operational and implementation levels in this setting is shared with the intent of providing evidence and useful advice in support of institutions and teachers who want to implement and continually improve the teaching of SL in their own contexts. In preceding chapters, a model for implementing rigorous SL experiences within a university setting and across disciplines has been presented and a number of cases describe how teachers and teaching teams have taught SL credit-bearing subjects. Forthcoming chapters

J. M. Csete (✉)
Educational Development Centre, The Hong Kong Polytechnic University, Hunghom, Hong Kong
e-mail: josephine.csete@polyu.edu.hk

D. T. L. Shek et al. (eds.), *Service-Learning for Youth Leadership*, Quality of Life in Asia 12, https://doi.org/10.1007/978-981-13-0448-4_16

will present hard-learned principles that have been identified through multiple years and extensive experience in implementing SL. And still, other chapters will describe the outcomes for students participating in SL as derived through carefully constructed evaluations that have collected data from thousands of students across several years.

The main aim of this chapter is to bridge the gap between the preceding chapters detailing individual case studies of teachers' experiences in SL and preparing teachers to plan and conduct their own scholarly investigations into the SL contexts they are involved in. References useful to supporting claims on the value and relevance of this form of scholarship as well as practical "how to" information are provided. Sections will respond to the following questions:

- What are my main motivations for engaging in scholarly work on SL?
- What kinds of studies might I do related to SL?
- What are the key concepts from the discipline of the Scholarship of Teaching and Learning (SoTL) and how might they assist me in my own studies?
- What must I pay attention to in planning and carrying out a scholarly study on teaching SL?

16.2 Benefits of Conducting Scholarly Work on Service-Learning

Do you often have the opportunity to think about how you spend your time on your work? Which tasks are more rewarding for you personally? Which are more valued by the organization you work for? It is important for your personal satisfaction and your potential for career advancement that you are aware of your answers to these questions. You should periodically review your responses to these questions as the answers are likely to change over the years for both you and your context.

It is particularly beneficial to reflect on how your work in SL relates to your personal motives and career goals. The vast majority of our own teachers report that teaching an SL subject takes much more time and energy than a "traditional" subject in their disciplinary area. Many also describe in glowing terms how much they enjoy working with students in this type of subject and the personal rewards their involvement in SL brings. Some describe how involvement in SL supports highly held personal values that other areas of their work do not address. All these are good reasons and rewards for becoming involved in teaching SL, but to stay involved for the long run and maximize the benefits for yourself as well as the learning outcomes for your students, it pays off to make sure you are also expending effort in ways that are recognized by your organization and further your career goals. Taking a scholarly approach to your teaching of SL can help you be more strategic and achieve even more with your efforts.

What does it mean to be "scholarly"? What are the kinds of work that academics do and how does SL fit within their work? Let us start with a bit of history. Career questions like those opening this section were asked of academics in the USA in surveys over several decades in the National Survey of Faculty conducted by the Carnegie Foundation. In 1990, Ernest Boyer published *Scholarship Reconsidered: Priorities of the Professoriate* (Boyer, 1990). It contains results of the 1989 survey answered by thousands of academics across hundreds of institutions in the USA. More importantly, it also contains a very influential eighty-page manuscript that draws on survey results as well as the other literature about higher education to propose a broader definition of scholarship to address concerns from academics about what is expected from their work, how their work is rewarded, and what is ultimately more important for higher education to focus on to make a contribution to society.

Boyer's definition of scholarship is much broader than prevalent definitions that usually rely on doing research and publishing. Boyer presents four forms of scholarship that he argues both more accurately capture the range of things academics do as well as the areas of contribution that society is looking for from higher education (see Fig. 16.1). These four forms of scholarship are: *Discovery*—which is engaging in original research to advance knowledge. Discovery can be represented by bench research and is the kind of scholarship people think of first and describe as "research." A second form of scholarship is *Integration*—which involves making connections across disciplines and relating findings from discovery scholarship to a larger context. A third form of scholarship is called *Application*—which connects theory to practice to address real-world problems. This is also often called "scholarship of engagement." This is very different from activities such as serving on committees and doing administrative tasks that are often labeled "service" in higher education. This engagement or application scholarship is more closely related to consultancy in that it requires using specialty knowledge from the disciplines. And the fourth form of scholarship is called *Teaching*—which involves making new forms of knowledge understandable to others so that it endures. Think about it.

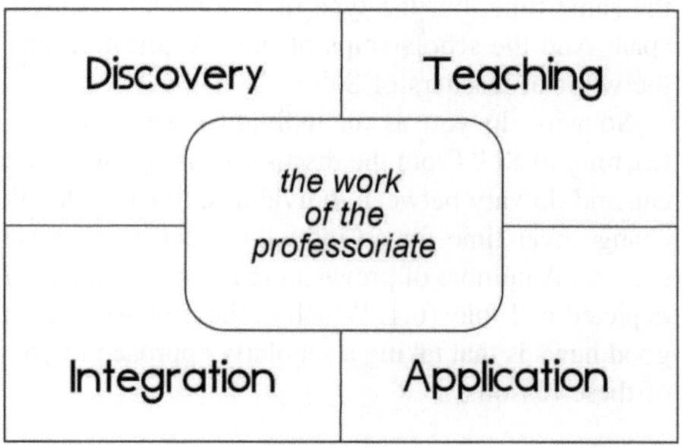

Fig. 16.1 Boyer's forms of scholarship

Teaching is essential to passing on the knowledge and skills that others have worked so hard to discover and develop. Teaching is key to both sustaining what we already know and for preparing future generations to make new contributions. Thus, the scholarship of teaching also involves drawing future scholars into the disciplines. In fact, many of us have chosen career paths because of inspiring teachers.

Boyer asserts that these four forms of scholarship are interdependent and also work synergistically. The four scholarships comprise "the work of the professoriate." *Discovery* is the investigation of new knowledge and may be described as "contributing to the field." It is relatively easy to think of scholars who are known for discovery. Marie Curie who conducted research on radioactive elements is an example. *Integration* transcends disciplinary boundaries, connects knowledge, and gives meaning to isolated facts. Integration creates new perspectives and can make ideas meaningful to non-specialists. The new disciplinary area of neuroscience is an integration of traditionally hard sciences such as anatomy, physiology, biochemistry, and molecular biology with social science fields in behavior and learning. Stephen Hawking, author of *A Brief History of Time* (1998) is known for his contributions as a scholar of integration both for incorporating ideas from different fields to develop new knowledge and for making this knowledge more accessible to lay people. Boyer describes *Application* as the rigorous application of academic expertise to "consequential problems" that affect individuals, institutions, and society. In the nineteenth century, higher education in the USA was expanded to focus on helping farmers increase the food supply for a growing population. Service-learning is strongly associated with this form of scholarship. *Teaching* is the means by which the knowledge we already possess is transmitted to the next generation. But scholarly teaching goes beyond simply transmitting knowledge. It also prepares learners to transform and extend existing knowledge into new areas. Scholarly teaching prepares future professionals to excel in their calling and to contribute new advancements. John Dewey and his contributions to education in books such as *How We Think* (1910) can be considered a scholar of teaching. In summary, each form of scholarship has an important contribution to make and society ultimately benefits when all four forms of scholarship are being pursued. An individual academic is unlikely to be participating in all four forms of scholarship at the same time, but the type of scholarship focused on may change over a career span. And the scholarships of both Application and Teaching provide support for the work of teachers of SL.

So why do you as an individual want to take a scholarly approach to your teaching of SL? From the discussion above, it can be assumed not only that reasons can and do vary between individuals, but also that the primary reasons are likely to change over time for an individual and in response to what is also valued in the context. A number of prevalent reasons accompanied by illustrative descriptions are depicted in Table 16.1. Which of these reasons are currently of interest to you? The good news is that taking a scholarly approach to your teaching of SL can benefit all of these reasons.

Table 16.1 Reasons for taking a scholarly approach to teaching SL

To understand what is happening to my students in a given situation
This is often an early exploratory stage that turns into a sustained scholarly investigation. The teacher gathers and analyzes evidence in order to gain a better understanding of the students' perspectives, problem areas, etc. It is particularly useful in subjects the teacher is new to teaching and/or when teaching and learning methods differ substantially from other subjects and is therefore very helpful in SL situations which often incorporate active learning methods
To address a particular problem or challenge
Most teachers have encountered situations where it becomes painfully obvious that the students "just are not getting it." Perhaps, many students are not working well together in project teams, or reflective essays are unfocused and poorly written. Teachers often undertake scholarly studies in which they trial a method that is new to them with the intent of improving a problem situation
To check for improvements to students' learning outcomes
The main goal of teaching is to facilitate student learning. So, teachers conduct studies to see if the methods they are currently using in their teaching are actually helping students learn. Note that this goal goes far beyond student expressions of satisfaction with the learning situation or method being investigated. Evidence is gathered and analyzed to look for actual gains in learning
To improve my teaching
This is part of a good teacher's continuous improvement philosophy. Teachers collect and analyze data to identify areas of strength as well as those that could be improved. The teacher then "closes the feedback loop" by choosing something to do differently and implements it in future teaching. Note that the data does not necessarily only come from students. Peer reviewers are another source
To gather evidence of the quality of my teaching
This goes beyond activities conducted to improve teaching (as described above) to more rigorously collect evidence that will be convincing to others. Evidence of the effectiveness of teaching is a useful component in teaching portfolios and for performance reviews. In particular, if the institution only collects short quantitative surveys from students, the data collected and compiled by teachers can provide a more detailed description of what is going on in their teaching. In this situation, triangulation (corroboration of claims from different data sources through different methods) becomes important. Many teachers with the goals of improving their teaching or gathering evidence of their teaching have made use of techniques for gathering data on students' learning that are described by Angelo and Cross (1993)

(continued)

Table 16.1 (continued)

To inform a discipline (your own, service-learning, or education)
We expect that academics conduct research to contribute to their disciplines. Scholarly work on the teaching of SL has the possibility to contribute to one or more disciplines. Teacher/researchers can have study results that contribute to: Their own core discipline. The application of disciplinary knowledge and skills to solve real-world problems in context can help develop new knowledge that is useful to the discipline. An example is a teacher of nursing developing a more error-free or time-saving way for less experienced health practitioners to take a health history as part of an SL project The discipline of service-learning. What is learned in a specific context in which SL is being taught has the potential to be useful to the entire discipline. Later chapters in this book which provide evidence of gains in student learning outcomes as a result of completing SL subjects can be used to support initiating or broadening SL initiatives in other universities in the world The discipline of educational research. Useful education innovations that are trialed and refined by individual teachers can be much more widely disseminated to other teachers and across disciplines if they are able to demonstrate evidence of impact. An example is physics educator Eric Mazur's scholarly studies that led to his developing the peer instruction method (Crouch & Mazur, 2001)
To publish
If publishing is important in your context and/or you are interested in building your career in SL, publishing can of course help. To be publishable, the scholarly work needs to offer results that will contribute to a discipline. Trigwell (2013) describes three levels of investigation in which the lowest and simplest level is to inform oneself which results in "personal knowledge" which may be useful to inform your own teaching practice but is not publishable. The third and most difficult level to achieve is that of "public knowledge" which is used to inform a wider audience. This form of evidence is typically verified by people outside the context and usually through a peer review process such as reputable journals use

16.3 Types of Scholarly Work on Service-Learning

There are a variety of types of scholarly studies that are applicable to the teaching of SL. These types can be categorized into broad categories according to the overarching aim of the investigation. Hutchings' (2000) taxonomy of SoTL research questions is depicted with examples from SL in Table 16.2. If you already have an idea for a scholarly study, which category does it fall under in this taxonomy? If you do not have a specific study in mind yet, which of these types most interest you?

Table 16.2 Hutchings' taxonomy of SoTL research questions

What works?
Overarching aim: to assess the effects of new educational methods and/or tools What works studies are useful for teachers who are trying something new and want to know if it is effective. Effectiveness should include achievement of student learning outcomes (and not rely solely on student satisfaction measures) Example from the literature: Pre- and posttest scores on a number of surveys are reported for 142 students in an undergraduate SL subject. Findings suggest significant positive changes in social and personal outcomes Simons and Cleary (2006)
What is?
Overarching aim: to accurately describe the current teaching and learning situation What are studies match up particularly well with a teacher's motivation to understand what is happening in a given situation (as described in Table 16.1) Example from the literature: An evaluation conducted using largely qualitative techniques with ten graduate students participating in a semester-long SL advocacy project Murray, Pope, and Rowell (2010)
What is possible? Or what would it look like?
Overarching aim: to pilot/examine an entirely new educational practice This may be an entirely new way of teaching for an individual teacher or for a discipline. SL, as a form of experiential education, is often first implemented as a what is possible type of initiative Example from the literature: All of the subjects described in this volume have been accredited according to standards established when the university began its plan to implement SL as a requirement for all students. Criteria include: (a) clear academic objectives and student learning outcomes, (b) a significant amount of service activity (typically 40–45 h), and (c) a rigorous process for student reflection and assessment Chan, Ngai, Yuen, and Kwan (2013)
Theory building
Overarching aim: to propose a new educational theory or concept for improving teaching In the words of Hutchings, a theory building scholarly work "is not so much exploring an aspect of practice as it is formulating a new conceptual framework for shaping thought about practice" (2000, p. 5) Example from the literature: A 1996 article by Andrew Furco is often cited for its clarification of how SL is distinct from other forms of service programs (such as community service and internships) Furco (1996)

16.4 Applying SoTL Principles and Standards to the Teaching of SL

> When we describe teaching as serious intellectual work or scholarship, we need to prove that the products of teaching can also be rigorously evaluated for excellence by a community of peers.
> (Bernstein, 2008, p. 51)

Previous sections have introduced the concept that there is a range of forms of scholarship, all of which make valuable contributions to society. An individual interested in taking a scholarly approach to the teaching of SL is likely to focus more on the scholarships of Application and Teaching. And as quoted from Bernstein above, serious intellectual work or scholarship must be rigorously evaluated. But then the questions arise "How do we rigorously evaluate scholarship?" This in turn raises the question "What is the accepted definition of scholarship?" A current definition of scholarship specific to the area of teaching (SoTL) that is becoming widely accepted is presented in this section. Standards for assessing all forms of scholarship are also provided. Both can be applied (and cited as justifications in teaching grant applications and research proposals) by individuals wishing to take a scholarly approach to teaching SL.

Felten (2013) proposes five principles for assessing whether a piece of work qualifies as SoTL. Principles of good practice in SoTL provide guidance for teachers which they can flexibly apply to their own scholarly work in teaching and learning. With the guideposts presented in Table 16.3, teachers and reviewers can reflect on, assess SoTL studies, and develop aims for future investigations.

Felten states that it is essential to have a shared definition of SoTL that acts as a guiding vision for the discipline of SoTL and can be used to communicate what SoTL is to others. These principles of good practice are broad enough to be implemented in different ways in different contexts and can be used as standards for judging excellence. Reviewing these principles when planning your own scholarly study can improve both the quality of your study and the likelihood that it will be recognized as scholarly work by others.

16.5 Applying Six Standards of Scholarly Work to Teaching and Learning

In conducting quality investigations into teaching and learning in SL that are truly scholarly, you should ascribe to the same standards as are expected for other forms of scholarship. As described in Section Two scholarship can take any of four forms: discovery, integration, application, and teaching. It is important that regardless of

Table 16.3 Felten's five principles of good practice in SoTL

Inquiry focused on student learning
The focus is on students and how they learn. The types of learning studied are broadly interpreted and include areas such as: • Disciplinary knowledge • Skills development • Broader learning issues (such as motivation or working in teams) and even • How teachers influence student learning However, theoretical discussions that do not include collecting some form of data from students are unlikely to be considered SoTL
Grounded in context
Both the broader scholarly and the local contexts are important. To be scholarly, investigations should build upon prior research and draw on relevant theory. Since teaching contexts vary widely, the local context in which the study is conducted should be identified so that others can determine whether the results are applicable in their own context. For example, studies conducted with extremely large classes may not directly apply to smaller groups or online settings
Methodologically sound
At first glance, the principle that an SoTL study must be methodologically sound seems obvious. Upon consideration, this may be harder to practice than expected. Firstly, since SoTL is conducted by teachers of all disciplines, each teacher may be more familiar with research practices in his or her own discipline. These differing disciplinary styles influence the types of questions asked about learning, as well as the methods chosen to collect and analyze data. In particular, hard science teachers may be less familiar with methods used in the social sciences and SoTL studies often include qualitative methods
Conducted in partnership with students
At a minimum, human subjects research rules must be followed and the students we are studying must be treated ethically and understand their rights. In addition, over recent years there is a growing trend to plan and carry out SoTL studies in a way that involves students in the inquiry process
Appropriately public
It is widely acknowledged that it may not be appropriate to judge SoTL studies by the more traditional approach accepted by many disciplines of publishing in a peer-reviewed journal. At this point in the (relatively early) development of the discipline of SoTL, what is most important is that both the methods used and the results are shared so that others can learn from them. Going public is a key distinction between a scholarly teacher who is conducting evidence-based enquiries and reflecting upon the results in order to make changes to his or her own teaching practices and the SoTL practitioner who lets others know what he/she has been doing

Table 16.4 Glassick, Huber, and Maeroff's six standards of scholarly work*

Clear goals • Does the scholar state the basic purpose of his or her work clearly? • Does the scholar define objectives that are realistic and achievable? • Does the scholar identify important questions in the field?
Adequate preparation • Does the scholar show an understanding of existing scholarship in the field? • Does the scholar bring the necessary skills to his or her work? • Does the scholar bring together the resources necessary to move the project forward?
Appropriate methods • Does the scholar use methods appropriate to the goals? • Does the scholar apply effectively the methods selected? • Does the scholar modify procedures in response to changing circumstances?
Significant results • Does the scholar achieve the goals? • Does the scholar's work add consequentially to the field? • Does the scholar's work open additional areas for further exploration?
Effective presentation • Does the scholar use a suitable style and effective organization to present his or her work? • Does the scholar use appropriate forums for communicating the work to its intended audiences? • Does the scholar present his or her message with clarity and integrity?
Reflective critique • Does the scholar critically evaluate his or her own work? • Does the scholar bring an appropriate breadth of evidence to his or her critique? • Does the scholar use evaluation to improve the quality of future work?

*Wording for standards and questions reproduced verbatim from Glassick et al. (1997)

the focus of the research, scholarly standards are applied. In 1997, Glassick, Huber, and Maeroff (1997) published the book *Scholarship Assessed: Evaluation of the Professoriate* presenting the six standards of scholarly work that should apply to all forms of scholarship. The six standards and accompanying questions are depicted in Table 16.4.

You can significantly increase the quality of your study by answering the questions presented under each of these six standards several times during your scholarly investigation. When planning your study, realistically assess your plan against these standards and modify in places where you detect weaknesses. Reviewing these questions during your study, especially if it spans many months or years, can help you detect and correct for drift in goals or methods. And finally, paying careful attention to these standards when preparing your findings for dissemination can increase your chances of your results being accepted by your peers. Compare the review criteria for a journal you are interested in publishing in to these standards and you are likely to notice significant overlap. For a cogent (four-page) overview of these standards that is often cited, see Glassick (2000).

16.6 Key Steps in Carrying Out a Scholarly Study

16.6.1 Overview of a Five-Stage Process

There are a multitude of approaches to designing and carrying out a study as well as many lengthy books that go into detail on how to carry out specific data collection and analysis methods. It is beyond the scope of a single chapter to cover all of these topics. In this chapter a five-step approach for planning an SoTL study (Bishop-Clark and Dietz-Uhler 2012) is used to illustrate how to begin planning a study related to teaching an SL subject. The five steps are:

1. **Generating a research question**—to transform the hunches and ideas you've had about your teaching and student learning into research questions and hypotheses that can be answered empirically;
2. **Designing the study**—to consider which type of research design best matches your research question;
3. **Collecting the data**—to collect data that will provide you with an answer to your question;
4. **Analyzing the data**—to look carefully at the data to arrive at substantiated results that include answers to your research question;
5. **Presenting and publishing your SoTL project**—to share your results with peers within your institution and/or at conferences or in journals.

16.6.2 Step One: Generating the Research Question

Identifying your research question is the most important part of starting your study, which will define and influence other aspects of your investigative process. According to the five-step approach for planning an SoTL study, there are three key questions to help you generate your research question(s).

- What type of research question do you want to study?
- What objectives do you want to achieve?
- How important is your research question in the field?

What type of research question do you want to study?

In Section Three, Pat Hutchings' four types of SoTL research questions (1) what works; (2) what is; (3) what is possible; and (4) theory building were introduced. As discussed in Section Two, your research question should be modified to bring better balance between your research interests and valued topics in your organization and between your research interests and valued topics in your discipline.

When you are looking for information and ideas for your scholarly investigation, library databases will give you access to authoritative resources already published. In addition to referring to these publications, you can use citation databases such as Web of Science and Scopus to help trace and search for additional resources using citations.

What objectives do you want to achieve?

Clear objectives specify your target problem and represent what you plan to achieve. Browning (2014) suggests using the S.M.A.R.T. method for writing your objectives. Make your objectives Specific, Measurable, Attainable, Realistic, and Time-bound. According to Carlson and O'Neal-McElrath (2008), objectives should:

- Be stated in quantifiable terms.
- Be stated as outcomes, not process.
- Specify the results of an activity.
- Identify the target audience or community served.
- Be realistic and capable of being accomplished within the period of the investigation.

How important is your research question in the field?

You must also explain why your research question is important and worthy of investigation in the field. Your study findings must be of interest to at least one community of scholars. An advantage of investigations into the teaching of SL is that they have the potential to appeal to more than one audience. Depending upon the focus of your study, results may be generalizable to SL, teaching and learning in your discipline and/or more broadly across education (see Table 16.2 for examples). Your research question is likely to be of some interest to peers and considered important if it fulfills at least one of the aims listed by Creswell (2002):

- Improve practice.
- Add to knowledge.
- Address gaps in knowledge.
- Expand knowledge—extending what we know in ways we never previously conceived of.
- Replicate knowledge—verifying previous findings.
- Add voices of individuals to knowledge—adding special perspectives to current practices.

Remember you are most probably already interested in your research question. However, you should take steps to ensure that others will also be interested in your results. And finally, the processes of identifying your research question cannot be completed in a single round. Expect to repeat this process several times before generating a version you are satisfied with.

16.6.3 Step Two: Designing the Study

After drafting your research question, the next stage is to figure out the most appropriate research design to address the question. Returning to key questions in the five-step approach for planning an SoTL study from Bishop-Clark and Dietz-Uhler (2012), below are responses to three key questions to help you start designing your study.

Quantitative, qualitative, or mixed methods?

Briefly, there are three general categories of research designs: quantitative, qualitative, and mixed methods. Asking "What?", "How?", and "Why?" questions helps scholars choose an appropriate research design. Here are brief descriptions of these three categories of research designs:

- *Quantitative studies*—Require numerical data to solve "What?" questions. Descriptive and inferential statistics are often used.
- *Qualitative studies*—Require word and image data to answer "How?" and "Why?" questions. Descriptions and thematic analyses are often employed.
- *Mixed methods studies*—Require both numerical data and word/image data to address a variety of kinds of research questions. Findings may be reported with both statistics and descriptions and thematic analysis.

Will you do a pilot?

A pilot is a study typically done on a small scale to help you try out study processes and collect preliminary data. Pilots can also identify unforeseen challenges as well as opportunities. It is particularly useful to conduct pilots: (1) in which new instruments are designed, (2) that will shape a further experiment or teaching method, and (3) that are small-scale versions of future experiments or teaching methods (Light, Singer, & Willett, 1990). One approach is to conduct a pilot in an SL subject one semester, and then after refining the instrument or method based upon what has been learned, conduct a fuller implementation the next time the SL subject is taught. No design is so complete that it cannot be improved by a pilot study. Pilots can last an hour, a day, a week, or a semester.

What specific research approach(es) will you use?

One challenge in doing scholarship in teaching SL is that answering your research question may require using some methods that you are less familiar with and/or are not commonly used in your native discipline. In particular, qualitative methods are often beneficial.

Bishop-Clark and Dietz-Uhler (2012) describe five qualitative and three quantitative approaches that are often used in SoTL studies. Descriptions of each approach are depicted in Table 16.5 with some examples of SL studies using these approaches. Read over this list and consider which methods you are familiar with and could comfortably carry out right now, and which are new to you and would require developing new knowledge and skills.

And about mixed methods

Each of the methods described above has its own strengths and weaknesses. The main idea behind using more than one method in a study or "mixed methods" is to increase confidence in study findings. Combining methods in a study is also referred to as triangulation. For more information on mixed methods studies, refer to Creswell and Plano Clark (2011).

16.6.4 Step Three: Collecting the Data

After identifying your research design approach, the next step is to collect your data. Returning to key questions in the five-step approach for planning an SoTL study from Bishop-Clark and Dietz-Uhler (2012), here are three key questions to help you collect your data.

What data will you collect?

The type of data you collect will depend upon the methods you have selected. Eight methods have been presented in Table 16.5. Among these methods, five tend to be more qualitative and three more quantitative. Case studies, interviews, and surveys are commonly used in more qualitative educational research approaches, and numerical responses, verbatim responses, and numerical recording are popular in quantitative educational research approaches. When considering data types keep in mind that the assignments your students are completing in your subject are a resource. In particular, many studies on the teaching of SL use students' reflective journals as a data source. If you are using a rubric to grade student work, these results can also provide data on student achievement of the intended learning outcomes. Adequately answering the research question is likely to require multiple methods and thus the collection of both qualitative and quantitative data.

When will you collect the data?

Normally, data is collected in at least three stages: before or at the start of the study, during the study, and at the end or after the implementation period has completed. For example, data on students' backgrounds can be collected as part of a pre-study survey. Students' attitudes toward a learning experience can be investigated via a mid-study survey, interview, or focus group session. And a combination of pre- and posttests of knowledge or skills can be used to assess students' learning performance.

When to collect the data depends on the needs of your study. And the answer usually is "at several different points in time over the course of the study."

Who will collect the data?

Bishop-Clark and Dietz-Uhler (2012) have suggested the teacher/researcher can involve students in collecting data in an SoTL study. And Felten (2013) goes even

Table 16.5 Overview of qualitative and quantitative approaches

Descriptive studies (Qualitative) Describe a current situation, issue, or topic Descriptive SoTL projects on SL ask questions like "What are the main themes that students write about in their reflective journals in my subject?" An example is Lai et al. (2015) which identified four main themes through content analysis of nursing students' reflective journals. Lin et al. (2017) also conducted a descriptive study through analyzing students' reflective journals, but the study was different in that the journals were examined for instances of student comments related to the hospitality education subject's intended learning outcomes Strength(s): Allow for observing with minimal impact on the situation. Useful for describing innovative teaching practices and student reactions Weakness(es): Cannot suggest causal relationships or may be difficult to broadly generalize
Case studies (Qualitative) Describe a specific event, person, or group in detail within the natural environment. Tend to collect data from multiple sources and across time (e.g., a student's pretest and posttest scores, interview responses, analysis of assignments, exam grades) Case study SoTL projects on SL describe a situation in a real-life context with enough detail to provide useful information for others. For example, Lo et al. (2016) describe using a shipping container to set up a community learning center in Cambodia as an example of a successful short-term effort from a foreign team leading to a sustainable model for enhancing access to technology education in a developing country Strength(s): Allow for observing with minimal impact on the situation; are rich in detail (often combining data from multiple sources) Weakness(es): Cannot suggest causal relationships or be broadly generalized; can be time consuming to conduct and analyze
Observations Gather information on a situation to develop a more holistic picture of teaching and/or learning. Best conducted by trained observers using a format for taking notes to both describe situation (e.g., types of questions students ask) and count instances of items of interest (e.g., how often students consult team members) Observation SoTL projects on SL would ask questions about how often students exhibit a behavior of interest, such as demonstrating listening or leadership skills when working with teammates, or demonstrate empathy with the people they are serving through verbal and nonverbal methods Strength(s): Allow for observing with minimal impact on the situation; may allow for collecting feelings or concerns from students that they would not normally reveal; useful for identifying unanticipated outcomes Weakness(es): The observer must be as unobtrusive as possible to avoid altering the situation being observed; cannot suggest causal relationships or may be difficult to broadly generalize

(continued)

Table 16.5 (continued)

Interviews (Qualitative) Gather detailed information on interviewee perspectives. Formats range from unstructured (no predetermined questions) through semi-structured (predetermined questions but mostly open ended) to highly structured (predetermined questions and response categories—similar to a written survey) Interview SoTL projects on SL ask questions like "What are students'/teachers'/service recipients' perceptions of 'X'?" For example, Pechak and Thompson (2011) interviewed educators to identify common program structures and processes in international service-learning programs in physical therapy Strength(s): Allow for detailed understanding of interviewee perspectives; allow for probing of open-ended questions, appropriate for complex and detailed research questions, and allow unanticipated responses to emerge Weakness(es): The interviewer must be skilled to avoid biasing responses the situation being observed; cannot suggest causal relationships or may be difficult to broadly generalize
Focus groups (Qualitative) Small groups of people discuss questions about their perceptions, beliefs, and attitudes. Similar to interviews but with people reacting to each other's comments SoTL projects on SL using focus groups ask questions like "What are students' perceptions of the SL course that they are participating in?" For example, Deeley (2010) conducted focus group sessions with students both before and after their service placements and semi-structured in-depth interviews in an inductive approach to identify the effects of service-learning on the students Strength(s): Allow for gathering a large amount of information within a short time frame; can show how participants arrive at conclusions; allow for exploration of unanticipated topics Weakness(es): The moderator must be skilled to avoid biasing responses; individual participants can dominate the conversation; data not as rich in detail as may be collected in interviews
Surveys/Questionnaires (Tends toward Quantitative) Interviews and focus groups are also a form of survey. In this instance, the focus in on questionnaire-type surveys that can contain open-ended, closed-ended, partially opened-ended, and Likert rating scales SoTL projects on SL using questionnaires ask questions like "What are students'/service recipients' perceptions of the service?" An example is Lam and Au (2018) use of a questionnaire survey with ex-offenders who had been involved in textile arts and fashion creativity workshops in a project associated with an SL subject Strength(s): Allow for collection of data from a large number of respondents; can be administered in paper-based, online, or interview formats Weakness(es): Low response rates can lower the reliability of findings; how questions are asked can bias answers; difficult to capture unexpected responses; data not as rich in detail as may be collected through more qualitative survey methods such as interviews and focus groups

(continued)

Table 16.5 (continued)

Experiments
(Quantitative) Involve experiment and control groups. Require keeping as much of the situation (variables) the same between groups as possible to isolate the effect of the treatment being studied. Include random assignment to groups SoTL projects on SL designed as experiments ask questions like "Does experiential learning method 'X' lead to improvement in students' learning outcomes?" For reasons described under weaknesses, it is difficult to identify a true "experiment" conducted on the teaching of an SL subject. Instead, a quasi-experimental design is much more likely Strength(s): Considered a "powerful" research design because can potentially prove a causal relationship. "Significant" results can allow a conclusion that a particular treatment actually results in a change. Useful to prove a teaching method helps students learn more, change a behavior or attitude, etc. Weakness(es): Experiments are very hard to implement in educational settings (i.e., students may not be randomly assigned; teacher "enthusiasm" may bias results toward the treatment group; treatment group students may share information with control group students, etc.)
Quasi-experiments
(Quantitative) Involve experiment and control groups in which random assignment to groups is not possible or ethical. Requires keeping as much of the situation the same between groups as possible to isolate the effect of the treatment being studied. Variants include single-group posttest only, single-group pre- and posttest, two-group posttest only, and two-group pre- and posttest Single-group posttest only: Data is collected after the treatment has been implemented. Example-type question: "Have students achieved the intended learning outcomes of this SL subject?" measured by performance on a final report (weakest design) Single-group pre- and posttest: Using an instrument that measures knowledge or attitude both before and after a teaching method (the treatment) strengthens the design to remove some (but not all) other potentially confounding variables. Better able to measure "change." An example is use of pre- and postservice project surveys for students in an ecotourism service-learning course by Mak et al. (2017) as one method for measuring the development of students' generic competencies Two-group posttest only: An improvement over single-group posttest only by introducing a second group as a comparison. Still lacks random assignment and cannot rule out potentially confounding variables (e.g., if two sections of the same subject are studied, perhaps the evening class is composed of differently motivated students than the daytime class) Two-group pre- and posttest: Data is collected twice from two groups, one receiving the treatment and the other not. One of the most powerful designs that can be reasonably used in studies into teaching and learning

further suggesting that "good practice requires that inquiry into learning be conducted in partnership with students" (p. 123).

However, care should be taken to consider when it may or may not be appropriate for students to be involved in data collection. Students can help to distribute and collect data such as surveys or questionnaires, keep the completed instruments in a sealed envelope, and make it clear to the students providing the responses that the data will only be delivered to the teacher/researcher after grades have been published. For other methods, such as reviewing essays, feedback on assignments or examination scores, involving current students in the collection or review process could bring privacy and confidentiality concerns into question.

And certainly, at a minimum all research that involves collecting data from students should apply for ethics clearance and follow all the rules to make sure students are not harmed and are informed of their rights. McKinney (2007) identifies three key criteria for ethics clearance that are particularly relevant when studying teaching and learning situations:

- Informed consent;
- Right to privacy;
- Protection from harm.

Therefore, you should apply for ethics clearance for studies related to teaching SL. This expectation is growing globally, and journals are requiring proof of ethics clearance prior to accepting a manuscript for publication. Institutions of higher education across the world have ethics offices and/or committees, and many now have online application and approval processes. If you are already applying for ethics clearance in your native discipline, also apply for clearance for your teaching and learning studies. If you are new to applying for ethics clearance, start now.

16.6.5 Step Four: Analyzing the Data

Labeling data analysis as a step that follows data collection is somewhat misleading. Do not wait until you have collected all of your data to begin analyzing it. If you are using multiple methods, you can analyze each data set after you have collected it. Also, educational settings make it particularly easy to have several rounds of data collection from students in different semesters or terms. This approach allows you to modify later stages of your study to follow up on areas in which perhaps less data than was desired was collected using an earlier method, or to begin to follow up on interesting new questions. Data analysis can be very exciting as you begin to answer to your research question. Returning to the five-step approach for planning an SoTL study from Bishop-Clark and Dietz-Uhler (2012), here are four key questions to help you analyze your data.

Quantitative and/or Qualitative Data Analysis?

Depending upon your experience as a scholar in your discipline, you may already be familiar with quantitative approaches, qualitative approaches, both, or neither. It is not possible to explain how to analyze all forms of data in a single chapter—instead, this chapter is intended to get you started. As has been previously presented, studies of teaching and learning are strengthened by using mixed methods, so even if you are familiar with one approach, you may be less so with another. You can conduct a teaching and learning study using methods you are less familiar with if you keep it simple and get help from others who do have expertise. In our context, more teachers have indicated that they know less about qualitative methods, so that is the primary focus.

Bishop-Clark and Dietz-Uhler (2012) suggest the following five steps in conducting qualitative data analysis:

- Spend time getting to know your data.
- Be mindful of your research question.
- Look for categories or themes in your data.
- Examine the data for patterns and connections between themes and categories (constant comparative method).
- Interpret and explain your data.

(p. 88)

Does the data set need to be coded for further analysis?

Quantitative data is typically analyzed using descriptive and inferential statistics. Qualitative data provides a valuable addition or alternative to more traditional quantitative data for studies on teaching SL. Qualitative data is valuable for interpreting what is happening in a complex setting and can help the researcher identify important themes or categories within a body of content, and provide a rich description of the social reality created by those themes/categories as they are lived out in a particular setting. Through careful data preparation, coding, and interpretation, the results of qualitative content analysis can support the development of new theories and models, as well as validate existing theories and provide thick descriptions of particular settings or phenomena.

How will you code the data set?

Categories and a coding scheme can be derived from three sources: the data itself, previous related studies, and theories. Coding schemes can be developed both inductively and deductively. Previous related studies and the theories that support them can be found from searching the literature on teaching and learning. If you are new to conducting research on teaching SL, you will probably find it much easier to conduct your first study using an existing framework and theory. This is called deductive content analysis. When searching, remember that it is not necessary for the framework to have been developed within your own disciplinary area or within SL. One place to begin looking for an existing framework is Richardson, Abraham, and Bond (2012) meta-analysis of the psychological correlates of university student performance.

In studies where no theories are available, you must generate categories inductively from the data. Inductive content analysis is particularly appropriate for studies that intend to develop theory rather than those that intend to describe a particular phenomenon or verify an existing theory. When developing categories inductively from raw data, you are encouraged to use the constant comparative method (Glaser & Strauss, 1967), since it is not only able to stimulate original insights, but is also able to distinguish differences between categories. The essence of the constant comparative method is (1) the systematic comparison of each text assigned to a category with each of those already assigned to that category, in order to fully understand the theoretical properties of the category, and (2) integrating categories and their properties through the development of interpretive memos.

To ensure consistency of coding, especially when multiple coders are involved, you should develop a coding manual, which usually consists of category names, definitions, or rules for assigning codes and examples (Weber, 1990). Often, part of the data set is coded first and then the coders meet to determine whether they are coding consistently. Some coding manuals have an additional field for taking notes as coding proceeds. Using the constant comparative method, your coding manual will evolve throughout the process of data analysis and will be augmented with interpretive memos.

How will you analyze the data?

Data analysis methods tend to be more often used within a particular research tradition. Inferential statistics are used in quantitative research approaches. Narrative analysis and rubric analysis are more common in qualitative research approaches. Descriptive statistics are common to both approaches.

If you have never analyzed qualitative data before, there are many resources that can help you. Zhang and Wildemuth (2016) provide an accessible start that includes an eight-step process for a systematic and rule-guided approach to qualitatively analyzing textual data. It also references many of the famous qualitative analysis texts.

16.6.6 Step Five: Presenting and Publishing Your Study

After collecting and analyzing your data, it is time to pull together your findings and conclusions and decide where and how to share them with others. This fifth step is in itself a large area that has been described in many articles and books. But for now, here is just a bit of information for you to consider.

Where do you plan to present your findings?

A scholar has many options for presentation formats when presenting his or her study on the teaching of SL. It may be formal or informal, as an oral, paper or poster presentation, local or international, and so forth. In general, SoTL needs to be reported beyond our own department or institution. Presentations can be made to local, regional, national, or international audiences.

Where do you plan to publish your findings?

Scholarly studies on the teaching of SL can be considered for publication in several different categories of journals: (1) journals in the discipline of SL; (2) journals in the discipline of SoTL; (3) journals in your native discipline that accept articles about teaching the discipline; (4) educational journals which are focused on a particular theme related to your study (such as technology or the psychology of learning); and (5) general educational journals. Academics tend to be familiar with journals in their native discipline, but it can be a challenge to identify journals outside of your discipline that would be interested in your study of teaching SL. You may want to seek help from a librarian on how to identify journals with aims that match your study.

Do you satisfy the target requirements for presenting/publishing?

Before you start drafting your manuscript, spend time researching how you can write up your study in a way that suits the target conference/journal. Log in to the organization's Web site to learn about their aims and requirements. Check the detailed information for submission such as "Guidelines for Authors." Access and read previous paper(s) from the conference/journal for reference.

And, if submitting to a peer-reviewed journal, do not take a request for revision as a rejection. In fact, very few articles are accepted upon first submission. Take the reviewer comments seriously, once again look over your manuscript, and modify it to better address the six standards of scholarly work described by Glassick, Huber, and Maeroff (1997).

16.6.7 Summarizing the Five-Stage Process

Although these activities for conducting a scholarly study on teaching SL have been presented as stages or steps, bear in mind that studies involving people rarely follow the linear path that was initially planned. Scholarly investigations benefit from revisiting stages and making adjustments in response to what has been learned so far and to accommodate challenges or opportunities identified during the study.

You will find the process more rewarding if you keep sight of your own reasons for conducting the investigation. Remembering the benefits to you for doing this study (some of which were mentioned in Section Two) will give you extra energy to continue the study over the course of time and the confidence to push forward when challenges arise.

16.7 Making Your Own Contribution to the Discipline of Service-Learning

SL is about improving the quality of life of the people being served and the students involved in SL. The premise of this chapter is that taking a scholarly approach to the teaching of SL can also enhance the quality of life of the teachers who are committed to making SL happen. This chapter has provided central concepts from the field of SoTL that a teacher can use to plan, carry out, and share a study on the teaching of SL that is in line with the teacher's own personal and career goals. In support of this endeavor, useful resources and guiding questions have been provided. A summary checklist of the guiding questions is provided at the end of this chapter in Sect. 8.

Teaching SL presents many new challenges to teachers as its basis in experiential learning means how the subject is taught by teachers and learned by students is very different from more traditionally taught subjects. However, you should be encouraged and remember that many of your skills learned in your native discipline transfer to conducting scholarly studies on teaching SL. For example, if you already have experience in planning and carrying out research in your discipline, many of the same skills will be used in an SoTL study. If you know how to use online databases to search for articles in your field, your skills easily transfer to searching for useful SL and SoTL articles. Conversely, if you are not sure how to plan a study or your information literacy skills could use a refresher course, the good news is that conducting your first scholarly study on teaching SL will help you develop skills for scholarship that can transfer back to other forms of research you do in your native discipline.

16.8 Checklist for Conducting Scholarly Work on Service-Learning

Consider the Benefits
• Have you reflected on the ways in which working on SL is rewarding for you personally?
• Are you aware of how working on SL is valued in your context/organization?
• Is your current distribution of effort across Boyer's four kinds of scholarship a good fit for both you and your context? Or is there a way you can adjust your activities to enhance the benefits to you and your context?
• Can you name your main reason(s) right now for taking a scholarly approach to your teaching of SL? (see Table 16.1)
Types of Scholarly Work on Service-Learning
• What is the overarching aim of the scholarly work you are considering? Does it relate to one of the four types in Hutchings' taxonomy? (see Table 16.2) – What works – What is

(continued)

(continued)

– What is possible – Theory building • Have you identified SL studies with a similar aim in the literature?
Applying SoTL Principles and Standards to SL
• Have you considered each of Felton's five principles of good practice in SoTL? (see Table 16.3) – Inquiry focused on student learning – Grounded in context – Methodologically sound – Conducted in partnership with students – Appropriately public
• Have you considered Glassick, Huber and Maeroff's six standards of scholarly work? (see Table 16.4) – Clear goals – Adequate preparation – Appropriate methods – Significant results – Effective presentation – Reflective critique
Key Steps in Carrying Out a Scholarly Study
Step One: Generating the research question • What type of research question do you want to study? • What objectives do you want to achieve? • How important is your research question in the field?
Step Two: Designing the study • Quantitative, qualitative, or mixed methods? • Will you do a pilot? • What specific research approach(es) will you use? (see Table 16.5)
Step Three: Collecting the data • What data will you collect? • When will you collect the data? • Who will collect the data?
Step Four: Analyzing the data • Quantitative and/or qualitative data analysis? • Does the data set need to be coded for further analysis? • How will you code the data set? • How will you analyze the data?
Step Five: Presenting and publishing your study • Where do you plan to present your findings? • Where do you plan to publish your findings? • Do you satisfy the target requirements for presenting/publishing?
And finally …
• What knowledge and skills do you already possess that you can use in conducting a scholarly investigation on teaching SL? • What knowledge and skills do you need to develop to conduct a scholarly investigation on teaching SL?

References

Angelo, T., & Cross, K. (1993). *Classroom assessment techniques: A handbook for college teachers* (2nd ed.)., The Jossey-Bass higher and adult education series San Francisco, CA: Jossey-Bass.

Bernstein, D. J. (2008). Peer review and evaluation of the intellectual work of teaching. *Change: The Magazine of Higher Learning, 40*(2), 48–51.

Bishop-Clark, C., & Dietz-Uhler, B. (2012). *Engaging in the scholarship of teaching and learning: A guide to the process, and how to develop a project from start to finish.* Sterling, VA: Stylus.

Boyer, E. L. (1990). *Scholarship reconsidered. Priorities of the professoriate.* Princeton, NJ: Carnegie Foundation for the Advancement of Teaching.

Browning, B. A. (2014). *Grant writing for dummies* (5th ed.). Hoboken, NJ: Wiley.

Carlson, M., & O'Neal-McElrath, T. (2008). *Winning grants: Step by step* (3rd ed.)., Jossey-Bass nonprofit guidebook series San Francisco, CA: Jossey-Bass.

Chan, S., Ngai, G., Yuen, W., & Kwan, K. (2013). Institutional strategies to educate professionals for social responsibility through service-learning. In *The International Conference on Enhancement and Innovation in Higher Education.* Glasgow, United Kingdom.

Creswell, J. (2002). *Educational research: Planning, conducting, and evaluating quantitative and qualitative research.* Upper Saddle River, NJ: Merrill.

Creswell, J., & Plano Clark, V. (2011). *Designing and conducting mixed methods research* (2nd ed.). Los Angeles: SAGE Publications.

Crouch, C., & Mazur, E. (2001). Peer instruction: Ten years of experience and results. *American Journal of Physics, 69*(9), 970–977. https://doi.org/10.1119/1.1374249.

Deeley, S. J. (2010). Service-learning: Thinking outside the box. *Active Learning in Higher Education, 11*(1), 43–53.

Dewey, J. (1910). *How we think.* Boston: D.C. Heath.

Felten, P. (2013). Principles of good practice in SoTL. *Teaching and Learning Inquiry: The ISSOTL Journal, 1*(1), 121–125.

Furco, A. (1996). Service-learning: A balanced approach to experiential education. In B. Taylor, B. Taylor, & Corporation for National Service (Eds.), *Expanding boundaries: Serving and learning* (pp. 2–6). Washington, DC: Corporation for National Service.

Glaser, B., & Strauss, A. (1967). *The discovery of grounded theory: Strategies for qualitative research.* New York, NY: Aldine Publications.

Glassick, C. E. (2000). Boyer's expanded definitions of scholarship, the standards for assessing scholarship, and the elusiveness of the scholarship of teaching. *Academic Medicine, 75*(9), 877–880.

Glassick, C., Huber, M., & Maeroff, G. (1997). *Scholarship assessed: Evaluation of the professoriate.* San Francisco: Jossey-Bass.

Hawking, S. (1998). *A brief history of time (Updated and expanded tenth anniversary ed.).* New York, NY: Bantam Books.

Hutchings, P. (2000). Introduction: Approaching the scholarship of teaching and learning. In P. Hutchings (Ed.), *Opening lines: Approaches to the scholarship of teaching and learning* (pp. 1–10). Princeton, NJ: Carnegie Foundation for the Advancement of Teaching.

Lai, C., Chan, J., Wong, I., Fung, J., Pang, P., Fung, K., et al. (2015). Gains and development of undergraduate nursing students during a 2-year community service program. *Journal of Nursing Education, 54*(3 Suppl), S21–S25. https://doi.org/10.3928/01484834-20150218-06.

Lam, J., & Au, J. (2018). Impact on underprivileged people practising expressive textile arts: An exploratory study applied to ex-offenders in Hong Kong. *World Academy of Science, Engineering and Technology, International Science Index, Fashion and Textile Engineering, 12*(1), 127.

Light, R., Singer, J., & Willett, J. (1990). *By design: Planning research on higher education.* Cambridge, MA: Harvard University Press.

Lin, P. M., Kim, Y., Qiu, H., & Ren, L. (2017). Experiential learning in hospitality education through a service-learning project. *Journal of Hospitality & Tourism Education, 29*(2), 71–81. https://doi.org/10.1080/10963758.2017.1297716.

Lo, K. W., Chan, S. C., & Ngai, G. (2016). Using a recycled container to setup a community learning centre in rural Cambodia—A case study. In *2016 IEEE Global Humanitarian Technology Conference (GHTC)* (pp. 286–291). Seattle, WA. https://doi.org/10.1109/ghtc.2016.7857294.

Mak, B., Lau, C., & Wong, A. (2017). Effects of experiential learning on students: An ecotourism service-learning course. *Journal of Teaching in Travel and Tourism, 17*(2), 85–100. https://doi.org/10.1080/15313220.2017.1285265.

McKinney, K. (2007). *Enhancing learning through the scholarship of teaching and learning: The challenges and joys of juggling*. Bolton, Mass: Anker Publications.

Murray, C. E., Pope, A. L., & Rowell, P. C. (2010). Promoting counseling students' advocacy competencies through service-learning. *Journal for Social Action in Counseling and Psychology, 2*(2), 29–47.

Pechak, C., & Thompson, M. (2011). Going global in physical therapist education: International service-learning in US-based programmes. *Physiotherapy Research International, 16,* 225–236. https://doi.org/10.1002/pri.501.

Richardson, M., Abraham, C., & Bond, R. (2012). Psychological correlates of university students' academic performance: A systematic review and meta-analysis. *Psychological Bulletin, 138*(2), 353–387.

Simons, L., & Cleary, B. (2006). The influence of service learning on students' personal and social development. *College Teaching, 54*(4), 307–319.

Trigwell, K. (2013). Scholarship of teaching and learning. In L. Hunt & D. Chalmers (Eds.), *University teaching in focus a learning-centred approach*. Hoboken, NJ: Taylor and Francis.

Weber, R. (1990). *Basic content analysis* (2nd ed.)., Quantitative applications in the social sciences; no. 07–049 Newbury Park, CA: Sage Publications.

Zhang, Y., & Wildemuth, B. M. (2016). Qualitative analysis of content. In B. Wildemuth (Ed.), *Applications of social research methods to questions in information and library science* (pp. 318–329). Westport, CT: Libraries Unlimited.

Chapter 17
Developing an e-Learning Module to Prepare Students for Service-Learning

Eugene L. P. Cheung and Kam-por Kwan

Abstract Research has shown that students' learning from service-learning (SL) is strongly affected by how well they have been prepared for the experience. In this chapter, we explain how we addressed this issue through the development of an e-learning module on SL for students and evaluated its usefulness in helping students. Data was collected from 9147 students via an online post-experience survey. Results show that most students found the module quite effective in equipping them with the necessary knowledge, skills and attitude for conducting conduct meaningful services for the community, and learn the most from the experience. An analysis of students' scores in the end-of-module test also reveals that most students were able to master the content of the module and pass the test. We also reflect on our experience of implementing the module and identify a number of issues that need to be addressed.

Keywords Service-learning · e-learning · Student preparation

Service-learning (SL) is a form of experiential education which combines vigorous academic studies with meaningful community services and deep reflection to promote student learning and development. Reflection and reciprocity are the two key components of SL (Jacoby, 1996). For it to be effective, SL should focus equally on the service being provided, as well as the learning that is occurring, and benefit both the service recipients and the providers, i.e. the students (Furco, 1996).

However, being an experiential pedagogy, SL is rather demanding or even threatening to many students as it is new to them. It invariably requires students to link the academic content of the course to their service activities, apply what they have learned in class to deal with real-life problems, address genuine human and

---

E. L. P. Cheung (✉) · K. Kwan
Office of Service-Learning, The Hong Kong Polytechnic University, Hunghom, Hong Kong
e-mail: eugene.lp.cheung@polyu.edu.hk

K. Kwan
e-mail: kam.por.kwan@polyu.edu.hk

D. T. L. Shek et al. (eds.), *Service-Learning for Youth Leadership*, Quality of Life in Asia 12, https://doi.org/10.1007/978-981-13-0448-4_17

community needs and learn from their service experience through critical reflection. They are often expected to work collaboratively in small teams and engage in more independent learning. Furthermore, their performance in planning and delivering the service affects not only their own learning and grades, but also the well-being of the people or community they serve. The SL literature and anecdotal experience among instructors also reveal that students face a number of struggles in SL courses (Averett & Arnd-Caddigan, 2014), many of which are due to students' inadequate preparation for the SL experience or project.

17.1 The Importance of Preparing Students for Service-Learning

Research has shown that while SL can have powerful impact on a wide range of student learning outcomes (Celio, Durlak, & Dymnicki, 2011; Novak, Markey, & Allen, 2007; Warren, 2012; Yorio & Ye, 2012), the amount of learning that students gain from the experience depends very much on their preparation for service (Astin, Vogelgesang, Ikeda, & Yee, 2000).

Students have different capacities and limitations when they undertake SL for the first time (Averett & Arnd-Caddigan, 2014). Studies have shown that many students, particularly those who are required to take SL as a mandatory component of a course, programme or institutional requirement, do not understand the meaning or value of SL and see it as a hassle rather than a valuable learning opportunity (Jones, Segar, & Gasiorski, 2008; Lam et al., 2016). Eby (1998) found that some students merely see SL as a means to improve their curriculum vitae; they do not invest much effort in the experience and hence learn little from it. Eyler (2005) pointed out that SL students are often required to deal with ambiguous and complex issues in the service setting. Many of them, however, have not developed the capacity to do so when they start working on their SL projects. Averett and Arnd-Caddigan (2014) therefore argued that there is a need for SL teachers to equip students with not only theories and practice techniques to be used in their SL experience, but also practical knowledge and skills in solving difficult and ambiguous problems and wading through competing theories, research, experiences and values to arrive at workable and ethical solutions. Furthermore, while it is widely recognised that reflection is an important component of SL (Bringle & Hatcher, 1999), teachers reported substantive difficulties faced by students in reflection, particularly in describing and evaluating an experience, and relating it to multiple perspectives (Leijen, Lam, Wildschut, & Simons, 2009).

A common complaint raised by community partners is that some of the students are ill-prepared to serve because they lack the understanding of the community and the service recipients, and do not possess the appropriate skills to deliver the service effectively (Ferrari & Worrall, 2000). Meyers (1999) suggested that to prepare students for SL, it is crucial for them to understand clearly the agency or the service site, their roles and responsibility, and the population they are going to serve. They also need to know clearly what they are supposed to do as well as how, when, where and why they are to do it, and with whom.

The importance of preparing students for SL has been highlighted by Morris (n. d.), who stressed that before students enter the community to serve, they need to

> … know themselves; know their strengths and assets; believe they can make a difference; see their community as a positive place to live and believe the opportunities for involvement are meaningful to themselves and their community … (p.1)

In summary, in order to provide a high-quality SL that meets the genuine needs of the community and maximise students' learning from the experience, it is essential that the students are adequately prepared for the service. They need to be equipped with the appropriate knowledge, skills and attitude before embarking on their service, including:

(a) An understanding of what SL is, why this particular pedagogy is being adopted for the course, and what they will learn from it.
(b) Recognition of the academic as well as the civic and other learning outcomes of the course, and their connection to the service activities.
(c) An awareness of their roles and responsibilities in, and how they should conduct themselves during the service delivery.
(d) A deeper understanding of the people or community that they plan to serve, and the problems they are facing.
(e) The knowledge and skills required for planning and implementing a good SL project, e.g. developing project proposals, teamwork and problem-solving skills, and dealing with contingencies.
(f) An understanding of the risks associated with their SL project and safety precautions to take to ensure their own as well as the service recipients' safety.
(g) Skills for gleaning the learning from the service experience through critical reflection.

17.2 Development of the e-Learning Module for Students on Service-Learning

17.2.1 Context and Rationale

To achieve the goal of educating students into responsible global citizens who make meaningful contributions to their profession and the community, The Hong Kong Polytechnic University (PolyU) has, starting from the 2012/13 academic year, included a mandatory service-learning requirement in its new 4-year undergraduate curriculum. To qualify for graduation, students must successfully complete a 3-credit SL subject that requires them to:

- Participate in substantial community service or civic engagement activities (~40 hours) that will benefit the service recipients or the community at large in a meaningful way.
- Apply the knowledge and skills acquired from their major or other learning experiences at the university to the community service activities.
- Reflect on their service-learning experience in order to link theory with practice, and to develop an enhanced sense of ethical, social and national responsibility.

While the university has a long history of co-curricular community service, academic SL with credits is something rather new to both students and staff at PolyU. Most students do not know what SL is about or why or how they are required to do it.

To prepare students for SL and equip them with the knowledge, skills and attitudes needed for planning, conducting and learning from their SL experience, we have developed an e-learning module on the concept and practices of SL for students and made it available to all SL subject teachers since the 2012/13 academic year, for possible inclusion in the teaching and learning activities of their respective subjects. The development is also a response to the concerns raised by some teachers that while they possess the specific knowledge and skills in designing and implementing an SL subject within their respective discipline areas, they may not have the experience and expertise in teaching students the concept and practices of SL, or the more generic skills such as teamwork, problem-solving or reflection which are much needed for the success of the projects. It also ensures that the preparations in terms of content and instructions are consistent across subjects using the module, saves valuable class time for preparing the students, and allows more time to be spent on developing the discipline- or project-specific knowledge and skills of the students.

17.2.2 Efficacy of E-Learning

With the rapid advance in Internet-based technologies in the last few decades, e-learning has become a regular part of teaching and learning in most universities worldwide. Advocates cite a number of potential pedagogical benefits of e-learning for faculty and students, for example, increased flexibility both in course offerings and access to course resources, and enhanced learning experience through media-rich learning environment and increasing interactivity (Bell & Federman, 2013; Bishel, 2013). Other educators, however, argue that e-learning is just a pedagogical tool, and thus, its effectiveness depends on the extent to which it helps teachers and students to achieve the desired learning outcomes (Ross, Morrison, & Lowther, 2010).

Numerous studies have been conducted on the effectiveness of e-learning on learners' achievement of desired learning outcomes. The findings are mixed. While some studies showed that e-learning improved learning outcomes, some others found no significant differences or even negative impacts (Derouin, Fritzsche, & Salas, 2005). The results suggest that the effectiveness of e-learning is far from ubiquitous and must be studied in relation to the context and pedagogy of the particular course. As pointed out by Bell and Federman (2013, p. 277), "whether a particular e-learning program is effective in a given situation will depend on its capacity to create the conditions necessary for students to learn."

Kozlowski and Bell (2007) propose a typology that underlines four key categories of instructional features that affect the effectiveness of e-learning: content (level of richness of the information presented), immersion (sense of realism that e-learning can create), interactivity (interactions among learners, between learners and instructors, and between learners and the materials) and communication (richness and bandwidth). In a study of college students in Australia, Volery and Lord (2000) identified three critical success factors in e-learning, namely technology (e.g. ease of access and navigation, interface design and level of interaction), instructor (e.g. attitudes towards students, instructor's technical competence and classroom interaction) and students' prior use of technology in learning. Swan (2003) carries out a systematic review of the literature on the learning effectiveness of asynchronous online learning environments and concludes that the effectiveness of e-learning is largely affected by students' interactions with the course interfaces and content, instructors, classmates as well as other forms of vicarious interactions. Bernard et al. (2009) conduct a meta-analysis on the impacts of different forms of interactivity on learning. Results show that interactivity significantly influences the effectiveness of e-learning, particularly student–content and student–students interactions. These principles have been taken into consideration in designing and evaluating the efficacy of the e-Learning module.

17.2.3 Content and Features of the Module

The current module entitled "Concept and Practices of Service-Learning" has been offered since Semester 2 of the 2014/15 academic year, based on an earlier version developed in 2012/13. It consists of an introduction, five instructional units and an end-of-module test. The module has been developed and offered through Blackboard, the learning management system (LMS) adopted by the university. The total student study effort expected for completing the module is 10 hours. We intend that, upon completing this module, students will be able to:

- Explain what SL is, and distinguish it from other forms of experiential learning or community service programmes.
- Recognise the benefits of SL to the students, the community and the university.
- Be more aware of the appropriate attitudes towards, and the responsibilities and other ethical considerations in SL, and act accordingly.
- Develop a good proposal or plan for their SL project, and implement the project effectively, demonstrating effective teamwork and problem-solving skills.
- Apply Gibb's Reflective Cycle to engage in a deep, critical reflection on their SL experience.

A detailed description of the content and structure of the module is shown in Fig. 17.1.

To help students develop the knowledge and skills, and check their own understanding of SL, a variety of in-text learning activities are embedded in the five

Introduction

1. What is service-learning?

1.1 Definition of service-learning

1.2 Service-learning vs. other types of service activities

1.3 The experiential learning cycle

1.4 Myths about service-learning

1.5 Summary

2. Benefits of service-learning

2.1 Service-learning and desirable attributes of university graduates

2.2 Intended learning outcomes of service-learning

2.3 Benefits of service-learning to students

2.4 Benefits of service-learning to the community

2.5 Benefits of service-learning to the university

2.6 Further testimonial on benefits of service-learning

2.7 Summary

3. Responsibilities, attitudes and ethics in service-learning

3.1 Roles and responsibilities in service-learning

3.2 Developing a positive attitude towards service-learning

3.3 Ethics in service-learning

3.4 Summary

Fig. 17.1 Content and structure of the e-learning module on SL

4. Planning and delivering your service-learning project

4.1 Milestones of a service-learning subject

4.2 Developing an effective service-learning project plan

4.3 Effective strategies for implementing your service plan

4.4 Teamwork skills

4.5 Problem-solving skills

4.6 Common challenges in service delivery and ways to handle them

4.7 What constitutes good performance in service delivery

4.8 Summary

5. Reflecting on your service-learning experience

5.1 Reflection in service-learning: What is it and why do it

5.2 Types of reflective activities

5.3 Mastering your reflection skills

5.4 Depth of reflection

5.5 Summary

End-of-Module Test

Fig. 17.1 (continued)

instructional units to stimulate them to interact with the materials, providing opportunities for them to apply or think more deeply about the content. These included: short videos, concept tests, case studies, experience sharing by students having completed SL subjects. Some examples of in-text learning activities are shown in Fig. 17.2.

Example 1 A Video Case Study

Description: This exercise is intended to enable you to reflect on what you should do and what you should not do during the service.

Instruction: Please examine the case and answer the questions after watching the video.

Question 1:

Please list out Fanny's inappropriate behaviors in delivering the SL project and explain the reasons behind. Please suggest the corresponding good behaviors that Fanny should display.

Example 2 A Case Study

Description: This exercise aims to develop your problem-solving skills as a leader in dealing with team problems.

Instruction: Read the case about problems faced by a small team working on an SL project, and answer the question that follows.

Case:

The members of your team come from different departments. They did not know each other before, so the team spirit is very low. They are not serious about their service project. Some of them are often late for the group meeting, or even absent. They always miss some important decision-making meetings, but they will complain about the tasks assigned to them. They will fight with other members until the tasks are re-decided. In fact, it is very time-consuming and some members who are more disciplined may feel that they are being treated unfairly. This results in a poor relationship within the team.

Now, if you are a team member, what will you do? And why?

Fig. 17.2 Examples of in-text learning activities

Most of the subjects using the module require students to successfully complete the module before they start their service. This involves: (a) studying every page of the five instructional units and attempt all the learning activities embedded in the units, (b) attempting an end-of-module test (maximum three attempts) and (c) obtaining at least 9 out of 15 marks in the test. Failure to do so may lead to a failure grade for the whole subject.

At the time of writing this chapter (August 2017), of the 9891 students enroled in 173 subjects offered from Semester 2 of the 2014/15 to Semester 3 of the 2016/17 academic years, 9147 students from 148 subjects took this module, with overall usage rates of 92.5 and 85.6%, respectively, for the students and the subjects. The high usage rates suggest that the module has been welcomed by most SL teachers, especially those from outside the humanities and social sciences disciplines.

17.3 Evaluation of the e-Learning Module

To examine the extent to which the module is effective in helping students acquire the knowledge, skills and attitudes required for planning and conducting effective SL projects and learn from the experience, an evaluation was conducted using student feedback and assessment data. It was guided by the following three evaluation questions:

(a) To what extent did the module help students attain its intended learning outcomes?
(b) What was students' experience of studying the module?
(c) To what extent did the module equip students with the necessary knowledge, skills and understanding to complete and learn the most from the service-learning subject?

17.4 Methods

The evaluation was conducted in the form of a one-group posttest-only design, using questionnaire survey as the main method of data collection. Participants were 9147 students enroled in 148 subjects offered from Semester 2 of the 2014/15 to Semester 3 of the 2016/17 academic years. The survey questionnaire was developed by the Office of Service-Learning, with reference to the specific context in which the e-learning module was implemented, including its instructional objectives, content and pedagogy. The questionnaire contained, inter alia, the following two sets of questions pertaining to the evaluation questions:

- One set of questions asking students to rate, on a five-point scale (1 = little; 3 = adequate; 5 = much), the extent to which the e-learning module has enabled them to achieve the various intended learning outcomes of the module.
- One set of questions (Question 11–18) seeking to collect students' feedback on their experience of studying the module, including: depth of content, organisation and understandability, ease of navigation, amount and usefulness of in-text learning activities, difficulty level of English language used, time required for completing the module and its effectiveness in providing students with the necessary knowledge, skills and understanding to complete and learn the most from the service-learning subject. All items were rated on a 5-point scale (1 = strongly disagree; 3 = neutral; 5 = strongly agree).

The questionnaire was administered to the target participants through the embedded survey in the e-learning module. Students could complete the questionnaire at their own time, after completing the instructional units and the end-of-module test. Students' best scores from their three attempts in the end-of-module test were also collected from the learning management system for analysis.

Data was combined and cleaned before analysis, and the statistical analysis software SPSS was used to analyse the data.

17.4.1 Response Rate

A total of 6729 valid student feedback responses were received, making up an overall response rate of 73.6%. A detailed breakdown of the response rates by academic years is shown in Table 17.1.

In addition, 8783 student scores in the end-of-module test were obtained from the Blackboard LMS, with a response rate of 96.0%.

Table 17.1 Response rates

Semester and academic year	No. of subjects	No. of students enroled	No. of returns	Response rate (%)
2 and 3; 2014/15	35	2070	1499	72.42
1, 2 and 3; 2015/16	55	3448	2408	69.84
1, 2 and 3; 2016/17	58	3629	2822	77.76
Total	148	9147	6729	73.57

17.5 Results

The means and percentage distributions of students' ratings on each of the items with regard to the extent to which the e-learning module has enabled them to achieve the ten intended learning outcomes are shown in Table 17.2.

Students generally indicated that the e-learning module has been effective in helping them achieve the module's intended learning outcomes. The mean rating of each item was high, ranging from 3.70 to 3.83 (i.e. between 'adequate' and

Table 17.2 Student ratings on effectiveness of the module and their achievement of intended learning outcomes

Items		Mean	SD	Percentage distribution (%)		
				1–2 Little	3 Adequate	4–5 Much
1	Explain what service-learning is and how it differs from voluntary services or other forms of experiential learning	3.77	.870	5.0	31.5	63.5
2	Identify the benefits of service-learning to you as a student, and to the community and the university	3.80	.851	4.2	30.3	65.4
3	Develop a positive attitude towards service-learning	3.73	.922	6.8	31.8	61.3
4	Be aware of your ethical responsibilities in delivering ervice-learning projects	3.83	.870	4.3	29.2	66.4
5	Plan and execute appropriate service-learning projects to address identified community needs	3.74	.852	5.2	32.0	62.7
6	Apply teamwork skills in planning and carrying out service-learning projects	3.73	.886	6.0	32.4	61.7
7	Be aware of the real-life/potential challenges you may face in service-learning projects	3.74	.877	5.7	32.1	62.3
8	Apply problem-solving skills to deal with issues or problems encountered in your service-learning project	3.70	.877	6.3	33.2	60.5
9	Apply Gibb's model of reflective cycle to consolidate and reflect on your service-learning experience	3.71	.890	6.1	33.8	60.1
10	Distinguish between superficial and deep reflection	3.70	.870	5.9	34.1	60.0

$N = 6729$; rating scale: 1—little; 3—adequate; 5—much
Row percentage totals may not add up to 100% because of rounding of decimal values

'much'), with 93.1 to 95.7% of the respondents giving a rating of 3 (adequate) or above on all of the items. The following three items were most highly rated:

- Be aware of your ethical responsibilities in delivering service-learning projects (mean = 3.83; 95.6% of respondents rated adequate or above, and 66.4% gave a rating of 4 or 5).
- Identify the benefits of service-learning to you as a student, and to the community and the university (3.80; 95.7; 65.4%).
- Explain what service-learning is and how it differs from voluntary services or other forms of experiential learning (3.77; 95.0; 63.5%).

Students generally reported that the module has also enabled to "plan and execute appropriate service-learning projects to address identified community needs" (3.74; 94.7; 62.7%) and "be aware of the real-life/potential challenges (they) may face in service-learning projects (3.74; 94.4; 62.3%). They also opined that it helped them "apply teamwork skills in planning and carrying out service-learning projects" (3.73, 94.1, 61.7%), and "develop a positive attitude towards service-learning" (3.73, 93.1; 61.3%).

In contrast, the items on "apply problem-solving skills to deal with issues or problems encountered in your service-learning project" (3.70; 93.7; 60.5%) and "distinguish between superficial and deep reflection" (3.70; 94.1; 60.0%) received relatively lower (but still rather positive) ratings.

Students' views on their experience of studying the module were more diverse, with 30.2 to 48.5% of the respondents giving a rating of 3 (neutral) on the items (see Table 17.3). More students agreed than disagreed that:

- There are sufficient learning activities (e.g. case studies, videos, exercises) to stimulate them to think more deeply about the content (63.8% agreed/strongly agreed vs. 6.0% disagreed/strongly disagreed).
- The learning activities (e.g. case studies, videos, exercises) are useful to their learning (53.7 vs. 11.5%).
- The learning materials are well organised and easy to understand (52.9 vs. 11.0%).

The majority of students have found the content and the English used appropriate, with 89.4 and 82.8% indicated disagreement or neutral opinion about the statements that "The content is too easy or superficial" and "The English used is difficult to understand" respectively. Regarding students' study effort, while 31.1% agreed that it took them a lot more than 10 h to complete the module, 26.8% disagreed and 42.1% were neutral.

Students also expressed positive feedback on the overall usefulness of the module, with a mean rating of 3.61 and 59.5% agreeing with the item that "The module has provided me with the necessary knowledge, skills and understanding to complete and learn the most from the Service-Learning subject". Only 6.3% of students disagreed with the item.

Table 17.3 Student ratings on different aspects of their study experience

Items		Mean	SD	Percentage distribution (%)		
				1–2 Disagree	3 Neutral	4–5 Agree
11	The content is too easy or superficial	2.63	.855	40.9	48.5	10.6
12	The learning materials are well organised and easy to understand	3.48	.882	11.0	36.1	52.9
13	It is easy to find the buttons or links to navigate to different parts of the module	3.45	.975	14.8	33.7	51.5
14	There are sufficient learning activities (e.g. case studies, videos, exercises) to stimulate me to think more deeply about the content	3.74	.868	6.0	30.2	63.8
15	The learning activities (e.g. case studies, videos, exercises, etc) are useful to my learning	3.49	.915	11.5	34.9	53.7
16	The English used is difficult to understand	2.68	.943	44.1	38.7	17.1
17	It takes me a lot *more than* 10 h to study the materials and the two required assignments of this e-learning module	3.10	1.007	26.8	42.1	31.1
18	The module has provided me with the necessary knowledge, skills and understanding to complete and learn the most from the service-learning subject	3.61	.811	6.3	34.2	59.5

N = 6729; Rating scale: 1—strongly disagree; 3—neutral; 5—strongly agree
Row percentage totals may not add up to 100% because of rounding of decimal values

A detailed analysis of students' best scores in the end-of-module test reveals that most students were able to master the content of the module, with 8563 students (97.5%) obtaining 9 marks or above in the test and successfully completed the module (Table 17.4). Only 2.5% of the students failed the test.

17.6 Conclusion and Reflection

Previous research and anecdotal experiences of teachers suggest that students need to be properly prepared for participating in SL. The results of this study clearly demonstrate that a well-designed e-learning module on the theory and practices of SL can be an effective means to equip students with the necessary knowledge, skills and attitude to conduct meaningful services for the community and learn the most

Table 17.4 Percentage distributions of students' scores of the end-of-module test

Score range	No. of students	Percentage distribution (%)
14–15	562	6.40
11–13	4787	54.50
9–10	3214	36.59
7–8	171	1.95
4–6	41	.47
3 or below	8	.09
Total	8783	100.00

Passing score = 9 out of 15

from the experience. There is evidence that the module is welcomed by most teachers, and has been quite effective in achieving its intended learning outcomes, as attested by the positive student feedback on the usefulness of the module in helping them achieve the intended learning outcomes and the encouraging performance of the students in the end-of-module test.

Reflections on our experience of implementing the module in the past few years, however, suggest a number of issues that need to be addressed. Firstly, as the module is intended for students across different SL subjects, its content needs to be sufficiently generic to apply to all classes and, thus, may not cater for the specific nature and needs of the individual subjects or projects. It must therefore be augmented by additional inputs by the individual SL teachers, to provide students with a deeper understanding of the problems and needs of the clients or community they are going to serve, and equip them with the technical knowledge and hands-on skills to deliver the service. These may include briefing sessions, talks by the community partners, site visits and skills-based workshops that are customised according to the SL project. Secondly, we observed a disconnection between the module and the regular teaching and learning process in some classes where the teachers simply instructed students to do the e-learning module out of class without making any explicit attempt to link students' learning from the module to their planning and execution of, and reflection from, the service activities. We also noted a tendency for some teachers to focus their teaching on developing students' practical knowledge and skills for delivering the service, relying solely on the module to educate students about the meaning and purpose of SL, or the appropriate value and attitude towards the service and the recipients. These may greatly reduce the usefulness of the module as students do not see the link between the two, and fail to apply the theory and principles of SL espoused in the module in their actual practice. A more effective approach will be for the teachers to refer or require students to study the relevant sections or topics of the module right before they embark on a particular learning task (e.g. developing a project plan or writing up a reflective journal) in a 'just-in-time' manner, and to reinforce and emphasise in class, where appropriate and needed, the important knowledge, skill and attitudes about SL covered in the module.

Several limitations of the study should be noted. Firstly, it relied mainly on students' perceptual data, although students' performance in the end-of-module test was also examined. Secondly, the study adopted a one-group posttest design, which is a rather weak design for demonstrating impact. Thirdly, the data was drawn from the experience of a single university in Hong Kong; its applicability to other institutions or contexts is yet to be established. Future research might look into the actual learning outcomes attained by comparable groups of students after the SL experience, with and without completing the e-learning module.

To conclude, results of the study support that an e-learning module on SL can be an effective means to prepare students for SL. However, it should be fully integrated into the teaching and learning process of the subject, rather than being as a substitute for the teachers or the teaching.

References

Astin, A. W., Vogelgesang, L. J., Ikeda, E. K., & Yee, J. A. (2000). *How service learning affects students*. Los Angeles: University of California, Higher Education Research Institute.

Averett, P. E., & Arnd-Caddigan, M. (2014). Preparing BSW students for service-learning: Enhancing epistemological reflection. *Journal of Teaching in Social Work, 34*(3), 316–333.

Bell, B. S., & Federman, J. E. (2013). E-learning in postsecondary education. *The Future of Children, 23*(1), 165–185.

Bernard, R. M., Abrami, P. C., Borokhovski, E., Wade, C. A., Tamim, R. M., Surkes, M. A., et al. (2009). A meta-analysis of three types of interaction treatments in distance education. *Review of Educational Research, 79*(3), 1243–1289.

Bishel, J. (2013). *The state of e-learning in higher education: An eye toward growth and increaed access (Research report).* Louisville, CO: EDUCAUSE Center for Analysis and Research. Retrieved from https://www.educause.edu/ecar.

Bringle, R. G., & Hatcher, J. A. (1999). Reflection in service learning: Making meaning of experience. *Educaional Horizons, 77,* 179–185.

Celio, C. I., Durlak, J., & Dymnicki, A. (2011). A meta-analysis of the impact of service-learning on students. *Journal of Experiential Education, 34*(2), 164–181.

Derouin, R. E., Fritzsche, B. A., & Salas, E. (2005). E-learning in organizations. *Journal of Management, 31*(6), 920–940.

Eby, J. (1998). Why service-learning is bad. *Service Learning, General, 27.* Retrieved from https://digitalcommons.unomaha.edu/slceslgen/27/.

Eyler, J. (2005). Academic service-learning for effective civic engagement. *Diversity Digest, 9,* 16–17.

Ferrari, J. R., & Worrall, L. (2000). Assessments by community agencies: How 'the other side' sees service-learning. *Michigan Journal of Community Service Learning, 7*(1), 35–40.

Furco, A. (1996). Service-learning: A balanced approach to experiential education. *Service Learning, General, 128.* Retrieved from https://digitalcommons.unomaha.edu/slceslgen/128.

Jacoby, B. (1996). *Service-learning in higher education: Concepts and practices. The Jossey-Bass higher and adult education series*. San Francisco, CA: Jossey-Bass Publishers.

Jones, S. R., Segar, T. C., & Gasiorski, A. L. (2008). "A double-edged sword": College student perceptions of required high school service-learning. *Michigan Journal of Community Service Learning, 15*(1), 5–17.

Kozlowski, S. W., & Bell, B. S. (2007). A theory-based approah for designing distributed learning systems. In S. M. Fiore & E. Salas (Eds.), *Toward a science of distributed learning* (pp. 15–39). Washington: APA.

Lam, H. Y., Lau, C. K., Cheung, E., Chan, S. C., Ngai, G., & Kwan, K. P. (2016). *Qualitative analysis of students' expeience and outcomes of service-learning at PolyU. Unpublished manuscript.* Hong Kong: Office of Service-learning, The Hong Kong Polytechnic University.

Leijen, Ä., Lam, I., Wildschut, L., & Simons, P. R. (2009). Difficulties teachers report about students' reflection; Lessons learned from dance education. *Teaching in Higher Education, 14*(3), 315–326.

Meyers, S. (1999). Service learning in alternative education settings. *The Clearing House, 73*(2), 114–117.

Morris, J. J. (n.d.). *Preparing students for service learning and civic efficacy projects.* Council of Michigan Foundations, Learning to Give.

Novak, J. M., Markey, V., & Allen, M. (2007). Evaluating cognitive outcomes of service learning in higher education: A meta-analysis. *Communication Research Reports, 24*(2), 149–157.

Ross, S. M., Morrison, G. R., & Lowther, D. L. (2010). Educational technology research past and present: Balancing rigor and relevance to impact school learning. *Contemporary Educational Technology, 1*(1), 17–35.

Swan, K. (2003). Learning effectiveness: What the research tells us. In J. Bourne & J. C. Moore (Eds.), *Elements of quality online education: Practice and direction* (pp. 13–45). Needham, MA: Sloan Center for Online Education.

Volery, T., & Lord, D. (2000). Critical success factors in online education. *The International Journal of Educational Management, 14*(5), 216–223.

Warren, J. L. (2012). Does service-learning increase student learning: A meta-analysis. *Michigan Journal of Community Service Learning, 18*(2), 56–61.

Yorio, P. L., & Ye, F. (2012). A meta-analysis on the effects of service-learning on the social, personal, and cognitive outcomes of learning. *Academy of Management Learning & Education, 11*(1), 9–27.

Chapter 18
Engaging Teachers in Teaching Service-Learning Subjects: Critical Issues and Strategies

Grace Ngai and Stephen C. F. Chan

Abstract Our university faced a number of obstacles in the implementation of service-learning: the lack of experience in academic service-learning, the lack of a public service culture, and the perceived lack of appropriate recognition for good teaching. To tackle these obstacles, we designed carefully a financial and workload model to address the issues of motivation and recognition. We also set up an Office of Service-Learning to provide comprehensive operational support and staff development. These include the use of eLearning in blended learning environments. It includes workshops on all aspects such as subject development, project development, assessment, offshore project development, and perhaps most effectively, practical experiential learning. We aggressively develop our own research program on critical aspects of service-learning scholarship. We are also experimenting with innovative pedagogies such as an offshore base in Cambodia as a platform for international collaboration in service-learning.

Keywords Staff development · Motivation · Recognition · Pedagogy Strategy

18.1 Introduction

In mid 2010, the university set up a task force to investigate ways to integrate service-learning into our undergraduate curriculum. After half a year of research, internal discussions and consultations with various stakeholders, the task force

G. Ngai (✉)
Department of Computing, The Hong Kong Polytechnic University, Hunghom, Hong Kong
e-mail: grace.ngai@polyu.edu.hk

S. C. F. Chan
Office of Service Learning, The Hong Kong Polytechnic University, Hunghom, Hong Kong
e-mail: stephen.c.chan@polyu.edu.hk

D. T. L. Shek et al. (eds.), *Service-Learning for Youth Leadership*, Quality of Life in Asia 12, https://doi.org/10.1007/978-981-13-0448-4_18

produced a proposal to include a 3-credit academic service-learning requirement for all undergraduate students.

Previous work has studied critical factors for success in implementing service-learning in leading higher education institutions, particularly those in the USA. Despite the awareness of the learning gains that it offers for students—many of which have been verified in literature—the structures and cultures of many higher education institutions, including our own, are not conducive to large-scale participation in service-learning. Based on our observations, there are a number of critical factors or problems that are particularly detrimental to our ambitions.

1. Lack of experience and preparation—Service-learning is a relatively new academic pedagogy in most countries, and particularly in Hong Kong. If we simply wish to encourage students to participate in volunteer work, it may not be as much as a problem, as this could conceivably be "outsourced" to outside parties such as NGOs and youth development organizations. However, our vision is to adopt service-learning as a rigorous academic pedagogy across the university. The "academic" part implies that the ownership and directorship of the activities lies in the curriculum. This means that we need a critical mass of academics experienced in applying SL in a serious academic manner.
2. Good teaching not perceived to be sufficiently recognized—At the most obvious level, service-learning makes higher demands on time and effort than teaching wholly in the classroom. Higher education is often perceived as being increasingly competitive and performance-driven (Hazelkorn, 2015; Lewis, 2006), which makes instituting service-learning into higher-education institutions add to the already-existing tension between research and teaching. In many universities, even when the management has decreed that teaching and research are equally valued, many academic staff continue to perceive research as the relatively surer path toward career advancement. This means that many teachers are not particularly unwilling to put extra effort into learning and teaching service-learning.
3. Lack of a public service culture—It has been shown that, while, the institutional leadership may encourage the integration of service-learning (or other pedagogical innovations) into student learning experiences, it is more likely to be successful if the incentives are both intrinsic (i.e., building upon faculty members' personal values), and extrinsic (i.e., congruent with issues such as resources, and subsequently promotion and retention) (Abes, Jackson, & Jones, 2002; Eimers, 1997; Helm-Stevens et al., 2015; Serow, Brawner, & Demery, 1999). Unfortunately, such a culture of intrinsic desire for social engagement is not well developed in many universities. This means that to truly implement service-learning effectively necessitates nothing less than the development of a social engagement culture in the university.

To test the waters and to develop a set of long-term strategies to implement the vision, after the proposal was approved for implementation by the University Senate, the university called for interested colleagues to propose several pilot service-learning courses. Five proposals were approved and given permission to be offered as formal credit-bearing subjects during Summer 2011 and the 2011–12 academic year. The piloting was successful, with excellent student feedbacks and substantive demonstrated learning gains, and plenty of lessons for the teachers and administrators.

18.2 Strategies to Tackle the Critical Issues

From our observations of the first three service-learning subjects, it was obvious that we had a small number of teachers who were very well prepared to teach and conduct an excellent service-learning subject and project. They had substantive teaching experience, good rapport with students, extensive community connections, and a wealth of experience doing community service projects outside of the university.

This was a good start, but for the service-learning requirement to be realized at the university level at the scale, breadth and depth that we were aiming at, it was obviously not going to be possible to rely solely on the expertise currently existing in the university. With over 4000 incoming students (2800 freshmen and 1200 senior year/articulation) every year, we estimated from the first three pilot subjects that if each service-learning subject enrolled around 40 students, then we would need around 60 subjects to meet demand. Added to that was the diversity of subjects needed—the first three service-learning subjects were offered by the Department of Computing, the English Learning Center, Chinese and Bilingual Studies, Biomedical Engineering and Applied Social Sciences (Social Work). This is a very narrow slice of the 30 departments belonging to 8 faculties and schools that comprise the Hong Kong Polytechnic University. For service-learning to truly be deployed across the University, it is beneficial for service-learning to be adopted in as wide a range of the academic disciplines as possible.

We analyzed the successful implementation of service-learning in several leading universities. As a result, we identified the following strategies that could be adopted to dress the critical issues identified above:

(a) Motivation and incentives—for the teachers who might propose service-learning subjects and the management of their departments, to address the issue of recognition and reward;
(b) Staff development—for the teachers who would be interested in teaching service-learning, to prepare the academic staff with the needed expertise and skills;
(c) Teaching and operational support—for the subjects that would be offered, to encourage the academic to engage;
(d) Evaluation, feedback and continuous improvement—for the future outlook of the service-learning program and the development of a critical mass of expertise.

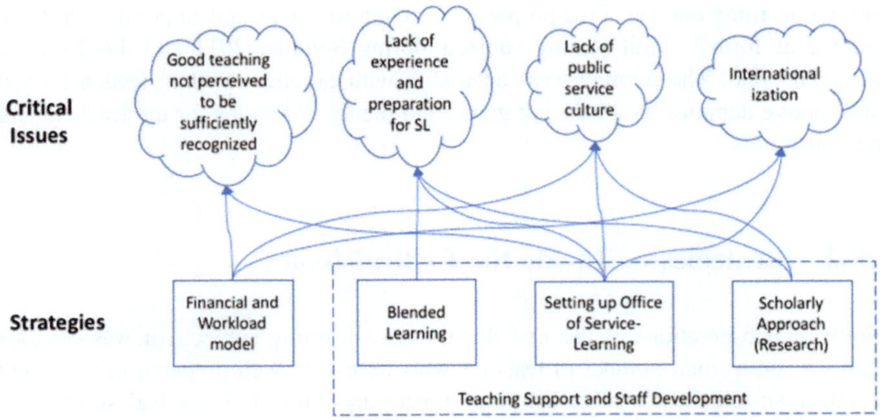

Fig. 18.1 Critical issues and strategies to address such issues

Figure 18.1 shows the critical issues and the strategies that were adopted to address these issues. The next sections will elaborate on our design and implementation of these strategies. The lessons we learned have been tremendously rewarding for us. We hope that the experience would also be of value for other universities who have similar visions and facing similar challenges.

18.3 Financial and Workload Model

Experiential learning pedagogies, such as service-learning, that involve activities that are undertaken outside of the controlled environment of a classroom, tend to be more labor- and resource-intensive than other forms of learning that involve mainly classroom learning activities. This raises concerns on both individual and departmental levels. Similar to many other research-led universities, individual faculty members constantly experience tension between the demands of teaching and research and thus are usually not too enthusiastic about teaching subjects that are known to have a higher workload than others. On another level, many academic departments are running on tight budgets and do not have a surplus of teaching staff. Department management, who need to balance the demands of all the subjects on their roster, will give priority to subjects that are key to the major programs offered by their department.

For teachers who had been active in coordinating student co-curricular activities, the recognition of SL as a subject was actually welcome. As a co-curricular activity, service-learning previously occupied an amorphous space between teaching and services. As they were extraneous to "regular" duties, SL projects were usually viewed as something that was "good to do," but certainly not crucial, particularly in relation to academic and career advancement. This meant that the effort put into coordinating students, training them, liaising with community partners, etc., was not fully recognized. For these colleagues, the recognition of SL as a formal subject meant that it counted into workload calculations for teaching. Properly done, it would also contribute to performance appraisals for promotion and retention.

To address the concerns of department management, the University made revisions to the funding allocation model for courses offered by departments. Basically each course is allocated a certain amount of funds, and the more students in a course, the more is the funding. The main difference between "regular" subjects and service-learning subjects is the experiential service project component, which was mandated to be at least 40 hours, or roughly a third of a 3-credit subject. Recognizing that this component was the part that would incur the most additional cost, the University funding model allocates a premium to service-learning subjects. This premium, which is directly proportional to the number of students enrolled in the subject, works out to approximately a third of the total amount "paid" to a department for offering a service-learning subject, and is designated specifically for the support of the project. Our teachers have used this funding in a variety of ways, ranging from hiring additional teaching assistants to help them supervise the student projects, or to guide students to reflect upon their experiences, or to assess student performance; to paying for student transportation to the service sites; or purchasing equipment to be used on projects.

18.4 Teaching and Operational Support

Unlike the North American (primarily the USA) context, service-learning in Hong Kong and Asia is very much a novel pedagogy. While service to the community is common and encouraged, it usually comes in the form of voluntary community service projects that are done in students' (and teachers') spare time, or as "voluntourism" holidays organized by NGOs or government bodies. The majority of teachers, therefore, do not have experience with this mode of learning. In addition, most of PolyU's disciplines are focused on the "hard" sciences of engineering, construction, mathematics, physics, etc., which traditionally rely on objective, deterministic measures of student learning. Some teachers have experience bringing students on projects in the community, but their focus generally centers on preparing students technically to carry out the projects. For example, a project that brings students to build solar power solutions for rural villages would focus on ensuring that the students understand the elements of basic electricity and circuitry and how the various components of a solar power solution (panels, controllers, batteries) are connected. Another project on promoting healthy eating might focus on ensuring students understand the food pyramid, calorie counting, and basic health measurements. These types of training ensures that students are prepared to carry out an impactful project, but does little to ensure their learning about social responsibility, or indeed their ability to learn via reflection.

When the service-learning requirement was approved, the University developed a well-formed set of guidelines and requirements that define an service-learning subject at PolyU. These requirements appear logical and straightforward: The subject has to link to academic concepts that are relevant to the students' learning and require critical thinking; the service has to be reciprocal and bring the community real benefit in return for being a classroom for our students; the service project needs to be feasible, coherent within itself and with the academic focus of the class; there have to be opportunities to understand and empathize with the underprivileged; and students need to be guided to reflect on and learn from the experience.

Somewhat disappointingly, we found that these requirements are not always easy to grasp or fulfill. Some colleagues were experienced teachers, but were not experienced in designing a new academic subject. Some other colleagues were experienced in leading student community service projects, but had trouble articulating their learning objectives, or identifying valid and relevant academic concepts. Finally, some proposals are closer to community-based learning, with projects that are closer to "study tours" or "experiences" which do not provide real benefit to the community.

In discussions with individual colleagues, we noted that many were not familiar with the concept of service-learning, or indeed, with experiential learning in general. Many colleagues perceived service-learning as difficult to teach and to manage. They were concerned about the unpredictable nature of out-of-classroom activities. They were worried about assessing student learning of concepts such as social responsibility and empathy. Given all this, it was most important that we reassure worried colleagues and provide guidance, training, and support to empower them and build their self-confidence. In other words, we wished to build an "if others can do it, then so can I" mentality. Simultaneously, we needed to "win hearts and minds" by showing colleagues the impact and transformations in students that had been made possible through service-learning, and which had so touched and convinced many others.

18.4.1 A Blended Learning Approach to Educate and Convince

Service-learning is well established and supported in the literature as an effective pedagogy, and there are numerous studies addressing different aspects, from the principles and theories to assessments and reflections. In-house at PolyU, there were also colleagues who had previously led students on service and therefore would have valuable experience to share. There were also colleagues who had a good sense of the local NGO scene in Hong Kong and the needs of the communities that they were serving.

We felt that all of these would be valuable information with which to educate and convince colleagues about the value and feasibility of academic service-learning. Some of these topics are relatively static and generic (e.g., concepts of service-learning), while others are more dynamic and contextual (e.g., liaising with NGOs).

This called for a mixed approach combining online and face-to-face sessions. We secured some funding support from the United Board for Higher Education in Asia to develop a 3-hour e-Learning module for teachers that aimed to cover some of the core theoretical aspects online. This module contained the following components:

- Principles of Service-Learning
- Impacts/Benefits of Service-Learning
- Myths and Positive Attitudes toward Service-Learning
- Developing a Service-Learning Subject at PolyU
- Self-reflection in Service-Learning

This module was taken by over 100 colleagues. It also served as the prototype for an extended, 10-hour, student e-Learning module that is now integrated into most of the service-learning subjects at PolyU in a "flipped classroom" mode (Chap. 17).

In parallel, a series of face-to-face seminars and workshops were also organized. Initially, these workshops were given by external experts, such as visiting professors from overseas institutions, or community partners. Between 2011 and 2018, over 60 workshops and seminars were offered. Topics included introducing service-learning as a pedagogy, planning and designing service-learning subjects, assessing students in experiential learning activities, exploring opportunities for collaboration between academia and community agencies, risk management, etc. As time went on, and more colleagues gained the necessary expertise and experience, more and more of these seminars were given by our own teachers. With experience, the content for these seminars were also gradually adapted to the PolyU and East Asian context. To inspire other colleagues, service-learning teachers were also invited to share their subjects as a case study.

We also made use of Hong Kong government funding for educational development purposes. In 2013, we formed a team consisting of members from all 8 University Grants Committee (UGC)-funded institutions to secure funding for a Collaborative Forum on Service-Learning. This allowed us to organize two guest seminar series, which brought international experts from the USA to give a series of in-depth workshops on doing research in service-learning, facilitating and assessing critical reflection, and taking service-learning to the next level.

These seminars, workshops, and e-Learning courses educate colleagues with intellectual knowledge about service-learning, which is important. However, in the same way as experiential learning is impactful for students, we felt that winning over "hearts and minds" would benefit from an immersive approach. From our own experience, we believed that nothing would be more persuasive than actually seeing how things work, experiencing what we experience, and watching our students learn. To this end, we opened *COMP2S01: Technology Beyond Borders*, one of our flagship service-learning courses, to colleagues to experience, explore, and learn. From 2013 to 15, this class incorporated on-site staff development activities that bring academic staff on-site to our Cambodia project. Colleagues are invited to observe every part of the execution, from visiting students as they serve, to sitting in on the debriefings and reflection sessions, even the internal team meetings with the teaching assistants every night. The idea was to be transparent and authentic with the challenges and rewards associated with teaching a service-learning class. For the participating colleagues, this seems to have been a powerful experience, and at least three new subjects and two new offshore projects have resulted from this. In 2016 and 2017, this staff development activity was expanded into a staff service-learning project that brought academic and administration colleagues to Cambodia, to serve and learn alongside the students, such that they would also get to experience the transformative experience for themselves. To date, two additional new subjects have resulted from this staff project. In 2018, with funding from UGC, we will start a staff service-learning course, with sessions in both Hong Kong and Cambodia, and which will be open to colleagues from all 8 UGC-funded institutions in Hong Kong (Table 18.1).

18.4.2 A Dedicated Unit for Institutional Support

Previous work has suggested that the presence of a dedicated unit on university campuses is helpful toward fostering a culture and a campus-wide commitment to community engagement (Antonio, 2000). Hence, PolyU set up the Office of Service-Learning (OSL) in 2011, soon after the decision to make service-learning a requirement.

The Office was tasked with the following mandate:

1. Support and assist in the development and implementation of high-impact credit-bearing service-learning subjects at PolyU;
2. Promote effective service-learning pedagogies that enhance students' learning and development as a civic-minded professional;

Table 18.1 Capacity-building activities on service-learning for teachers

Activity	Years	Number of participants
e-Learning module for teachers	2011, 2012	131
Workshops and seminars	2011–	Over 1000
Collaborative forum on SL	2014	Over 300
On-site course observation	2013–15	8
Staff service-learning project	2016, 2017	27
Staff SL development course	Summer 2018	

3. Solicit and sustain community support for service-learning at PolyU;
4. Provide further opportunities and support for students' continual engagement in meaningful community services beyond credit-bearing service-learning subjects;
5. Advance the scholarship and research in service-learning through rigorous evaluation studies of impacts and community-based research; and
6. Foster inter-institutional collaboration in service-learning, both locally and internationally.

In other words, the Office would not be responsible for hosting the subjects. The subjects would be "housed" in the academic departments. This meant that the Office would need to have an intimate understanding and connection with the academic departments. To this end, instead of hiring a person from outside the university, it was decided that OSL should be headed by a faculty member on secondment from the academic departments. That gave the Office an understanding of the culture and procedures of the University, and a rapport and working relationship with the colleagues, that would otherwise have taken years to achieve.

The collaboration between OSL and the academic departments take takes forms, depending on the needs of the department, and the objectives that the university wishes to achieve. OSL can give advice in the writing of subject proposals, give occasional guest lectures and workshops, co-teach in a long-term arrangement, take charge of student teams in service, etc. Through close and dynamic collaboration, PolyU, through OSL, not only supports the academic departments, but also achieves long-term strategic objectives through gentle guidance and nurturing. These include the important monitoring and ensuring of academic quality in teaching. It includes experimenting with innovative pedagogies such as eLearning and virtual classes through video-conference. It also includes creating innovative opportunities for international exchange for our own as well as students from foreign universities. These help to form and strengthen strategic alliances with other universities and organizations.

Over the last several years, the Office has steadily built up its presence at the University. It has endeavored to have a voice in many University proceedings at multiple levels. Colleagues from the Office were often invited to sit on various University committees to offer their input on various University initiatives, some of them only tangentially related to service-learning. Most of the University policies and guidelines concerning service-learning were devised with significant input from the Office. Over the years, some of these policies and guidelines were extended to cover other student learning activities, such as overseas exchange and internships.

Teaching can sometimes be a challenging and stressful activity, and many teachers often feel very "lonely" as they face the challenges of managing a classroom of students without peer support. Previous work has shown that collegial support is instrumental in encouraging adoption of innovative teaching practices (Furco & Moely, 2012). The Office thus made cultivating and nurturing a like-minded community of SL teachers at PolyU one of its top priorities. With funding from UGC, this was realized through the setting up of a Community of

Practice (CoP) on Service-Learning (CoP-SL), with the goal of establishing a network of colleagues with a common interest in service-learning. This was a statement of intent from the university leadership: that service-learning is an important initiative of the university, and staff participation is encouraged. In practice, CoP-SL provides a forum for sharing of experience, development of expertise, and mutual support. It organized seminars and workshops for colleagues who were teaching service-learning subjects to develop their expertise in the subject area. For more experienced colleagues who were interested in taking a scholarly approach to their teaching, small amounts of funding were also made available for members, who could apply to use it for staff development, such as going to an overseas conference, or running a small-scale action research project. As of 2017, CoP-SL has a membership of over 100 colleagues.

The Office of Service-Learning has also made one of its imperatives to support and encourage international service-learning. Many of PolyU's students come from working-class backgrounds and do not have the privilege of international immersion prior to enrolling at PolyU. From our own experience, we also find that when students are immersed into a context away from their comfort zone, they are more open to new experiences and receptive to learning. We want more students to benefit and learn from this impactful form of experiential learning, and more teachers to experience the power of bringing students into a challenging environment, provide the right instruction at the most "teachable" moment, share the joy of watching them transform, and the reward of bringing benefit to a community.

In the past several years, we have developed a team at OSL experienced in exploring, setting-up, and expanding foreign sites for service-learning. This team has been invaluable in collaborating with academic staff in developing innovative international service-learning projects, which has increasingly been recognized as a strength of the service-learning program at PolyU. The impact of this team is evidential in the number of offshore projects and participating students, which has grown from the 20 students, in one subject, going to Cambodia in 2010 to almost 250, from 8 subjects, who will serve in Cambodia, Myanmar, Vietnam, Rwanda, and Kyrgyzstan in 2018. This is in addition to over 600, from around 15 subjects, who will serve in the Chinese mainland.

Our experience has shown us that the process of exploring a potential overseas project site, identifying a suitable partner, and building up a sustainable project, is time-consuming and tedious. At the same time, community needs are very rarely ever only one-dimensional; the best solutions are usually multi-faceted and interdisciplinary. It therefore makes sense to build up "umbrella" sites in which multiple teachers and subjects can contribute and collaborate in different ways for the betterment of the community. The Office of Service Learning has been taking steps to identify and build up such "umbrella" sites. This involves understanding the needs of the local community in a broad sense, building rapport with community leaders and local universities, exploring logistical and financial solutions, and training the capability and readiness of colleagues.

This effort has paid off with our first "umbrella" site in Kampong Speu in Cambodia. Collaborating with the Royal University of Phnom Penh (RUPP) and a handful of local organizations, 2017 saw the first Cambodia Summer School in Service-Learning and Leadership organized in conjunction with RUPP. In 2018, 130 PolyU students will travel to Cambodia. Together with 100 local RUPP students, they will enroll in 2 leadership subjects and complete 5 service-learning projects. These projects, mostly targeting the same community, will create digital storytelling social media services for the local NGOs, perform basic health and nutritional counseling for rural families, build solutions for providing clean filtered water and basic electricity for rural communities, and build a zero-carbon computer laboratory for a local primary school. Similar efforts are underway, and we target to have at least 3 similar summer schools by 2022.

18.5 Encouraging a Scholarly Approach to Service-Learning

As academics, research and a scholarly approach should be integral to our work. As teachers, we have a responsibility to learn from best practices, reflect upon our own efforts, to document and share what we have learned, for dialogue with other academics for mutual benefit. As academics, it is important to take an evidence-based approach to our own teaching, to disseminate what worked and what did not work, for our own learning as well as for the betterment of the service-learning community.

In 2013, the *numerical* target in service-learning was being close to fulfilled. That year, we commenced a project targeted at evaluating and enhancing the quality of credit-bearing SL subjects at PolyU. We examined all major aspects of service-learning that are important to us—learning outcomes, community impact, and international experience.

The project has revealed several interesting findings. For example, one study looked at the learning outcomes of service-learning subjects and involved over 2000 students with almost 700 valid responses. Findings show that service-learning substantively, positively impacted the learning of students—even those who were "passive participators" or even "hostile negatives" before taking the subject. In addition, evidence shows that among all the factors considered, including prior experience in community service, a personal belief in serving and helping others, or even interest in the subject matter—there is one single variable that most significantly correlates with students' learning gains—the student learning experience in the subject.

Another study performed a multivariate analysis correlating student learning outcomes with the pedagogical factors. Again, it was a large-scale study involving over 2800 students enrolled in a collection of over 50 courses. Findings showed that the most impactful pedagogical factors were: requiring students to work on challenging and meaningful tasks, their perception of the benefit of their project to the community, preparing students properly and adequately for their service, and having adequate interaction with the community. Most of these findings are not unexpected, but at the same time, there were also some surprises, as it was also found that student autonomy was not particularly impactful upon student learning. This appears to contradict some prior studies (mostly in the West) about the impact of "student voice" on student learning outcomes, and more investigation will be done in future work to explore the causes behind this phenomenon.

These results are not just for publication, but are of real imports as they help to build up a model for service-learning as it pertains to the Hong Kong, and Asian, culture and tradition. The results were disseminated to relevant university committees for deliberation to guide evidence-based improvements in policies and practices.

We wish also to facilitate and encourage other colleagues into taking an evidence-based, scholarly approach to service-learning. Since PolyU does not have a School of Education, many colleagues have never previously done educational research. To facilitate these colleagues, we have organized, through the Community of Practice, a series of seminars and workshops on conducting scholarly work in service-learning. These include workshops on action research, qualitative evaluation, using library citation indexes to search for potential publication venues, etc. In 2017, we took one more step and secured funding for a collaborative action research project on investigating student learning outcomes from 9 international service-learning projects over the next 2 years.

It is also important to give colleagues a platform to share about the work that they are conducting. In 2014, PolyU hosted an International Conference on Service-Learning. This conference encouraged many colleagues to collate and publish their experiences and lessons learned. In April 2016, a service-learning research salon was organized internally at the university. The research salon involved posters and short talks with the target of brainstorming and sharing projects and ideas. The second International Conference on Service-Learning was organized in December 2016, and planning is currently underway for the third conference to be organized in December 2018. These international conferences attract participants from Hong Kong, Mainland China, Taiwan, and many other countries, particularly from East and South East Asia. Together with other initiatives involving cross-country collaboration, they are helping to promote an increasingly active service-learning movement across Asia.

18.6 Looking Ahead

Going forward, we intend to further develop and expand our vision of global service-learning. Our dream is nothing short of a global classroom—to have multicultural student teams to work together on projects in international contexts that focus on global issues, taught by teachers with backgrounds from multiple disciplines and ethnicities. Through these projects, we hope to do our part in fostering cross-cultural sensitivity and international collaborations, as well as sharing and transferring of expertise between institutions.

These efforts have already started. Over the last several years, as we strove to build up our own service-learning program, we learned a lot from other people's experiences, through reading, researching, visiting other institutions, and hosting visitors. Extending and molding these different models and methods into a service-learning framework and paradigm that works for the unique context at PolyU has taught us a lot of lessons along the way, and, in a full circle, that others see as valuable and want to learn. Where we once visited other universities to learn how they did service-learning and strove to copy their model (and we still do), we are now being invited to other institutions to speak about service-learning, and to hold workshops for them as the build up their own service-learning program. We are also hosting visitors from foreign universities who wish to learn about our experiences.

Partially as a result of the success of the service-learning program, PolyU started a University Social Responsibility Network in 2015. This network, which links together 14 universities with track records in various social responsibility initiatives, regularly meets to share know-how. 2015 also saw the launch of the University Social Responsibility Global Service-Learning Scheme in which we accepted students from Beijing Normal University, Sichuan University, and Peking University into our Cambodia and Rwanda projects, to learn and serve together with our students. This was followed in 2016 and 2017 by students from Washington University in St Louis and Haifa University in Israel, joining our Cambodia projects. So far, 19 students have participated in various service-learning courses, contributing to the global learning of our students as well as the social responsibility mindset of their home institutions. We anticipate this to continue in 2018 and onward, expanding to other projects.

As we move forward, we target to both broaden and deepen our impact. In 2017, we commenced a multi-institutional project to build capacity for service-learning among all the higher education institutes in Hong Kong. As part of this project, we will design an online e-Learning course to cover basics and principles of service-learning. This e-Learning course will be open to all higher education institutes in Hong Kong, and eventually we target to open it up to other institutions in Asia and globally. Another deliverable of this project is a teachers' development course in service-learning, which blends together online and face-to-face modules, which will also be open to colleagues from all higher-educational institutions in Hong Kong and potentially in Asia. Through these two modules, we hope to share our knowledge and experience with others, and at the same time, to build up and strengthen our leading role in service-learning and civic engagement at the higher-educational level. Simultaneously, a planned cross-institutional Community of Practice in Service-Learning, and several multi-institutional, multidisciplinary courses will facilitate the sharing of experience and expertise between teachers at the participating institutions.

18.7 Conclusions

Over the last eight years of teaching, coordinating, and promoting service-learning at PolyU, it has become very apparent to us that, just like any other educational initiative, teachers are the critical factor in a successful service-learning program. This is supported by our evaluation results (Chap. 19), which have revealed that the single most impactful factor in students' learning from service-learning is not their motivation to serve, their prior experience in community service, or indeed even their interest in the subject matter—but rather, their learning experience from the subject. Out of all the factors that we investigated, this is the only factor that teachers have control over. The qualitative analyses into students' perceived challenges during their service-learning experience also suggest that teacher competency and, by extension, capacity building are critical.

PolyU has been very fortunate in having a strong, sizeable community of teachers and colleagues who are passionate about service-learning—indeed, passionate enough to teach the subject and project year after year, and expanding and building on it. Many of our teachers have gone on to become ambassadors of service-learning, exciting and motivating other colleagues to get involved; still others have parlayed their service-learning experiences into scholarly work. This community of teachers is truly the biggest asset to the university.

References

Abes, E. S., Jackson, G., & Jones, S. R. (2002). Factors that motivate and deter faculty use of service-learning. *Michigan Journal of Community Service Learning, 9,* 5–17.

Antonio, A. L. (2000). Community service in higher education: A look at the nation's faculty. *The Review of Higher Education, 23*(4), 373–397.

Eimers, M. T. (1997). The role of intrinsic enjoyment in motivating faculty. *Thought and Action, 13*(2), 125–142.

Furco, A., & Moely, B. E. (2012). Using learning communities to build faculty support for pedagogical innovation: A multi-campus study. *Journal of Higher Education, 83*(1), 128–153.

Hazelkorn, E. (2015). *Rankings and the reshaping of higher education: The battle for world-class excellence*. London: Palgrave Macmillan.

Helm-Stevens, R., Rawlings, M. A., Hutchinson, J., Tsai, A., Duke, R., & McPhee, C. W. (2015). Examining faculty motivations for engagement in service-learning at a faith-based institution: A comparison of service-learning faculty versus non-service-learning faculty. *International Education Research, 3*(3), 1–15.

Lewis, H. R. (2006). *Excellence without a soul: Does liberal education have a future?*. New York: Public Affairs.

Serow, R. C., Brawner, C. E., & Demery, J. (1999). Instructional reform at research universities: Studying faculty motivation. *The Review of Higher Education, 22*(4), 411–423.

Chapter 19
Instituting a Service-Learning Requirement in Higher Education: Evaluation and Lessons Learned

Grace Ngai, Cindy H. Y. Lam, Kam-por Kwan and Stephen C. F. Chan

Abstract We found that students generally perceived that they learned quite a lot from service-learning. Learning gains are strongly correlated to the student's interest and the learning experience, while the correlations to the student's grade and whether they took service-learning primarily to fulfil the requirement are weak. It can be considered an encouraging affirmation of the decision to make service-learning compulsory. On the other hand, some students found the physical hardship tougher than expected. Some also have difficulties when the realities in the field were different from their expectations, when their preparations were inadequate, etc. Cultural and other factors seem to pose interesting challenges different from what is commonly presented in literature. Some lessons may be relevant to global adoption of service-learning as an educational pedagogy.

Keywords Mandatory service-learning · Higher education · Impacting factors
Student learning experience · Perceived challenges

G. Ngai (✉)
Department of Computing, The Hong Kong Polytechnic University,
Hunghom, Hong Kong
e-mail: grace.ngai@polyu.edu.hk

C. H. Y. Lam · K. Kwan · S. C. F. Chan
Office of Service Learning, The Hong Kong Polytechnic University,
Hunghom, Hong Kong
e-mail: hy.lam@polyu.edu.hk

K. Kwan
e-mail: kam.por.kwan@polyu.edu.hk

S. C. F. Chan
e-mail: stephen.c.chan@polyu.edu.hk

D. T. L. Shek et al. (eds.), *Service-Learning for Youth Leadership*,
Quality of Life in Asia 12, https://doi.org/10.1007/978-981-13-0448-4_19

19.1 Introduction

In the 2012–13 academic year, the Hong Kong Polytechnic University (PolyU) introduced service-learning (SL) as a graduation requirement for all undergraduate students. Up to 2017, more than 60 credit-bearing SL subjects have been approved and over 4000 SL places are offered to students every year. The previous chapters have described the philosophy, design and implementation of the program. This chapter will evaluate the impact of the requirement and investigate some emerging issues for lessons learned. Service-Learning was made a requirement because it was expected to nurture the students' sense of civic responsibility, an important part of an all-rounded education. It is also a critical aspect of youth leadership, enabling the students to fulfil their potential as a person, enriching their own quality of life. While they help to meet the needs of the underprivileged, it also improves the quality of life of those that they serve.

19.2 Background and Previous Work

Previous studies have revealed that SL generally has a positive—and at the very least, neutral—impact on student learning outcomes (Lambright & Lu, 2009). These positive outcomes have been re-affirmed by several meta-analyses (Celio, Durlak, & Dymnicki, 2011; Conway, Amel, & Gerwien, 2009) and can be broadly categorised into four main areas: academic learning (Novak, Markey, & Allen, 2007; Vogelgesang & Astin, 2000; Warren, 2012), personal development (Eyler & Giles, 1999; Simons & Cleary, 2006), social development (Conway et al., 2009; Eyler & Giles, 1999) and civic or citizenship development (Celio et al., 2011; Eyler & Giles, 1999).

Having said that, there has been scant empirical evidence about the impact of mandatory service-learning. Proponents (Cambell, 2000) argue that service-learning has been shown to successfully promote students' intellectual, social, personal, career and most important civic development, and if these are deemed to be important attributes for students, mandatory service-learning has the advantage of reaching all students, including those who would ordinarily not participate willingly in it. In this sense, they argue that a mandatory service-learning requirement is not that different from the mandatory language, mathematics or capstone requirements that are found in many college curricula.

Opponents (Brock, 2001; Marks & Jones, 2004; Stukas, Snyder, & Clary, 1999), on the other hand, argue that mandatory service-learning is akin to "involuntary servitude". They argue that while it is possible to force students to serve the community, it is not possible to force a caring attitude and civic mindedness, and indeed, mandating service learning may well undermine the whole experience, for the unwilling students as well as their peers, and potentially causing harm to the community.

In previous work (Chan, Ngai, & Kwan, 2017) undertaken in 2014, two years after the requirement was instated, we investigated the impact of the mandatory requirement upon students' learning, particularly those who were initially less-inclined to take part in it. The study found that all students reported substantive learning gains from the SL course, and the less-inclined students learned almost as much as those who were more positively inclined towards SL. In addition, the main factors impacting students' learning and development from SL were their total learning experience in the class, which outweighed other factors such as their interest in the SL project or their prior experience (or lack thereof) in SL or community service.

There are multiple impacting factors within the SL experience. The National Service Learning Cooperative (NSLC), for example, identified 11 key elements of effective SL practice (National Service-learning Cooperative, 1999), including "clear educational goals", "cognitively challenging tasks", "assessment", "clear goals", "youth voice", etc. Some of these factors have been corroborated by other researchers, including Billig, Root, and Jesse (2005), who also showed that cognitive challenge associated with specific increases in academic and civic outcomes.

Results from our other study (Ngai, Chan, Wong, & Kwan, 2016) support a portion of those findings. We investigated a cross section of 55 subjects offered in the 2014/15 academic year and the almost 3000 students enrolled in these subjects. "Challenging and meaningful tasks" had a significant predictive value on personal, intellectual, social and civic learning outcomes, and "Challenge students to try new things" had significant impact on personal, intellectual and civic outcomes. Contradicting previous work, however, "student autonomy in service tasks", which is linked to "youth voice in selecting, designing, implementing and evaluating service-learning projects" (a key element identified by NSLC), was not found to be a statistically significant factor for our students.

Combining our results with previous work, it appears to be clear that challenging projects, which are linked to the "competence" factor in the Self-Determination Theory (Deci & Ryan, 1985), form part of a successful pedagogy for impactful student learning. However, when designing "challenging" projects, we usually consider the "challenge" from the teachers'—our—own point of view. Whether this view is congruent with students' perceptions of challenge is as yet unexplored.

In this chapter, 6 years into the requirement, and with two graduated cohorts, we will revisit the impact of service-learning to student learning, both on motivated and less-inclined students. We will also present a qualitative study into student-perceived challenges and conclude with some lessons learned and good practices.

19.3 Do Students Learn from the Mandatory SL Requirement?

Our first study re-examines students' learning gains (or lack thereof) from the mandatory SL requirement, using data from the latest cohort of students completing the SL courses. In particular, given the fact that PolyU institutes a SL graduation requirement, we are interested in the learning gains of the less-inclined students. To put it simply, does a student's initial attitude towards service-learning bias his/her learning from the subject? And what do students perceive that they have learned from taking a mandatory service-learning subject?

19.3.1 Setting and Participants

This study adopted a post hoc correlation study design and involved 4002 students in 67 courses offered in the 2016/17 academic year. Participants were asked, at the end of the service project, to complete a questionnaire developed by the research team. Valid responses were received from 2670 students, giving us a response rate of 66.7%.

The questionnaire comprises, among other things, the following questions:

- One question (Question I (a)–(l)) asking students to rate, on a 7-point scale (1 = very little; 4 = a fair amount; 7 = very much), their attainment of intellectual learning outcomes (four items), social learning outcomes (two items), civic learning outcomes (five items) and personal learning outcomes (one item).
- One question (Question II (b)–(r)) inviting students to rate, on a 7-point scale (1 = strongly disagree, 4 = neutral; 7 = strongly agree), their level of agreement with items on the following:
  - Whether they took the subject because they were interested in the service project (one item).
  - Various aspects of their learning experience of the service learning subject/project they had completed (16 items).
- Questions on students' initial inclination towards service learning as measured by their responses to the items on the following:
  - Whether their main reason for taking the subject was to fulfil the graduation requirement (Question II (a)).
  - Whether they had ever engaged in community service at university before enrolling in the service learning subject (Question III (a2)).

In addition, students' overall subject grades were obtained from students' record with the approval of the University.

19.3.2 Data Analysis and Results

The data was analysed using the Statistical Package for Social Sciences (SPSS) software. The students' grades were converted into the numerical subject GPA equivalent, ranging from A+ at 4.5 down to D at 1 and F at 0, with a step size of 0.5 between half-grades. Students' individual scores on their attainment of the different learning outcomes and their total learning experience in studying the service-learning subject were computed by the mean of the corresponding items. For measures which involved more than one survey item, the student's response for that measure was counted only if valid responses were available for all the items. Discarding invalid responses gave us over 2200 valid responses for each of the dependent variables being investigated.

The descriptive statistics of the variables included in the study give an overall picture of students' self-perceived gains from studying the service-learning subject.

From Table 19.1, it can be seen that students generally perceived that they had learned quite a lot from the experience, with mean scores of the four learning outcomes ranging from 5.45 to 5.67 on a 7-point scale (i.e. between "very much" and "a fair amount"). The scores on the learning outcomes have increased from the 2014 study, suggesting that students' self-perceived gains have increased. The mean subject grade for SL subjects (mean = 3.29) was halfway between a B ("good") and a B+ ("very good"). This is a slight decrease from the 3.47 from the 2014 study and may be due to teachers' being more objective in grading SL as they gain more experience.

Table 19.2 shows the correlations between the different variables. As expected, there are strong correlations between the students' self-reported gains in the four different dimensions. Furthermore, moderate to strong positive correlations were noted between the four self-reported learning gains with the students' interest (INTEREST) and their total learning experience (LEARN_EXP) in the subject. There is a weak positive correlation between students' subject grades (GRADE), their learning experience and their interest in the subject. There is also a very weak, albeit statistically significant, negative correlations between students' grade, their self-reported learning gains, and whether they took the subject primarily to fulfil the SL requirement (MEET_REQ).

These results are consistent with those from our 2014 study and suggest that students' initial inclination has negligible impact on their learning and development from service-learning. However, these results do not control for the presence of multiple confounding variables. A series of univariate multiple regression analyses on the data was therefore carried out to examine the independent effect of each variable after controlling for the variations in other factors (Table 19.3).

With regard to students' self-reported learning gains, the regression models are statistically significant, with R^2 values equal to 0.55 or above. Similar to the 2014 study, LEARN_EXP had the strongest statistically significant impact on students' four self-reported learning outcomes (INTELLECT, SOCIAL, CIVIC, PERSONAL, β values from 0.788 to 0.859). INTEREST had a much weaker, albeit still

Table 19.1 Descriptive statistics of variables included in the study

Variable	Description	Mean	SD	Min.	Max.	No. of items	Cronbach's alpha
INTELLECT	Intellectual learning outcomes	5.45	0.908	1	7	4	0.898
SOCIAL	Social learning outcomes	5.67	0.954	1	7	2	0.852
CIVIC	Civic learning outcomes	5.46	0.907	1	7	5	0.912
PERSONAL	Personal learning outcomes	5.67	0.992	1	7	1	NA
MEET_REQ	Main reason for enrolling in subject is to fulfil the graduation requirements	4.85	1.498	1	7	1	NA
INTEREST	Taking the subject because of interest in the SL project	4.97	1.236	1	7	1	NA
LEARN_EXP	Different aspects of their learning experience of the SL project	5.55	0.810	1	7	16	0.945
GRADE		3.29	0.514	0	4.5	NA	NA
PRE-ENGAGE	Engagement in community service at university prior to enrolling in the subject	0.13	0.332	0	1	1	NA

statistically significant impact, on the learning outcomes (β values from 0.035 to 0.081). MEET_REQ had a negative impact on the INTELLECT ($\beta = -0.033$) and CIVIC ($\beta = -0.045$) learning outcomes, but this impact was very weak.

As for students' subject grade, the regression model is also statistically significant ($R^2 = 0.026$, $p < 0.001$), but could only explain less than 3% of the total variance. LEARN_EXP had a significant positive impact on grade ($\beta = 0.079$, $p < 0.001$), whereas MEET_REQ had a significant negative impact ($\beta = -0.019$, $p = 0.003$). The impact of INTEREST on GRADE was not statistically significant at 0.05 level.

Taken together, the results suggest that students who took the course primarily to fulfil the SL requirement—i.e. those who are not particularly inclined to participate in service-learning—learned almost as much, at least according to their own perception—as their more-inclined counterparts.

Finally, a series of analysis of covariance (ANCOVA) tests were conducted to examine the effects of students' previous engagement in community service at university (PRE_ENGAGE) on their learning outcomes from service-learning, and

Table 19.2 Intercorrelation of the study variables

	GRADE	INTELLECT	SOCIAL	CIVIC	LEARN_EXP	PERSONAL	MEET_REQ	INTEREST	PRE_ENGAGE
GRADE	1	0.109[b]	0.125[b]	0.086[b]	0.146[b]	0.081[b]	−0.058[b]	0.114[b]	0.007
INTELLECT		1	0.774[b]	0.812[b]	0.761[b]	0.750[b]	−0.066[b]	0.502[b]	0.038
SOCIAL			1	0.757[b]	0.741[b]	0.712[b]	−0.028	0.458[b]	0.036
CIVIC				1	0.782[b]	0.775[b]	−0.072[b]	0.527[b]	0.039
LEARN_EXP					1	0.738[b]	0.002	0.566[b]	0.031
PERSONAL						1	−0.032	0.461[b]	0.015
MEET_REQ							1	−0.147[b]	−0.050[b]
INTEREST								1	0.018
PRE_ENGAGE									1

[a]Significant at 0.05 level (two-tailed)
[b]Significant at 0.01 level (two-tailed)

Table 19.3 Results of univariate multiple regression analyses

Dependent variable	Independent variable	Standardised coefficients		Model Summary			
		β	Sig.	R^2	Adjusted R^2	F	Sig
INTELLECT (n = 2610)	MEET_REQ	−0.033	<0.001[a]	0.589	0.589	1246.514	<0.001[a]
	INTEREST	0.068	<0.001[a]				
	LEARN_EXP	0.788	<0.001[a]				
SOCIAL (n = 2624)	MEET_REQ	−0.014	0.090	0.552	0.551	1074.953	<0.001[a]
	INTEREST	0.035	0.005[a]				
	LEARN_EXP	0.831	<0.001[a]				
CIVIC (n = 2262)	MEET_REQ	−0.045	<0.001[a]	0.627	0.626	1263.968	<0.001[a]
	INTEREST	0.081	<0.001[a]				
	LEARN_EXP	0.800	<0.001[a]				
PERSONAL (n = 2605)	MEET_REQ	−0.019	0.028	0.550	0.549	1058.631	<0.001[a]
	INTEREST	0.048	<0.001[a]				
	LEARN_EXP	0.859	<0.001[a]				
GRADE (n = 2438)	MEET_REQ	−0.019	0.003[a]	0.026	0.025	22.008	<0.001[a]
	INTEREST	0.011	0.263				
	LEARN_EXP	0.079	<0.001[a]				

[a]Significant at 0.01 level (two-tailed)

their subject grades, with their interest and learning experience in the service-learning subject as covariates.

Table 19.4 shows the results. Similar to the 2014 study, students' previous engagement in community service at university had a statistically significant, but small, impact on their PERSONAL learning outcome from service-learning ($p < 0.001$), after controlling for their interest and total learning experience in the class. Again, LEARN_EXP was found to have a statistically significant impact on all four self-reported learning gains ($p < 0.001$, $\eta^2 p = 0.415$ to 0.468), and a smaller impact (though still statistically significant impact) on their subject GRADE ($p < 0.001$, $\eta^2 p = 0.011$). Students' INTEREST in the subject had a smaller statistically significant impact on all four learning outcomes ($p < 0.001$, $\eta^2 p = 0.006$ to 0.029), but not on their GRADE.

19.3.3 Discussion and Implications

In summary, our results clearly show that, after controlling for students' interest and total learning experience of the subject:

Table 19.4 Results of univariate ANCOVA

Dependent variable	Factors and covariates	F	Sig.	Partial eta square.
INTELLECT (n = 2449)	INTEREST	14.305	<0.001[a]	0.017
	LEARN_EXP	1922.570	<0.001[a]	0.440
	PRE_ENGAGE	1.547	0.214	0.001
SOCIAL (n = 2463)	INTEREST	7.168	0.007[a]	0.003
	LEARN_EXP	1851.978	<0.001[a]	0.430
	PRE_ENGAGE	1.582	0.209	0.001
CIVIL (n = 2133)	INTEREST	61.161	<0.001[a]	0.029
	LEARN_EXP	1874.558	<0.001[a]	0.468
	PRE_ENGAGE	5.891	0.015	0.003
PERSONAL (n = 2448)	INTEREST	14.650	<0.001[a]	0.006
	LEARN_EXP	1734.510	<0.001[a]	0.415
	PRE_ENGAGE	0.002	<0.001[a]	0.000
GRADE (n = 2439)	INTEREST	3.024	0.082	0.001
	LEARN_EXP	26.122	<0.001[a]	0.011
	PRE_ENGAGE	1.637	0.201	0.001

[a]Significant at 0.01 level (two-tailed)

1. Students' initial motivation for taking the service-learning subject had negligible impact on their self-reported intellectual, civic, personal and social development gains attained from completing the mandatory service-learning requirement.
2. Students who were more inclined to service-learning (i.e. those who did not take the subject primarily just to fulfil the requirement) did tend to perform better than their less-inclined counterparts who took the subject simply because it was required. However, the difference was very small.
3. Whether students' previously engaged in community service at university had a very small impact upon their self-reported personal learning gains from service-learning, but did not have any significant impact upon their other (intellectual, social and civic development) learning outcomes.
4. The main overriding factor affecting students' learning and development from service-learning was students' total learning experience in the service-learning subject. Their interest in the subject also had an impact, but to a much lesser extent.

These results re-confirm the conclusions from the 2014 study. This is significant as one of the limitations that was noted in that study was that it was done only two years into the introduction of the policy, when enthusiasm and novelty were still at a rather high level. In contrast, by the time this study was done, the university already had five years of experience running the service-learning requirement, which is more than enough time for service-learning to become "routinized" as an academic subject. Our evaluation results suggest that as a whole, the mandatory aspect of service-learning did not harm students' learning from service-learning (given a positive learning experience). In fact, these results reinforce the argument for mandatory service-learning, since, if left completely to themselves, the less-inclined students—the ones who would most likely benefit from the experience—would not take a service-learning course of their own volition.

In addition, in 2014/15, the University started admitting its first cohort of senior year, or articulation, students, who entered the university at the third-year level. The University's decision to include the service-learning requirement for these students was not without controversy, as these students only had two years to complete all the requirements, including service-learning. The argument for mandatory service-learning would also apply to many of the senior year students, as the pressure of finishing a degree in two years would likely encourage them to gravitate towards the more conventional and "predictable" courses that comprise mainly of classroom-based learning activities, as opposed to service-learning courses that bring them into the community and require them to deal with the complexities and the messiness that come along with real world, real-life contexts.

19.4 Student-Perceived Challenges During the Service-Learning Experience

Our latest results and those from our earlier 2014 study confirm that students' initial inclination and experience in service-learning do not matter much in their learning gains—provided that the learning experience is positive. It also affirms the role of the teacher in the course, as the most consistent impactful factor on students' learning is their learning experience in the course. This is encouraging as, compared with the other variables (students' interest, students' inclination, etc.), the learning experience in the course is a factor in which we, as teachers, have the most control.

In this study, we investigate student challenge, one significant aspect within the student learning experience, and an aspect which has been identified as a key element for impactful student learning. Our research question is: what do students find to be the most challenging aspects of the service-learning experience? And do these challenges negatively impact their learning from service-learning?

The study takes the form of a retrospective post hoc design and adopted a qualitative approach using semi-structured individual interviews. The target participants were students who had completed one of 20 selected service-learning subjects offered during the 2012/13 and 2013/14 academic years. The students were selected through a two-stage purposive sampling. A total of 20 subjects (out of 32) offered in the said period were selected based on the subject-offering department, the nature of the subject, the location of service and the intended beneficiaries of their projects to ensure a broad coverage of different types of subjects. Secondly, three students—one each from the high-, average- and low-performance groups—were chosen randomly from each of the selected subjects based on their subject grades. For subjects with skewed grade distributions, one more student would be selected from the group of the average performers to replace the higher or lower performer missing in the sample. Students were invited by email to attend an interview and were asked to reply within seven days. Non-respondents would be replaced by other selected students.

The interview protocol included prompts to solicit demographic and background information about the students and invited students to identify their most frustrating or dissatisfying experience, to discuss the challenges, difficulties and/or problems they had encountered. Students were also asked if they perceived any negative impact from the SL experience.

The semi-structured interviews were conducted in the student's preferred language (Cantonese or Putonghua) and audio-recorded with the permission from the participants. A total of 49 interviews were conducted and transcribed verbatim in Chinese. The grounded theory approach (Charmaz, 2014; Corbin & Strass, 2008; Glaser & Strauss, 1967) was adopted to categorise, code and analyse the data. The analysis was performed independently by two experts to identify the major categories and themes. Any different opinions between the two members about the categorisation were discussed until an agreement was reached. Detailed coding was then done, and major themes that emerged from a detailed analysis of the data were identified. Direct quotes from the participants were selected to support and illustrate the identified categories and themes.

A total of 198 students were invited to take part in the study, and 49 of them accepted the invitation and attended the interviews. The take-up rate is 25%. Of the 49 respondents, 23 (47%) were male and 26 (53%) were female. While 46 (94%) participants were local students, the remaining three (6%) had come from the Chinese Mainland. Sixteen of them were from the high-performance, 26 from the average-performance and seven from the lower-performance groups.

19.4.1 Result and Discussion

In the interviews, students were asked to identify one or two most frustrating or dissatisfying experiences, as well as other problems, difficulties or challenges they had encountered in studying the SL subjects. All students responded to the questions, and most of the students mentioned more than one issue in their responses. A detailed analysis of the interview records reveals 11 major problems as follows.

- *Unexpected situations or hardships*

Nearly half of the students (n = 22) commented that the major challenge or problem for them was when they came across unexpected situations or hardships, mostly during the project. Most of the challenges mentioned were project-specific—for example, students participating in overseas projects in developing countries often complained about harsh living environments. Other problems included: impracticable service plans, teammates falling sick, shortage of service materials or equipment, etc. Unexpected circumstances were also mentioned as another source of challenge. For example, the weather was mentioned in more than one instance.

> The most dissatisfying (experience) was, first of all, that the secondary school required us to do things different from what we had planned. We were supposed to build lamp poles, teach the students some relevant knowledge and involve them in the building process, that's all. But it was completely different after we arrived. All of a sudden, (we needed to prepare for) the farewell night, PE lessons, attending ceremonies, etc. It was annoying to have these additional things, and yet they (the school) had many opinions on the building of the lamp poles, (so we) needed to amend, I was really… particularly when they had scheduled for the farewell night to be held soon after we had finished building the lamp poles. If my memory is correct, we were only told at around 7 or 8 pm that evening that we would have the farewell night the next day… our classmate fell sick, it was my teammate. Moreover, in actual operation, building lamp poles on rainy days was a challenge. We had to think about how to set up a tent to cover the lamp poles as they carried electricity and couldn't get wet. [Student #1]

- *Difficult interactions with clients*

Many students (n = 22) who were involved in teaching-related services found it difficult to interact with their service recipients effectively. Classroom management, discipline and motivation were common issues:

> The secondary school students didn't really listen to us… Actually, we couldn't follow our teaching plan; they were playing (in class) and we didn't know how to make them concentrate, we felt helpless. [Student #48]

Tension among students and service recipients was also reported; for example, one senior left during the service session, two children and their parents had a quarrel, students and recipients had disagreements. One student reported that a service recipient contacted him frequently, which was annoying.

- *Inadequate knowledge, skills or practice*

Over one-third of the students (n = 18) were concerned about not having adequate knowledge, skills or practice to deliver the service. For example, one Business student taking a Chemistry and Biology subject felt she did not have enough background in biology [*Student #45*].

Some of these comments were raised by students who took service-learning courses outside of their discipline. However, quite a number of students who chose a subject offered by their own or a related academic department also commented that there was no or insufficient training/practice/observation to prepare them for the service. For instance, three engineering students enrolled in an engineering course mentioned that they did not know how to program, use the software or build the product as required:

> (My most frustrating experience was) definitely about programming. I really knew nothing, so I just followed the YouTube video; I watched 10 seconds and followed the steps. There were lots of codes we needed to input, but we had no idea at all about what we had done, so it turned out to be full of errors. [Student #29]

- *Insufficient communication*

A number of students ($n = 14$) mentioned poor communication and unclear guidelines. One student mentioned additional requirements from the service partner that the teacher did not know about and blamed communication of the teacher with the service partner. Some students expressed that they found the guidelines unclear and thus were not sure if they were on the right track when preparing for the service:

> Overall speaking, I dislike the lecturer. He sometimes expected us to think of a solution by ourselves, or do the job by ourselves. But there were many things that we were not sure about: whether we could do it this way, or should we do it another way. Also, we had many small teams, and each team had its own opinions. We couldn't group these opinions together, but the lecturer just asked us to figure it out by ourselves. It finally turned out okay, because all four groups had become one big group. [Student #41]

On a similar note, some students ($n = 13$) mentioned that they lacked sufficient information and thus could not plan effectively. For example, some commented that they did not know about the backgrounds or profiles of the people they were serving, or that even the service schedule was not confirmed until a very late stage:

> We were not sure what we were going to do, how many days were for the service, when to do the service, when we could take rest, or when to do what. There was no concrete schedule, and it's all very unclear. It seemed like going there without any preparation. [Student #10]

Other examples included: students were unsure of the needs of their visually impaired elderly clients, the health status of their elderly service recipients, the level of science knowledge of the secondary school students they were about to teach, or even the age and grade of the children.

- *Teamwork Challenges*

Some students ($n = 10$) found that working in teams was quite challenging because of the following reasons: teammates being free riders or not serious about their work, different opinions among members in the team, unclear or uneven work distribution, etc. Some teachers put students from different disciplines in one team; this made their communication difficult as it was hard to schedule a time which was convenient for the whole team to work together. For example, when students were left to work out the schedules with the community partners by themselves, timetable clashes among teammates added to schedule constraints with community partners to create additional challenges.

- *Inadequate resources*

Quite a number of students ($n = 8$) indicated that inadequate resources posed some difficulties to their SL projects. Two students said they needed to find sponsorship for organising the service project, which was quite challenging to them. Some felt that there were not enough supporting resources for the projects. Examples included limited technical support, having to borrow or purchase the service equipment themselves, insufficient materials for practice and no space for storing service materials, etc.

- *Heavy workload*

Several students ($n = 6$) pinpointed that heavy workload was another challenge. Three of these students enrolled in the same subject. They had to interview members of an ethnic minority group during the day and spend a long time in the evening transcribing the interview records. A student from another subject said he had spent lots of time every week to collect information for doing the assignments [*Student #2*]. A student who had joined an overseas project said the workload before the trip was heavy because they had to attend intensive training sessions while preparing for their final examination in June [*Student #24*]. Similarly, another student said that most of the tasks were assigned at the last minute, and the training and course work of the service-learning subject clashed with her own busy study schedule; all these made her feel tired [*Student #34*].

- *Unclear Assessment*

A minority of students ($n = 5$) expressed concerns related to assessment. Two students said they were not clear about the assessment methods or the criteria. A few of them felt that the assessment methods or the assigned group tasks were not fair or too stressful:

> A free rider always wins. This is the most frustrating thing that I must mention. If you are committed to the project, you will try all your best to do an excellent job. If one only wants to take a free ride, there's nothing you can do to motivate him. What we could do then was to finish his (the free rider's) tasks. I knew he got an A grade, and I felt that was totally unfair because he was an outright free rider. [Student #46]

> The most difficult part was the presentation at the end. It contributed 30% to the subject assessment. I think it was all about bluffing. We normally wrote reflective journals, but this time it was verbal presentation, it was very different and very difficult. It couldn't be too brief, or there was no reflection. But I didn't really know how to present reflection verbally. [Student #2]

- *Poor Planning*

Several students ($n = 7$) encountered challenges that were related to planning of the project. Five students, who took part in a service project in another country in which they did not know the language, revealed that they had no access to interpreters, which made communication with their clients very difficult. One student mentioned that the published class schedule did not match with their actual service schedule [*Student #9*]; they were asked to reflect on their service delivery when only part of the class had started on their service project. Another student said the resources provided for each group in the subject were not equal [*Student #20*].

Other students reported that they were given inadequate time for writing the reflective journals.

- *Others*

Some other students mentioned it was very difficult to get enrolled in a service-learning subject because of the very many different enrolment methods and timetable clashes. A few students were doubtful if their service for the clients or their learning from and reflection about the experience was worthy or meaningful. One student disagreed with the subject teacher on how to teach the secondary school students and found it difficult to follow his advice or instructions [*Student #41*].

19.4.2 Did These Challenges Have Any Negative Impact on Students?

Although all students mentioned challenges, problems or difficulties, when they were asked about negative impacts or consequences, about half (24 out of 49) clearly indicated that the service-learning experience, challenges and all had no negative impact. Some even remarked that the challenges and problems made them learn more, and that had become a positive experience for them [*Students #32, #36*]. Likewise, a student commented that in spite of all the problems and difficulties, the service-learning subject had provided her with a very good learning experience [*Student #40*]. Another student said she had developed a better understanding and changed her original perception of the visually impaired even though she had encountered many difficulties during the service experience [*Student #49*].

22 of the 49 students did mention some negative impacts. However, some of the students were quick to point out that most of the negative impacts were quite minor and short-lived and challenged them to learn from the experience:

> (I) felt (I was) very emotional and needed to control my emotion… In fact, the negative emotion was not too serious, but I had learnt a lot from it, e.g. how to solve problems, and how to avoid letting your own emotion affect the whole process. Anger will not do any help, (and we) need to solve the problem. [Student #16]

Some students mentioned that their service-learning subject was time-consuming as they had to put a lot of effort in providing services and discussing the project with teammates and other stakeholders. These made it hard for them to balance between that subject and other courses, especially when service sessions were conducted in the evenings:

> Indeed the effect was not that serious; it just affected other subjects, as I would skip class if I got up late in the next morning. [Student #2]

A few students reported more long-lasting negative impacts. One student who taught LEGO workshops stated that she was sick of LEGO and would never touch it again [*Student #48*]. One student commented that he had become more pessimistic about life after serving the elderly.

> What (had affected me) most was, after seeing the elderly, I felt rather down sometimes… my view towards life become pessimistic. I would think about myself, when I'm old, I don't know what I will be. I would worry that I will be the one who needs others to take care of… like those elderlies who live alone, and wait for social workers to take care of them. [Student #38]

19.4.3 Limitations and Lessons Learned

The data that was collected in this study can serve as a useful reference for teachers who are interested in designing or refining a service-learning subject. However, it should be noted that the interviewed students came from different departments and studied different subjects, the challenges and difficulties are broadly reported independently of the context of the projects involved, and students' correlation with learning gains are not discussed. Hence, it needs to be noted that the described challenges may be very project-specific, and indeed, we noted that some were contradictory or inconsistent.

From the analysis of the data, it is obvious that service-learning subjects are very different from other academic subjects. As an experiential pedagogy, especially one that requires service back to the community as well as interaction with the community, some challenges, problems and difficulties are inevitable, inherent or even intentional. Unlike a classroom setting, service-learning requires students to interact with authentic people, learn in an authentic environment, and apply their hands-on skills to an authentic problem. Unlike classroom exercises, real-life contexts and situations are rarely ever simple. Since (most) undergraduate students have so far experienced only classroom problems, this complexity would obviously pose a challenge. This challenge may even be exacerbated by the Hong Kong (Asian) context, where students are expected to learn mainly by rote, and where teachers are expected to "have all the answers".

That said, some of these issues can definitely be addressed. Many of these challenges appear to arise from the uncertainty inherent in service-learning subjects —such as scheduling concerns or unclear expectations. From our experience, academia and community need to learn to work together; the first working experience does tend to be more chaotic and unpredictable as both sides learn each other's constraints and requirements. To this end, teachers are encouraged to work with the same community partner as much as possible. We have noticed that successive iterations of the same project tend to be smoother, perhaps because both parties have learned what to expect from each other, and thus the teacher is in a better position to support and guide his/her students. From the community side, this also makes possible more sustainable impact, as most real problems cannot be solved within the space of one subject or project.

Where possible, teachers should provide students with clear and adequate guidance about the service environment, deliverables and expectations from stakeholders. However, there are instances where this is not possible. An example could be a service project that collaborates with an NGO to run workshops for street children. The background, age or even the number of children may not be known in advance. In situations like these, teachers are encouraged to include sharing sessions from former students. The experiences of these students, coming from the students themselves, can often serve as examples that their peers can draw from, in a manner similar to example-based learning. This can set expectations accordingly and reassure their peers. Community partners can also play a part in equipping students with a deeper understanding of the service recipients and the community they are going to serve, which may complement the interactions during the service project to provide a deeper and more nuanced overview.

Another aspect of the challenges appear to be due to teachers' inexperience. The aforementioned challenges of poor planning, mis-scheduling and unequal allocation of resources can be attributed to oversights on the part of the teaching team while planning and coordinating the subject and project. This suggests that teacher training and capacity building are critical—certainly for all new pedagogies or initiatives, but even more so for service-learning because of the inherent complexity of the pedagogy.

Extending from the previous point, mentorship and community are important. A community of practice for service-learning practitioners and teachers, and staff development activities can serve to facilitate sharing and disseminating of good practices. This exchange of experience, and the "learning from examples" that it facilitates, could help practitioners and teachers to anticipate and avoid unintended challenges, direct students to focus on tackling the intended challenges and to improve their subjects and projects.

That said, it should be iterated that about half of the interviewees clearly indicated that the service-learning experience had no negative impact on them; a few even felt that the difficulties and problems they faced challenged them to learn more from the experience. Less than half of the students mentioned some negative impacts, but most of these were quite minor and short-lived. In that sense, the focus of this study is not aimed at providing a "how-to" for teachers to clear the obstacles for students, but, rather, for them to manage the experience, to identify and transfer the inevitable and inherent challenges into intended learning opportunities. Teachers should be aware of potential challenges and consider how to best prepare, train or support students who struggle with these challenges and make use of the challenges to foster positive learning outcomes.

19.5 Overall Conclusions and Looking Forward

The introduction of the service-learning requirement at PolyU in 2012 was, in a way, a big risk-taking step for the University. Much of the literature on the effectiveness and benefits of service-learning were situated in the West, in smaller schools, and with smaller groups (or even single classes) of students. The Hong Kong context and the background of PolyU as a state-funded institute with heavy emphasis on professional training create a very different environment and culture.

This difference in environment and culture creates a different set of challenges and expectations for students and teachers. Given how education and personal development are strongly influenced by culture and environment, it is not surprising that some of the commonly held assumptions may not be valid in our context. Indeed, some of the results in this study, together with previous published work, appear to contradict commonly held beliefs about best practices in service-learning.

We believe that this calls for more research into the cultural aspects of service-learning, and potentially the development of a model for service-learning that is more culturally sensitive, or even culture-specific. This will be required if service-learning is to become more accepted worldwide as a high-impact pedagogy.

19.6 Acknowledgements

The project was funded by the University Grants Committee of Hong Kong and The Hong Kong Polytechnic University. We would like to express our sincere thanks to all the students who participated in the surveys and interviews.

References

Billig, S. H., Root, S., & Jesse, D. (2005). The relationship between the quality indicators of service-learning and student outcomes. In S. Root, J. Callahan, & S. H. Billig (Eds.), *Improving service-learning practice: Research on models to enhance impact* (pp. 97–115). Greenwich, Connecticut: Information Age Publishing.

Brock, K. L. (2001). Promoting voluntary action and civic society through the state. *Isuma: Canadian Journal of Policy Research, 2*(2), 53–61.

Cambell, E. D. (2000). Social capital and service-learning. *Political Science and Politics, 23*(3), 641–646.

Celio, C. I., Durlak, J., & Dymnicki, A. (2011). A meta-analysis of the impact of service-learning on students. *Journal of Experiential Education, 34*(2), 164–181.

Chan, S. C., Ngai, G., & Kwan, K. (2017). Mandatory service learning at university: Do less-inclined students learn from it? *Active Learning in Higher Education*, 1–14. https://doi.org/10.1177/1469787417742019.

Charmaz, K. (2014). *Constructing grouded theory*. Los Angeles: SAGE.

Conway, J. M., Amel, E. L., & Gerwien, D. P. (2009). Teaching and learning in the social context: A meta-analysis of service learning's effects on academic, personal, social, and citizenship outcomes. *Teaching of Psychology, 36*(4), 233–245.

Corbin, J., & Strass, A. (2008). *Basics of qualitative research: Techniques and procedures for developing grounded theory*. Thousand Oaks, CA: SAGE.

Deci, E. L., & Ryan, R. M. (1985). *Intrinsic motivation and self-determinationn in human behavior*. New York: Plenum Press.

Eyler, J., & Giles, D. E. (1999). *Where's the learning in service-learning?*. San Francisco, CA: Jossey-Bass.

Glaser, B. G., & Strauss, A. L. (1967). *The discovery of grounded theory*. New York: Aldine.

Lambright, K. T., & Lu, Y. (2009). What impacts the learning in service learning? An examination of project structure and student characteristics. *The Journal of Public Affairs Education, 15*(4), 425–444. Retrieved from https://ssrn.com/abstract=2167980.

Marks, H. M., & Jones, S. R. (2004). Community service in the transitions: Shifts and continuities in participation from high school to college. *Journal of Higher Education, 75*(3), 307–339.

National Service-learning Cooperative. (1999). *Essential elements of service-learning*. St. Paul, MN: National Youth Leadership Council.

Ngai, G., Chan, S. C., Wong, W., & Kwan, K. (2016). *A multivariate study of factors influencing students' learning outcomes from service-learning*. New Orleans, LA: International Association for Research on Service-learning & Community Engagement.

Novak, J. M., Markey, V., & Allen, M. (2007). Evaluating cognitive outcomes of service learning in higher education: A meta-analysis. *Communication Research Reports, 24*(2), 149–157.

Simons, L., & Cleary, B. (2006). The influence of service learning on students' personal and social development. *College Teaching, 54*(4), 307–319.

Stukas, A. A., Snyder, N., & Clary, E. G. (1999). The effects of "mandatory volunteerism" on intentions to volunteer. *Psychological Science, 10*(1), 59–64.

Vogelgesang, L. J., & Astin, A. W. (2000). Comparing the effects of community service and service-learning. *Michigan Journal of Community Service Learning, 7*(1), 25–34.

Warren, J. L. (2012). Does service-learning increase student learning? A meta-analysis. *Michigan Journal of Community Service Learning, 18*(2), 56–61.

Chapter 20
Service-Learning at The Hong Kong Polytechnic University: Opportunities and Challenges Ahead

Daniel T. L. Shek

Abstract With the implementation of the new 4-year undergraduate curriculum, The Hong Kong Polytechnic University has used the extra year to launch the General University Requirements which includes Service-Learning (SL). In this chapter, the achievements in SL in the past few years are outlined. Several lessons have been learned in the implementation of SL, including the feasibility of offering a huge number of SL subjects across a wide range of disciplines and the importance of training and e-learning curriculum materials. Besides opportunities for developing SL initiatives, the major challenges are also highlighted. These include the issue of maintaining a competitive edge, sustainability in SL staff, promotion of the "we care" motivation behind SL, maintaining quality SL initiatives, integration across different disciplines, sectors and services, the need for strategic directions, and the importance of research and evaluation in SL in the promotion of quality of life.

Keywords Service-Learning · General University Requirements
Lessons learned · Challenges · Opportunities

20.1 Introduction

Service-Learning is still at its infancy in Hong Kong. With the opportunity of the higher education curriculum reform, universities in Hong Kong have changed from a three-year curriculum to a four-year curriculum. It is the wish of the University Grants Committee to broaden the mindset of undergraduate students and better equip them with the challenges of the changing global economy by adding more general education subjects for the extra year. By doing this, it is expected that university graduates can possess more generic skills conducive to holistic

D. T. L. Shek (✉)
Department of Applied Social Sciences, The Hong Kong Polytechnic University, Hunghom, Hong Kong
e-mail: daniel.shek@polyu.edu.hk

D. T. L. Shek et al. (eds.), *Service-Learning for Youth Leadership*,
Quality of Life in Asia 12, https://doi.org/10.1007/978-981-13-0448-4_20

development. At The Hong Kong Polytechnic University, the 30-credit General University Requirements (GUR) was developed to nurture different graduate attributes, including effective communication, innovative problem-solving, critical thinking, lifelong learning and ethical leadership (Shek, Yu, & Ng, 2016; Shek, Yu, & Merrick, 2017). Different components of GUR were constructed to provide diverse learning experience for the students. Among them, Service-Learning requirement is intrinsic to the GUR where graduates must take a 3-credit Service-Learning subject before graduation.

Several evaluation studies have demonstrated the positive impact of the 4-year programme on the holistic development of the students (Shek & Yu, 2016; Shek, Yu, & Zhu, 2016; Shek & Yu, 2017a, 2017b, 2017c; Shek, Yu, & Chai, 2017a, 2017b). In this chapter, the achievements, lessons learned, opportunities and challenges ahead are outlined. In particular, the challenges surrounding how SL may promote the quality of life of the students, service recipients and communities will be examined.

20.2 Achievements

There are several achievements regarding the development and implementation of the SL requirement at PolyU. The first achievement is the number of subjects developed. To successfully implement the SL requirement, there must be a sufficient large number of subjects available for the students to take. We have so far developed over 63 subjects involving a very wide range of fields (Table 20.1). The huge number of subjects means that students have sufficient choice in choosing SL subjects in line with their interest. This can also reduce their resentment and negative feeling on the mandatory nature of SL. Second, the number of students taking SL has grown from 189 in 2012–13 school year to 1894, 3124, 3745 and 3925 in 2013–14, 2014–15, 2015–16 and 2016–17 academic year, respectively. The provision of such a huge number of SL places is challenging because a lot of networking work has to be done with many service providers. Much effort is also needed to coach colleagues to write proposals. Third, PolyU has begun to build up a dedicated team of colleagues who are passionate about SL teaching. From a handful of teachers in 2012, we have more than 100 teachers in 2017. Furthermore, with the establishment of Office of Service-Learning, we have nurtured a group of passionate colleagues who are committed to SL.

Fourth, in terms of its vision and scale, PolyU leads all universities in Hong Kong and different parts of Asia. PolyU is the first university that makes SL a graduation requirement. This practice has been followed by two other universities in Hong Kong. An increasing number of credit-bearing SL subjects has also been developed by other universities in Hong Kong. Fifth, PolyU has won some prestigious teaching awards for Service-Learning subjects, including the University Grants Committee Teaching Award (Grace Ngai and Stephen Chan), Bronze Award (Social Enterprise) under QS Reimagine Education Awards 2016 (Daniel Shek)

Table 20.1 Examples of SL subjects

Faculty	Subject title
FAST	Community Engagement through Expressive Textile Arts and Fashion
	Educating Rural Farmers on Healthier Food Production
	Engaging Fashion as a Communication Media for the Needy
	Enhancing Scientific Literacy through Daily Physics
FB	Accounting and Internal Control in the Elderly Centre through Service Learning
	Business Project Development and Implementation for Underprivileged Communities
	Service Learning: Building Green Communities with Environmental NGOs
	Service-Learning: Financial Literacy for Low-income Youth in Hong Kong
FCE	Built Environment Enhancement for Underprivileged Communities
	Housing for the Community
	Science for Healthy and Sustainable Living Environments
	Social Justice in Private Housing Redevelopment
FENG	Assistive Technologies: Service Learning towards the Elderly and Disabled
	Reducing the Scientific Divide in Secondary Students through STEM (Science, Technology, Engineering and Mathematics) Projects
	Serving People with Special Needs through Assistive Technologies
	Technology Beyond Borders: Service Learning across Cultural, Ethnic and Community Lines
FH	Appreciating and Applying Chinese Literary Masterpieces in Modern Daily Life
	Empowering Teenagers through Teaching Workplace English
	Enhancing Biliteracy & Trilingualism through Language Service
	Language Arts for Community Projects: Teaching Chinese as a Service Learning experience
FHSS	Collaborative Care in School Health and Safety
	Promotion of Children and Adolescent Development
	Promotion of Healthy Ageing in the Community
	Public Health Optometry
SD	Communication Design for Sharing and Inheritance—'The Book of Life'
	Service-Learning through Design and Building for Remote Communities
SHTM	Accessible Tourism: Concepts, Challenges, and Practices
	Community Tourism: Tour, Training, Operator, and Event from and for the Community
	Ecotourism in Rural and Developing Regions
	Hospitality Management and Operations in Developing Regions

FAST faculty of applied science and textiles; *FB* faculty of business; *FCE* faculty of construction and environment; *FENG* faculty of engineering; *FH* faculty of humanities; *FHSS* faculty of health and social sciences; *SD* school of design; *SHTM* school of hotel and tourism management and Communist League Excellence Award (Daniel Shek). Sixth, PolyU is leading a huge Teaching Development Grant project (roughly HK$15 million) funded by the University Grants Committee. In the project, a series of studies will be conducted, such as the development of assessment scales and investigation of how SL might contribute to the well-being of students, service recipients and the organizations concerned. Finally, different evaluation findings showed that SL is making a positive impact on the students.

20.3 Lessons Learned

Several lessons can be learned after SL has been implemented for five years at PolyU. First, in contrast to the common myth that it would be impossible to offer SL subjects to a huge number of students, our experience shows that SL on a large scale is possible. In terms of the number of students, teachers, subjects, stakeholders, the related numbers are huge. Fortunately, with an orchestrated effort involving the Office of Service-Learning and support of the senior management as well as colleagues, the experience from PolyU shows that it is possible to cope with the "huge numbers". Hence, the PolyU experience is helpful to those universities with the intention to develop SL as a strategy to promote holistic development in students.

The second lesson learned is that training for teachers for SL teaching and engagement is important. As there are many myths about SL (e.g. wasting the time of students or only students of certain disciplines can perform SL tasks well), it is important to demystify them through systematic training where potential teachers are helped to acquire the basic knowledge of SL as well as to develop positive attitudes and mindset about SL. Most important of all, it is vital to develop a sense of mission in teachers so that they can implement SL in a dedicated manner. To train teachers in a systematic manner, we have developed a three-hour e-learning training package with different elements. The outline of the e-learning can be seen in Table 20.2. Preliminary evaluation shows that the e-learning package for teachers was well received (Shek & Chan, 2013a, 2013b).

The third lesson is that e-learning package facilitates the implementation of SL on a large scale. As a huge number of students are taking SL, there is a need to provide systematic training for them. As such, a 10-hour e-learning programme for students has been developed to ensure that students in different departments and faculties receive similar input about basic knowledge on SL. As seen in Table 20.3, an e-learning programme has been developed which covers different aspects of SL.

Fourth, our experience in the past few years shows that it is possible to develop credit-bearing SL subjects aiming at promoting holistic development of students from a wide range of disciplines. Traditionally, it is a myth that SL only applies to those disciplines in social sciences such as social work, social policy and psychology. However, in the past few years, we have witnessed that colleagues in different faculties have developed Service-Learning subjects across different faculties. Some examples are seen in the sections below.

Table 20.2 E-Learning module on SL (for staff)

Unit 1	**Introduction**
Unit 2	**What is Service-Learning?**
2.1	Definition of Service-learning at PolyU
2.2	Types of Service-learning
2.3	Four Models of Service-learning
2.4	Secondary/Additional Resources
2.5	Exemplary Projects of SL Subjects
2.6	Exemplary Projects and Service-learning Ideas across the Disciplines
2.7	Case Studies of Service-learning Projects
2.8	Learning Exercise
Unit 3	**Impact and Benefits of Service-Learning**
3.1	Learning Outcomes of Service-learning Curriculum
3.2	General Impacts/Benefits of Service-learning
3.3	Research Studies/Literature on Service-learning Outcomes
3.4	Secondary/Additional Resources
3.5	Evaluation Report at PolyU
3.6	Sharing and Models after Taking Service-learning Projects
3.7	Case Studies
3.8	Learning Exercise
Unit 4	**Myths and Positive Attitudes towards Service-Learning**
4.1	Myths of Service-learning
4.2	Attitudes towards Service-learning
4.3	Attitudes of Colleagues at PolyU towards Service-learning
4.4	Learning Exercise
Unit 5	**Developing a Service-Learning Subject at PolyU**
5.1	Milestones of Developing a Service-learning Subject at PolyU
5.2	Policies and Guidelines at PolyU
5.3	Components of a Well-Structured Service-learning Subject
5.4	Principles of Good Practice in Service-learning Pedagogy
5.5	Pedagogical Strategies for Service-learning Subjects
5.6	Additional Resources
5.7	Learning Exercise
Unit 6	**Self-reflection about Service-Learning**
6.1	What Is Self-Reflection about Service-learning?
6.2	Should I Formally Self-Reflect on a Service-learning Program?
6.3	Why Do You Need to Self-Reflect Critically after Service?
6.4	Sharing from the Academic Staff
6.5	Learning Exercise
Unit 7	**Concluding**

Table 20.3 E-Learning module on SL (for students)

Introduction	
Pre-experience Survey	
Unit 1	**What is Service-Learning?**
1.1	Definition of Service-learning
1.2	Service-Learning versus Other Types of Service Activities
1.3	The Experiential Learning Cycle
1.4	Myths about Service-learning
1.5	Summary
1.6	Reference
Unit 2	**Benefits of Service-Learning**
2.1	Service-Learning and the Desirable Attributes of PolyU Graduates
2.2	Intended Learning Outcomes of Service-learning Subjects at PolyU
2.3	Benefits of Service-learning to Students
2.4	Benefits of Service-learning to the Community
2.5	Benefits of Service-learning to the University
2.6	Further Testimonials on Benefits of Service-learning
2.7	Summary
2.8	Reference
Unit 3	**Responsibilities, Attitudes and Ethics in Service-Learning**
3.1	Roles and Responsibilities in Service-learning
3.2	Developing a Positive Attitude towards Service-learning
3.3	Ethics in Service-learning
3.4	Summary
3.5	Reference
Unit 4	**Planning and Delivering Your Service-Learning Project**
4.1	Milestones of a Service-learning Project
4.2	Developing an Effective Service-learning Project Plan
4.3	Effective Strategies for Implementing Your Service Plan
4.4	Teamwork Skills
4.5	Problem-Solving Skills
4.6	Common Challenges in Service Delivery and Ways to Handle Them
4.7	What Constitutes Good Performance in Service Delivery?
4.8	Summary
4.9	Reference
Unit 5	**Reflecting on Your Service-Learning Experience**
5.1	Reflection in Service-learning: What Is It and Why Do It?
5.2	Types of Reflective Activities
5.3	Mastering Your Reflection Skills
5.4	Depth of Reflection
5.5	Summary
5.6	Reference
End-of-Module Test	
Feedback on E-learning Module	

20.3.1 Subject Entitled "Technology Beyond Borders: Service-Learning Across Cultural, Ethnic and Community Lines" Developed by Department of Computing

Extracting from the course outline, the subject focuses on: (a) digital divide and how it influences the society; (b) relationship between culture and ethnicity and technology adoption and usage; (c) technology in social contexts, particularly the needs of the socially deprived and ethical, and proper uses of technology. The objectives of this subject are: "(a) to introduce the concept and practice of learning through community service to our students; (b) to increase our students' awareness and knowledge of communities that are culturally, ethnically or socially distinct from their own; (c) to acquaint students with significant issues of social needs, justice and ethics related to the information age, such as the concept of the information divide and how technology may be used to meet these needs; (d) to cultivate an awareness of information ethics and professional responsibility in our students; and (e) to nurture a sense of civic responsibility and engagement in our students". There are several intended learning outcomes of the subject. After taking the subject, students are expected to: "(a) demonstrate an awareness of the impact of the information/digital divide, and the linkage between social disadvantages and the availability of appropriate technology; (b) demonstrate an awareness of the impact of social status, culture and/or ethnicity, and empathy for the preconceptions, concerns and needs faced by disadvantaged individuals or community groups; (c) articulate the needs of the underprivileged in society, analyse complex issues in the service setting and design, implement or deploy appropriate and ethical technological solutions to meet the needs of the target recipients; (d) work effectively in teams to solve problems encountered in planning and delivering the service; (e) communicate effectively with clients and/or other stakeholders; (f) reflect on the relationship between their service-learning activities and experiences with the academic content of the subject, in particular, the needs of the underprivileged in society and their own discipline and sense of civic responsibility, especially pertaining to use and deployment of technological solutions".

20.3.2 Community Tourism: Tour, Training, Operator, and Event from and for the Community by School of Hotel and Tourism Management

This service-learning subject enables students to develop a Volunteer Community Ambassador (VCA) Programme. Students in this subject will design local community tour guided by VCAs, train local community residents as VCAs who are new arrival unemployed women, plan, organize community events to promote the community tourism project, create and operate a website to promote the community tourism project. There are several intended learning outcomes in this subject, including: (a) professional competence (demonstration and application of knowledge and skills to develop community tourism and event development); (b) critical thinking (demonstration of creative and analytical skills in designing community tourism project assignments); (c) effective communication (proactive dialogues and reaction to different stakeholders); (d) innovative problem-solving (showing higher-order thinking and problem-solving in proposal development and planning and justifying solutions to identified problems; discussing and explaining measures to satisfy requirements); (e) lifelong learning (showing reflection of oneself as a professional and a responsible citizen); (f) ethical leadership (showing empathy and civic responsibility).

The fifth lesson learned is that support from the senior management is indispensable. To facilitate the development of SL at PolyU, the University established the Office of Service-Learning which is supervised by the Associate Vice president (Undergraduate Programme) with the mission to "establish PolyU as a leader in service-learning (SL) and University Social Responsibility, and foster a campus culture of community service that benefits the students, the community and the University". The mission of OSL is "in partnership with staff, students and community, we are committed to advancing service-learning and community engagement at PolyU and preparing students to become civic-minded professionals with a heart to serve". Specifically, the OSL has the following duties: "(a) support and assist in the development and implementation of high-impact credit-bearing service-learning subjects at PolyU; (b) promote effective service-learning pedagogies that enhance students' learning and development as a civic-minded professional; (c) solicit and sustain community support for service-learning at PolyU; (d) provide further opportunities and support for students' continual engagement in meaningful community services beyond credit-bearing service-learning subjects; (e) advance the scholarship and research in service-learning through rigorous evaluation studies of impacts and community-based research; and (g) foster inter-institutional collaboration in service-learning, both locally and internationally". Besides the OSL, the University established the Sub-committee on Service-Learning under the Committee on General University Requirements which monitors and reviews SL subjects on offer, including their quality and implementation, and receives and considers the subject evaluation. To promote service-learning further, the University has also established the Committee on PolyU Community Service Fund which oversees the use, execution and administration of the Community Service Fund that supports community service-learning projects.

The sixth lesson is that multi-sectoral collaboration is necessary for the successful implementation of Service-Learning subjects. In the first place, many SL places take place in non-government organizations (e.g., elderly homes) and school settings (e.g., primary and secondary schools). Besides, for some SL projects, support from the Government is important. For example, without the Mainland Experience Scheme (Hong Kong) and the Ten Thousand People Scheme (China) which provide financial support for Hong Kong students to visit China, SL projects in China would not be possible. Finally, as SL (especially the offshore SL projects) requires much resources, donors, charities and the commercial sector play an important role in the success of SL projects.

The final lesson is that evaluation and research are important. Obviously, good intention underlying the use of SL to promote youth development alone is not enough. We have to demonstrate whether students have changed in a positive manner during and after taking SL subjects. For each subject, there are at least two routine evaluation methods. First, students respond to Student Feedback Questionnaire after completion of a subject. Second, students are typically asked to write reflective journals during and at the end of a subject. Besides these two routine evaluation strategies, other evaluation methods have been used. For example, in the longitudinal GUR study, focus groups are conducted to examine the views of the students on SL matters. In this book, chapters reporting the evaluation findings are included.

20.4 Opportunities and Challenges

There are several factors which promote the development of SL in higher education in Hong Kong. First, SL has been regarded as a strategy to promote youth development. As Hong Kong adolescents are seen as egocentric and their sense of social responsibility is declining, SL has been regarded as a good vehicle to promote personal maturity and social responsibility in students. Second, there has been growing effort among universities in the global context to use SL to promote civic engagement in students. Third, community and Government support for SL has been growing. In particular, there is a consensus that young people should attend to the needs of the vulnerable groups. Finally, the recent One Belt One Road initiative constitutes a good opportunity to develop offshore SL projects.

Despite the above opportunities and favourable conditions facilitating SL, there are several challenges that Service-Learning is facing at PolyU. First, although PolyU is the first university requiring students to take a Service-Learning subject before graduation, two other universities (Lingnan University and The Education University of Hong Kong) are having this graduation requirement now. For other sister universities, credit-bearing Service-Learning subjects are also increasing. In the Asian region, Singapore is also very enthusiastic in promoting SL initiatives. Hence, the fundamental challenge is how PolyU can maintain a leading role in the SL movement in Hong Kong. Besides, there is the question of differentiation. With the growing number of community service-learning projects (i.e., not credit-bearing service-learning subjects which are primarily related to voluntary service), how to help the public, colleagues and students understand the differences between the two modes of service and appreciate the value of credit-bearing SL subjects is an important question to be considered.

The second challenge is on the availability of colleagues with SL expertise. According to the 5P model, success in educational programmes depends on five critical factors—programme, policy, people, process and place. As far as "people" is concerned, although we have already trained and engaged more than 100 teachers for SL, the problem of succession and sustainability in vision is an issue to be considered. As SL competence is not inborn, how to help colleagues with high academic qualification (such as those with PhD degree) to develop passion in SL is important. With increasing demand placed on research such as getting grants from the Research Grants Council and publication in "high-impact" studies, dedicated colleagues will inevitably face the problem of burnout and the pressure of "publish or perish". Hence, new blood is needed. To help colleagues in research, how to sustain the motivation and SL research opportunities are important matters to be considered. Finally, engaging in the teaching of SL demands personal growth in the teachers. Hence, effort should be made to explore how we can help teachers to promote personal growth as a teacher and as a human being. In particular, how to help colleagues in the fields of science and engineering to reflect and appreciate the value of qualitative evaluation is an important task to be accomplished.

The third challenge concerns the motive behind offering SL subjects. As SL provides income for the departments, some departments may offer SL simply for the sake of earning money. In such cases, although departments can meet the threshold expectations, it would be difficult to expect sacrifice in colleagues and the department. While making money is not unacceptable, how to cultivate passion in the teachers is a very important task to be accomplished. Essentially, it touches on an important topic of how to develop the culture of "serving heart" at PolyU and articulate the spirit of "we serve, we care" in the DNA of PolyU culture.

The fourth challenge concerns the question of how the quality of SL subjects can be sustained and promoted. As far as quality assurance (QA) is concerned, we have different QA mechanisms in place, including the Senate, Academic Planning and Regulations Committee, Committee on General University Requirements and Sub-Committee on Service-Learning, where the quality of SL subjects offered are stringently scrutinized and their implementation are carefully monitored. However, with changing SL colleagues and departmental policies, fluctuation in the quality of SL subjects is expected and it should be actively responded to. In particular, how to work out fair, transparent and reasonable principles governing offering of SL subjects is an important area to be dealt with.

Besides QA issues, there are also concerns about how SL should be taught. As more students from a diverse background are taking SL, one possibility is to use e-learning strategies to ensure that students taking SL will have sufficient input in the basic knowledge and related skills. There are arguments for and against this approach. For those who support the use of e-learning, they believe that standardized curriculum would guarantee standard and it is an effective pedagogy. For those who are against the use of e-learning approach, they would argue that it is necessary to have face-to-face interaction experiential learning and e-learning may not help students to gain a thorough understanding of service-learning. Obviously, whether e-learning is helpful or not is an empirical question to be resolved. Besides, we should examine how technology-enhanced active learning (e.g., participatory/interactive lectures, games, peer instruction, case-based learning) can contribute to the effectiveness of service learning teaching.

Pedagogically, there is a need to review the issue of integration and collaboration which involves several levels. First, there is room for more inter-disciplinary collaboration in providing SL subjects. Although there are some inter-disciplinary SL subjects, they are on the low side at the present moment. Second, instead of having one-off SL projects, it is strategic to consider long-term collaborative projects with NGOs and communities so that accumulative benefits can be seen. One possibility is to have one to two district(s) with multiple SL subjects. Third, it would create more synergy in the impact of SL if we can involve different stakeholders, including the Government, commercial sector, the Third sector and the general public. Fourth, integration with different professionals such as social workers, teachers, engineers, politicians and district councillors would be desirable, especially when we wish to make things happen. Finally, integration of SL programmes in different regions and across the globe would be an exciting area for development.

The sixth challenge is how SL can be integrated into the Strategic Plan of PolyU, particularly the internationalization initiative related to "One Belt One Road" and "Engaging the Nation". Currently, we have many SL projects outside Hong Kong, such as the Belt (Kyrgyzstan and Xi'an) and maritime silk Road (Shanghai, Hangzhou, Vietnam, Cambodia). If SL further internationalizes, it means there will be more offshore SL subjects which will broaden the exposure and enhance the cultural competence of the students. This is also in line with the interest of young people to travel abroad. Of course, having more offshore SL subjects means reduction of local SL subjects. Besides, students have to bear the financial burden. It also constitutes additional strain for students and teachers because much more preparation work is associated with offshore service-learning. Besides securing donation, some existing schemes such as Mainland Experience Scheme administered by the HKSAR Government and the Ten Thousand People Scheme administered by the PRC Ministry of Education are helpful.

The seventh challenge is on research and evaluation. For research on SL, although much has been done in the West, there are still many knowledge gaps. This is particularly the case at PolyU (Table 20.4). First, predictors (i.e., causes) of SL engagement and outcomes remain to be identified. Second, we need to conduct research to look at the concomitants (i.e., correlates) of SL, such as the relationship between SL commitment and motivation of volunteer. Third, more work should be conducted to examine the outcomes (i.e., consequences) of volunteerism, such as how SL shapes the identity and social responsibility in the students. With SL implemented in different cultures, it is theoretically and practically important to look at cross-cultural similarities and differences in SL teaching and implementation. As far as the teaching of SL is concerned, it is important to ask what the best strategies for teaching SL and engaging the students are.

Regarding evaluation of SL, three common methods are employed, including pretest-posttest pre-experimental design, subjective outcome evaluation and

Table 20.4 Selected publications on SL

Chan, S. C. F., Ngai, G., & Kwan, K. P. (2017). Mandatory service learning at university: Do less-inclined students learn from it? *Active Learning in Higher Education*. https://doi.org/10.1177/1469787417742019.
Lo, K.W.K., Lau, C.K., Chan, S.C.F., & Ngai, G. (2017). When non-engineering students work on an international service-learning engineering project: A case study. Accepted for presentation at the 2017 IEEE Global Humanitarian Technology Conference (GHTC2017), San Jose, October 2017.
Chan, S.C.F., Ngai, G., Kwan, K.P., & Wong, W. (2016). A multivariate study of factors influencing students' learning outcomes from service-learning. In: International Association for Research on Service-Learning and Community Engagement. New Orleans, LA, 2016.
Lam, H.Y., Lau, C.K., & Cheung, E. (2016). Students' views of mandatory service-learning at university. In: Service-Learning Research Salon, Hong Kong, 2016.
Lau, C.K. (2016). Sustaining the impact of service-learning projects through community empowerment. In: Service-Learning Research Salon, Hong Kong, 2016.
Lau, C.K., Lo, K.W.K., Chan, S.C.F., & Ngai, G. (2016). From zero to one: Integrating engineering and non-engineering students in a service-learning engineering project. In: The 2nd International Conference on Service-Learning (pp. 186–191), Hong Kong, 2016.
Lo, K.W.K., Chan, S.C.F., & Ngai, G. (2016). Using a recycled container to setup a community learning centre in rural Cambodia: A case study. In: 2016 IEEE Global Humanitarian Technology Conference (GHTC2016), Seattle, USA, 2016.
Lo, K.W.K., Kwan, K.P., Chan, S.C.F., & Ngai, G. (2016). Cross-cultural validation of the Global Citizenship Scale for measuring impacts of international service-learning in Hong Kong setting. In: International Association for Research on Service-Learning and Community Engagement, New Orleans, LA, 2016.
Ngai, G., & Chan, S.C.F. (2016). A two-dimensional classification framework for service-learning. In: The 2nd International Conference on Service-Learning (pp. 55–59), Hong Kong, 2016.
Ngai, G., Chan, S.C.F., Chapman, N., & Spear, A. (2016). Learning to serve together: Creating an inter-continental classroom for service-learning. In: The 2nd International Conference on Service-Learning (pp. 198–203), Hong Kong, 2016.
Ngai, G., Chan, S.C.F., Kwan K.P., Csete, J. (2015). Designing, implementing and maintaining assessment policies and practices in support of an institution-wide initiative in service-learning. Presented at the International Conference on Assessment for Learning in Higher Education 2015, Hong Kong, 2015. http://www.cetl.hku.hk/conf2015/wp-content/uploads/2015/04/conf2015booklet-concurrent-sessions.pdf
Ngai, G., & Chan, S.C.F. (2015). How much impact can be made in a week?: Designing Effective International Service Learning Projects for Computing. In: The 46th ACM Technical Symposium on Computer Science Education (SIGCSE'15) (pp. 645–650). Kansas City, MO, 2015.
Chan, S.C.F., & Ngai, G. (2014). Service-Learning as a core academic component in undergraduate programmes: A brief introduction to The Hong Kong Polytechnic University model. In: The 1st International Conference on Service-Learning (pp. 87–96). Hong Kong, 2014.
Kwok, T.C.K., Yeung, T.S.W., & Lo, K.W.K. (2014). 2-Year experiences of deploying eResources in developing countries. In: The 1st International Conference on Service-Learning (pp. 324–325). Hong Kong, 2014.

(continued)

Table 20.4 (continued)

Lee, J.K.Y., Ling, S.L., & Lo, K.W.K. (2014). Case study: Essential elements of organizing a student-initiated service-learning project in developing countries. In: The 1st International Conference on Service-Learning (pp. 20–21), Hong Kong, 2014.
Lo, K.W.K., Kwan, K.P., Ngai, G., & Chan, S.C.F. (2014). An initial exploration of the cross-cultural validity of the Global Citizenship Scale in the Hong Kong setting. In: The 1st International Conference on Service-Learning (pp. 126–131), Hong Kong, 2014.
Tam, W.C., Lau, C.K., Ngai, G., Yuen, W.W., Chan, A.T.S., Lu, Q., & Chan, S.C.F. (2014). Problem-based learning: A teaching method to enhance learning experience for students in service-learning. In: The 1st International Conference on Service-Learning (pp. 271–279), Hong Kong, 2014.

qualitative evaluation. For evaluation based on pretest-posttest design, although it is easily done, there are many alternative explanations. For subjective outcome evaluation, it is the most popular evaluation design where the participants are invited to indicate the degree of satisfaction with the programme. While this method is easily conducted, its validity depends on the availability of objective measures. For qualitative evaluation, while it has been commended as being able to understand the subjective experiences of the stakeholders, it has been criticized as subjective and non-representative. In future, several directions of development are recommended. Primarily, randomized trials should be conducted to look at the effect of SL on the developmental outcomes in students. In particular, an effort to explore the long-term effects of SL using longitudinal research designs would be helpful. Besides, there is a need to develop more validated psychosocial assessment tools to capture the experience and consequences of SL.

With reference to the above challenges, what is (and should be) our vision about SL? In the long run, we have the vision of establishing PolyU as the centre of excellence in Service-Learning, at least in Asia. Within this centre of excellence, we pursue excellence in teaching, training, research, evaluation, dissemination and leadership development in SL. In particular, we should document more evidence on how SL contributes to the quality of life of the service providers (i.e., students), service recipients and the organization and/or community where the service project is carried out. While work has been done to examine how SL contributes to the quality of life of students who provide the service, comparatively fewer studies have been carried out to examine how SL among university students might promote the quality of life of the service recipients and the organization/community where the service is carried out. Obviously, these research directions are exciting opportunities for scholars and practitioners in the field of Service-Learning.

References

Shek, D. T. L., & Chan, S. C. F. (2013a). Development of an e-learning package on service-learning for university teachers: Experience from Hong Kong. *International Journal of Adolescent Medicine and Health, 25*(4), 441–448.

Shek, D. T. L., & Chan, S. C. F. (2013b). Service-learning from the views of university teachers: A qualitative study based on focus groups. *International Journal of Adolescent Medicine and Health, 25*(4), 385–393.

Shek, D. T. L., & Yu, L. (2016). Student feedback on a subject on leadership and intrapersonal development for university students in Hong Kong. *International Journal on Disability and Human Development, 15*(3), 339–346.

Shek, D. T. L., Yu, L., & Ng, C. S. M. (2016). Evaluation of a general education program in Hong Kong: Results based on multiple evaluation strategies. *International Journal of Child and Adolescent Health, 9*(2), 263–273.

Shek, D. T. L., Yu, L., & Zhu, X. (2016). Evaluation of a leadership and intrapersonal development subject for university students in Hong Kong: Findings based on two years. *International Journal on Disability and Human Development, 15*(1), 101–109.

Shek, D. T. L., & Yu, L. (2017a). General university requirements and holistic development in university students in Hong Kong. *International Journal of Adolescent Medicine and Health, 29*(1), 41–48.

Shek, D. T. L., & Yu, L. (2017b). The impact of 3-year and 4-year undergraduate programs on university students: The case of Hong Kong. *International Journal of Adolescent Medicine and Health, 29*(1), 49–55.

Shek, D. T. L., & Yu, L. (2017c). An evaluation study on a university general education subject in Hong Kong. *International Journal of Adolescent Medicine and Health, 29*(1), 103–109.

Shek, D. T. L., Yu, L., & Merrick, J. (2017). *University students: Promotion of holistic development in Hong Kong*. New York: Nova Science.

Shek, D. T. L., Yu, L., & Chai, W. (2017a). Evaluation of the general university requirements: What did students say? *International Journal of Adolescent Medicine and Health, 29*(1), 75–82.

Shek, D. T. L., Yu, L., & Chai, W. (2017b). Qualitative evaluation of a new general education program at a university in Hong Kong: Teachers' experiences. *International Journal of Child and Adolescent Health, 10*(1), 73–89.

Author Index

D. T. L. Shek et al. (eds.), *Service-Learning for Youth Leadership*,
Quality of Life in Asia 12, https://doi.org/10.1007/978-981-13-0448-4

Subject Index

D. T. L. Shek et al. (eds.), *Service-Learning for Youth Leadership*,
Quality of Life in Asia 12, https://doi.org/10.1007/978-981-13-0448-4

Experience, 6, 8, 10, 13–15, 21, 24–29, 31, 35, 38, 43–45, 65, 69, 71–73, 75, 77, 84, 110, 114, 118, 121, 122, 128, 133, 134, 139, 146, 148, 150–152, 155, 157, 159, 160, 166, 168, 175, 178, 182, 186, 187, 191, 193, 194, 196, 200–202, 204–209, 216, 220–222, 224, 230, 231, 235, 241, 244, 250, 252, 253, 255, 257–260, 262, 263, 265, 268, 285, 288, 293–297, 299, 301–307, 309–316, 318, 319, 321, 322, 324, 325, 327, 331–334, 337–339, 346, 348, 350, 353, 355

MIX
Papier aus verantwortungsvollen Quellen
Paper from responsible sources
FSC® C105338

If you have any concerns about our products,
you can contact us on
ProductSafety@springernature.com

In case Publisher is established outside the EU,
the EU authorized representative is:
Springer Nature Customer Service Center GmbH
Europaplatz 3, 69115 Heidelberg, Germany

Printed by Libri Plureos GmbH
in Hamburg, Germany